PROGRESS IN CLINICAL AND BIOLOGICAL RESEARCH

RECENT TITLES

Vol 350: **Uro-Oncology: Current Status and Future Trends,** H.G.W. Frohmüller, Manfred Wirth, *Editors*

Vol 351: **Taurine: Functional Neurochemistry, Physiology, and Cardiology,** Herminia Pasantes-Morales, David L. Martin, William Shain, Rafael Martín del Río, *Editors*

Vol 352: **The Biology of Hematopoiesis,** Nicholas Daniak, Eugene P. Cronkite, Ronald McCaffrey, Richard K. Shadduck, *Editors*

Vol 353: **Neoadjuvant Chemotherapy in Invasive Bladder Cancer,** Ted A.W. Splinter, Howard I. Scher, *Editors*

Vol 354: **Effects of Therapy on Biology and Kinetics of the Residual Tumor,** Joseph Ragaz, Linda Simpson-Herren, Marc Lippman, Bernard Fisher, *Editors*. Published in two volumes: *Part A: Pre-Clinical Aspects. Part B: Clinical Aspects.*

Vol 355: **Radiolabelled Cellular Blood Elements,** Helmut Sinzinger, Mathew L. Thakur, *Editors*

Vol 356: **Molecular Biology and Differentiation of Megakaryocytes,** Janine Breton-Gorius, Jack Levin, Alan T. Nurden, Neil Williams, *Editors*

Vol 357: **EORTC Genitourinary Group Monograph 7: Prostate Cancer and Testicular Cancer,** Donald W.W. Newling, William G. Jones, *Editors*

Vol 358: **Treatment of Post Surgical Adhesions,** Gere S. diZerega, L. Russell Malinak, Michael P. Diamond, Cary B. Linsky, *Editors*

Vol 359: **EORTC Genitourinary Group Monograph 8: Treatment of Prostatic Cancer—Facts and Controversies,** Fritz H. Schröder, *Editor*

Vol 360: **Molecular Genetics of Chromosome 21 and Down Syndrome,** David Patterson, Charles J. Epstein, *Editors*

Vol 361: **Current and Future Trends in Anticonvulsant, Anxiety, and Stroke Therapy,** Brian S. Meldrum, Michael Williams, *Editors*

Vol 362: **The Molecular Biology of the Retina: Basic and Clinically Relevant Studies,** Debora B. Farber, Gerald J. Chader, *Editors*

Vol 363: **Information Processing in Medical Imaging,** Douglas A. Ortendahl, Jorge Llacer, *Editors*

Vol 364: **The Hepatitis Delta Virus,** John L. Gerin, Robert H. Purcell, Mario Rizzetto, *Editors*

Vol 365: **Clinical and Experimental Approaches to Dermal and Epidermal Repair: Normal and Chronic Wounds,** Adrian Barbul, Michael D. Caldwell, William H. Eaglstein, Thomas K. Hunt, David Marshall, Eli Pines, Greg Skover, *Editors*

Vol 366: **Advances in Neuroblastoma Research 3,** Audrey E. Evans, Giulio J. D'Angio, Alfred F. Knudson, Jr., Robert C. Seeger, *Editors*

Vol 367: **Bacterial Endotoxins: Cytokine Mediators and New Therapies for Sepsis,** Augueste Sturk, Sander J.H. van Deventer, Jan Wouter ten Cate, Harry R. Büller, Lambertus G. Thijs, Jack Levin, *Editors*

Vol 368: **Fragile X/Cancer Cytogenetics,** Ann M. Willey, Patricia D. Murphy, *Editors*

Vol 369: **Chemically Induced Cell Proliferation: Implications for Risk Assessment,** Byron E. Butterworth, Thomas J. Slaga, William Farland, Michael McClain, *Editors*

Vol 370: **EORTC Genitourinary Group Monograph 10: Urological Oncology: Reconstructive Surgery, Organ Conservation, and Restoration of Function,** Philip H. Smith, Michele Pavone-Macaluso, *Editors*

Vol 371: **Operations Research: Helping Family Planning Programs Work Better,** Myrna Seidman, Marjorie C. Horn, *Editors*

Vol 372: **New Horizons in Biological Dosimetry,** Barton L. Gledhill, Francesco Mauro, *Editors*

Vol. 373: **The Morphogenesis of Down Syndrome,** Charles J. Epstein, *Editor*

Vol 374: **Relevance of Animal Studies to the Evaluation of Human Cancer Risk,** Robert D'Amato, Thomas J. Slaga, William H. Farland, Carol Henry, *Editors*

Vol 375: **New Developments in Fatty Acid Oxidation,** Paul M. Coates, Kay Tanaka, *Editors*

Vol 376: **Comparative Molecular Carcinogenesis,** Andres J.P. Klein-Szanto, Marshall Anderson, J. Carl Barrett, Thomas J. Slaga, *Editors*

Vol 377: **Advances in Bone Marrow Purging and Processing,** Diana A. Worthington-White, Adrian P. Gee, Samuel Gross, *Editors*

Vol 378: **EORTC Genitourinary Group Monograph 11: Recent Progress in Bladder and Kidney Cancer,** Fritz H. Schröder, *Editor*

Vol 379: **Down Syndrome and Alzheimer Disease,** Lynn Nadel, Charles J. Epstein, *Editors*

Vol 380: **Essential and Toxic Trace Elements in Human Health and Disease, Vol. II,** Ananda S. Prasad, *Editor*

Vol 381: **Gynecologic Surgery and Adhesion Prevention,** Michael P. Diamond, Gere S. diZerega, Cary B. Linsky, Robert L. Reid, *Editors*

Vol 382: **Hepatitis Delta Virus: Molecular Biology, Pathogenesis, and Clinical Aspects,** Stephanos J. Hadziyannis, John M. Taylor, Ferruccio Bonino, *Editors*

Vol 383: **Limb Development and Regeneration, Parts A and B,** John F. Fallon, Paul F. Goetinck, Robert O. Kelley, David L. Stocum, *Editors*

Vol 384: **The Phenotypic Mapping of Down Syndrome and Other Aneuploid Conditions,** Charles J. Epstein, *Editor*

Vol 385: **Advances in Neuroblastoma Research 4,** Audrey E. Evans, June L. Biedler, Garrett M. Brodeur, Giulio D'Angio, Akira Nakagawara, *Editors*

Vol 386: **EORTC Genitourinary Group Monograph 12: Benign Prostatic Hyperplasia: Recent Progress in Clinical Research and Practice,** Karlheinz Kurth, Donald W.W. Newling, *Editors*

Vol 387: **Receptor-Mediated Biological Processes: Implications for Evaluating Carcinogenesis,** Hugh L. Spitzer, Thomas J. Slaga, William F. Greenlee, Michael McClain, *Editors*

Vol 388: **Bacterial Endotoxins: Basic Science to Anti-Sepsis Strategies,** Jack Levin, Sander J.H. van Deventer, Tom van der Poll, Augueste Sturk, *Editors*

Vol 389: **Advances in Bone Marrow Purging and Processing: Fourth International Symposium,** Adrian P. Gee, Samuel Gross, Diana A. Worthington-White, *Editors*

Vol 390: **Molecular Neurobiology: Mechanisms Common to Brain, Skin, and Immune System,** Gerald D. Fischbach, Nobutaka Hirokawa, Steven E. Hyman, Tatsuya Ozawa, *Editors*

Vol 391: **Growth Factors and Tumor Promotion: Implications for Risk Assessment,** R. Michael McClain, Thomas J. Slaga, Robert LeBoeuf, Henry Pitot, *Editors*

Vol 392: **Bacterial Endotoxins: Lipopolysaccharides From Genes to Therapy,** Jack Levin, Carl R. Alving, Robert S. Munford, Heinz Redl, *Editors*

Vol 393: **Etiology and Pathogenesis of Down Syndrome,** Charles J. Epstein, Terry Hassold, Ira T. Lott, Lynn Nadel, David Patterson, *Editors*

Vol 394: **Cellular and Molecular Mechanisms of Hormonal Carcinogenesis: Environmental Influences,** James Huff, Jeff Boyd, J. Carl Barrett, *Editors*

Vol 395: **Genetics and Cancer Susceptibility: Implications for Risk Assessment,** Cheryl Walker, John Groopman, Thomas J. Slaga, Andres Klein-Szanto, *Editors*

Please contact the publisher for information about previous titles in this series

GENETICS AND CANCER SUSCEPTIBILITY

Implications for Risk Assessment

GENETICS AND CANCER SUSCEPTIBILITY

Implications for Risk Assessment

Proceedings of the Eighth International Conference on Carcinogenesis and Risk Assessment, Held in Austin, Texas, November 30 – December 3, 1994

Editors

Cheryl Walker
University of Texas
M.D. Anderson Cancer Center
Science Park - Research Division
Smithville, Texas

John Groopman
Department of Environmental Health Sciences
School of Hygiene and Public Health
Johns Hopkins University
Baltimore Maryland

Thomas J. Slaga
University of Texas
M.D. Anderson Cancer Center
Science Park - Research Division
Smithville, Texas

Andres Klein-Szanto
Fox Chase Cancer Center
Philadelphia, Pennsylvania

WILEY-LISS

A JOHN WILEY & SONS, INC., PUBLICATION
NEW YORK • CHICHESTER • BRISBANE • TORONTO • SINGAPORE

Address All Inquiries to the Publisher
Wiley-Liss, Inc., 605 Third Avenue, New York, NY 10158-0012

Printed in the United States of America.

Library of Congress Cataloging-in-Publication Data

International Conference on Carcinogenesis and Risk Assessment (8th : 1994 : Austin, Tex.)
Genetics and cancer susceptibility : implications for risk assessment : proceedings of the Eighth International Conference on Carcinogenesis and Risk Assessment, held in Austin, Texas, November 30–December 3, 1994 / editors, Cheryl Walker ... [et al.].
p. cm. — (Progress in clinical and biological research ; 395)
Includes bibliographical references and index.
ISBN 0-471-13777-4 (alk. paper)
1. Cancer—Genetic aspects—Congresses. 2. Cancer—Epidemiology--Congresses. 3. Health risk assessment—Congresses. 4. Carcinogenesis—Congresses. I. Walker, Cheryl, 1955– II. Title. III. Series.
[DNLM: 1. Neoplasms—genetics—congresses. 2. Disease Susceptibility—genetics—congresses. 3. Risk Assessment--congresses. 4. Carcinogens—congresses. W1 PR668E v.395 1996 / QZ 200 I6046g 1996]
RC268.4.I58 1996
616.99'4042—dc20
DNLM/DLC
for Library of Congress 96-5969
CIP

The text of this book is printed on acid-free paper.

10 9 8 7 6 5 4 3 2 1

Contents

Contributors

C. Marcelo Aldaz, Department of Carcinogenesis, University of Texas, M.D. Anderson Cancer Center, Science Park - Research Division, Smithville, TX 78957 [**1**]

Joe M. Angel, Department of Carcinogenesis, University of Texas, M.D. Anderson Cancer Center, Science Park - Research Division, Smithville, TX 78957 [**23**]

Alaa F. Badawi, Food and Drug Administration, National Center for Toxicological Research, Jefferson, AR 72079 [**109**]

Diane F. Birt, Eppley Institute for Research in Cancer, Department of Biochemistry and Molecular Biology, University of Nebraska Medical Center, Omaha, NE 68198-6805 [**223**]

Allan Bradley, Institue for Molecular Genetics and Howard Hughes Medical Insititute, Baylor College of Medicine, Houston, TX 77030 [**1**]

Reynaldo A. Carabeo, McArdle Laboratory for Cancer Research, University of Wisconsin Medical School, Madison, WI 53706 [**33**]

Teresa A. Chiaverotti, McArdle Laboratory for Cancer Research, University of Wisconsin Medical School, Madison, WI 53706 [**33**]

Claudio J. Conti, Department of Carcinogenesis, University of Texas, M.D. Anderson Cancer Center, Science Park - Research Division, Smithville, TX 78957 [**47**]

Norman R. Drinkwater, McArdle Laboratory for Cancer Research, University of Wisconsin Medical School, Madison, WI 53706 [**33**]

Lawrence A. Donehower, Division of Molecular Virology, Baylor College of Medicine, Houston, TX 77030 [**1**]

Lucy A. Godley, Varmus Laboratory, National Cancer Institute, Bethesda, MD 20892 [**1**]

Tamra L. Goodrow, Department of Pathology, Fox Chase Cancer Center, Philadelphia, PA 19111 [**57**]

Nancy J. Gorelick, Miami Valley Labs, Proctor & Gamble Company, Cincinnati, OH 45253-8707 [**81**]

The numbers in brackets are the opening page numbers of the contributors' articles.

Joe Gray, Division of Molecular Cytometry, Department of Laboratory Medicine, University of California at San Francisco, San Francisco, CA 94143 [**1**]

John D. Groopman, Department of Environmental Health Sciences, The Johns Hopkins University School of Hygiene and Public Health, Baltimore, MD 21205 [**211**]

Barbara S. Hulka, Department of Epidemiology, The University of North Carolina, Chapel Hill, NC 27599-7400 [**159**]

Fred F. Kadlubar, Office of Research, Food and Drug Administration, National Center for Toxicological Research, Jefferson, AR 72079 [**109**]

Paul Kleihues, International Agency for Research on Cancer, 69372 Lyon Cedex 08, France [**201**]

Nicholas P. Lang, Department of Surgery, Arkansas Cancer Research Center, University of Arkansas Medical Sciences, Little Rock, AR 72205 [**109**]

Denise Lepley, Eppley Institute for Research in Cancer, Department of Biochemistry and Molecular Biology, University of Nebraska Medical Center, Omaha, NE 68198-6805 [**223**]

Daniel Medina, Department of Cell Biology, Baylor College of Medicine, Houston, TX 77030 [**1**]

Satish Nair, Eppley Institute for Research in Cancer, Department of Biochemistry and Molecular Biology, University of Nebraska Medical Center, Omaha, NE 68198-6805 [**223**]

Gilbert S. Omenn, School of Public Health and Community Medicine, University of Washington, Seattle, WA 98195-7230 [**235**]

Jill C. Pelling, Eppley Institute for Research in Cancer, Department of Biochemistry and Molecular Biology, University of Nebraska Medical Center, Omaha, NE 68198-6805 [**223**]

Dan Pinkel, Division of Molecular Cytometry, Department of Laboratory Medicine, University of California at San Francisco, San Francisco, CA 94143 [**1**]

Therese M. Poole, McArdle Laboratory for Cancer Research, University of Wisconsin Medical School, Madison, WI 53706 [**33**]

Ruth Pyle, Division of Molecular Virology, Baylor College of Medicine, Houston, TX 77030 [**1**]

Ellen R. Richie, Department of Carcinogenesis, University of Texas, M.D. Anderson Cancer Center, Science Park - Research Division, Smithville, TX 78957 [**23**]

Eugene M. Rinchik, Biology Division, Oak Ridge National Laboratory, Oak Ridge, TN 37831 [**23**]

Peter Scholl, Department of Environmental Health Sciences, The Johns Hopkins University School of Hygiene and Public Health, Baltimore, MD 21205 [**211**]

Yu-Ping Shi, Division of Molecular Cytometry, Department of Laboratory Medicine, University of California at San Francisco, San Francisco, CA 94143 [**1**]

Peter G. Shields, Molecular Epidemiology Section, Laboratory of Human Carcinogenesis, National Cancer Institute, Bethesda, MD 20892 [**141**]

Mariana C. Stern, Department of Carcinogenesis, University of Texas, M.D. Anderson Cancer Center, Science Park - Research Division, Smithville, TX 78957 [**47**]

Scott J. Stern, Department of Otolaryngology, University of Arkansas Medical Sciences, Little Rock, AR 72205 [**109**]

Bernard W. Stewart, Children's Leukemia and Cancer Research Centre, University of New South Wales Children's Hospital, Sydney, New South Wales 2031, Australia [**201**]

Larry H. Thompson, Biology and Biotechnology Research Program, Lawrence Livermore National Laboratory, Livermore, CA 94551 [**175**]

Harold E. Varmus, Office of the Director, National Institutes of Health, Bethesda, MD 20892 [**1**]

Cheryl Walker, Department of Carcinogenesis, University of Texas, M.D. Anderson Cancer Center, Science Park - Research Division, Smithville, TX 78957 [**13**]

Jia-Sheng Wang, The Johns Hopkins University School of Hygiene and Public Health, Baltimore, MD 21205 [**211**]

Preface

Contributors to this volume were participants at the Eighth International Conference on Carcinogenesis and Risk Assessment, "Genetics and Susceptibility: Impact on Risk Assessment." Participants included individuals from academia, industry, and government, who met to discuss issues related to incorporating emerging information about genetic susceptibility to cancer into the risk assessment process. Risk characterization is an integral part of the risk assessment process, and must take into account external factors such as dose and route of exposure that can modulate the probability for a given population of developing cancer following exposure to a carcinogenic agent. In addition to extrinsic factors that can modify cancer risk, it is now clear that there are also intrinsic factors that can contribute to the probability of cancer developing in an exposed individual. The degree to which individuals are able to metabolize certain chemical carcinogens and inheritance of defects in tumor suppressor genes are both examples of intrinsic determinants of cancer susceptibility that are genetic in origin and that can lead to an increased risk of developing this disease.

Recent advances in molecular genetics have made it possible to identify individuals in a population who are predisposed to the development of various types of cancer due to inherited genetic traits. How this information can be used to identify those individuals who are the most sensitive to potentially carcinogenic agents in the environment or workplace, and therefore at greatest risk of developing carcinogen-induced tumors, was a central theme of the meeting. Work currently being conducted to identify genetic determinants of cancer susceptibility using *in vitro* and animal model systems was discussed within the context of how this information can be extrapolated to humans. Recent data on cancer susceptibility obtained from human studies using molecular, genetic, and epidemiological approaches was also discussed, and this information was placed within the framework of how it can be used to better characterize individual risk to carcinogenic agents.

How best to incorporate genetic data into the risk assessment process will require additional information. Several common themes emerged from discussions among the participants at this meeting that will be useful in the design of future studies in this area. One recurring theme was that genetic determinants of susceptibility will be specific in their action. Species-specific and cell type-specific factors will need to be taken into account when factoring genetics into the risk assessment equation. A gene that predisposes to breast cancer may have little effect on an individual's risk of developing other types of cancer, and a gene responsible for carcinogen metabolism that produces an increased risk for the development of one type of cancer may actually protect against the development of another. Important questions relating to how to extrapolate carcinogenicity data obtained from sensitive indicator strains, such as transgenic mice, to humans must also be answered. Whether carcinogenicity data obtained from such animal studies is predictive of the action of carcinogens in humans must be determined before this type of information can be fully utilized. Ethical issues related to the use and protection of private information regarding an individual's genetic makeup that may predispose him or her to cancer are also important considerations that our society must begin to address.

Cheryl Walker
John Groopman
Thomas J. Slaga
Andres Klein-Szanto

Acknowledgments

The Chairs of this meeting, Drs. Cheryl Walker and John Groopman, were assisted in the planning and organization of the conference by Program Committee members Drs. Bill Farland, Andres Klein-Szanto, Tom Slaga, and Hugh Spitzer. The Conference was supported in part by grants from the National Institute of Environmental Health Sciences, the National Cancer Institute, and the Environmental Protection Agency. Other sponsors of the meeting were Proctor and Gamble, Rohm and Haas, the University of Texas M.D. Anderson Cancer Center–Science Park Research Division, the American Petroleum Institute, the ILSI-Health and Environmental Sciences Institute, Allied Signal, E. I. Dupont De Nemours, the American Industrial Health Council, Hoffman-LaRoche, Merck Research Laboratories, Bristol-Myers Squibb Pharmaceutical Research Institute, and Dermigen. Special thanks go to Carrie McKinley for her work on this volume and to the Conference staff, Karen Engel, Mary Lou Fendley, Judy Ing, LeNel Rice, and Michelle Gardiner.

Genetics and Cancer Susceptibility:
Implications for Risk Assessment, pages 1–11

THE ROLE OF p53 LOSS IN GENOMIC INSTABILITY AND TUMOR PROGRESSION IN A MURINE MAMMMARY CANCER MODEL

Lawrence A. Donehower, Lucy A. Godley, C. Marcelo Aldaz, Ruth Pyle, Yu-Ping Shi, Dan Pinkel, Joe Gray, Allan Bradley, Daniel Medina, and Harold E. Varmus

Division of Molecular Virology, Baylor College of Medicine, Houston,TX 77030 ; (L.A.D., R.P.); Varmus Laboratory, National Cancer Institute, Bethesda, MD 20892 and Department of Biochemistry and Biophysics, University of California, San Francisco, CA 94143 (L.A.G.); Department of Carcinogenesis, University of Texas M.D. Anderson Cancer Center-Science Park, Smithville, TX 78957 (C.M.A.); Division of Molecular Cytometry, Department of Laboratory Medicine, University of California at San Francisco, San Francisco, CA 94143 (Y.-P.S., D.P., J.G.); Institute for Molecular Genetics and Howard Hughes Medical Institute, Baylor College of Medicine, Houston, TX 77030 (A.B); Department of Cell Biology, Baylor College of Medicine, Houston, TX 77030; (D.M.); Office of the Director, National Institutes of Health, Bethesda, MD 20892 and Department of Microbiology and Immunology, University of California, San Francisco, CA 94143 (H.E.V.)

INTRODUCTION

The p53 gene is often mutated or lost in human tumors, including about 30% of all breast cancers (Greenblatt et al., 1994). In addition, germ line mutations in the p53 gene are linked with an inherited early cancer predisposition called Li-Fraumeni syndrome (Malkin et al., 1990, Srivastava et al., 1990). The p53 gene encodes a tumor suppressor protein which can mediate G1 arrest of the cell cycle following DNA damage (Finlay et al., 1989; Kastan et al., 1992). In some contexts, p53 appears to induce apoptosis as a result of DNA damage or an intracellular imbalance in growth signals (Yonish-Rouach et al., 1991; Clarke et al., 1993; Lowe et al., 1993a). Loss of p53 in cells has been associated with a loss of cell cycle checkpoint control and increased genomic instability (Livingstone et al., 1992; Yin et al., 1992). Absence of normal p53 function in a tumor cell is correlated with a poorer clinical prognosis and a resistance to treatment with various anticancer agents (Lowe et al., 1993b; Lowe et al., 1994).

TUMORIGENESIS IN p53-DEFICIENT MICE

To investigate the role of p53 in mammalian tumorigenesis, we have utilized gene targeting techniques to generate mice with one or two disrupted germ line p53 alleles (Donehower et al., 1992). These disrupted alleles are null for p53, as they are incapable of producing intact functional p53. Over 90% of mice nullizygous for p53 (p53-/-) are developmentally normal, but are highly susceptible to early onset tumors

(Table 1). Heterozygous mice (p53+/-) were also susceptible to tumors but at a significantly delayed rate compared to the nullizygotes (Harvey et al., 1993) (Table 1). Wild type (p53+/+) littermates of the p53-deficient mice rarely developed tumors during monitoring.

Table 1. Tumorigenesis in p53-Deficient Mice[a]

Genotype	50% Tumor Incidence	Tumor Types (No. observed)	% of Total	Mean Time of Onset
p53-/-	19 weeks	Lymphomas (59)	64%	20 weeks
		Soft Tissue Sarcomas (24)	26%	21 weeks
		Osteosarcomas (2)	2%	
		Carcinomas (1)	1%	
		Other (6)	7%	
p53+/-	76 weeks	Osteosarcomas (31)	35%	66 weeks
		Lymphomas (25)	28%	64 weeks
		Soft Tissue Sarcomas (24)	27%	68 weeks
		Carcinomas (6)	7%	73 weeks
		Other (2)	2%	

[a] 92 p53-/- and 184 p53+/- mice of mixed inbred genetic background (75% C57BL/6 and 25% 129/Sv) were monitored up to two years of age.

The tumor types observed in the p53-deficient mice were predominantly lymphomas and sarcomas, with a small number of carcinomas and other tumor types (brain tumors, testicular tumors). One p53-/- and one p53+/- mouse each developed a mammary adenocarcinoma, indicating that this particular tumor type rarely occurred spontaneously.

THE EFFECTS OF p53 LOSS ON TUMORIGENESIS IN A MURINE MAMMARY CANCER MODEL

The diversity of tumor types and relatively long time to tumor onset for the p53+/- mice complicates mechanistic studies of the role of p53 in tumorigenesis. To study the role of p53 loss in tumor development in a single tissue, we crossed the p53-deficient mice to mammary tumor-susceptible *Wnt-1* transgenic mice (Tsukamoto et al., 1988). Our rationale was that the effects of the presence or absence of p53 on the development of mammary cancer could be studied more readily in the offspring of these crosses.

The *Wnt-1* transgenic (*Wnt-1 TG*) mice contain additional copies of the murine *Wnt-1* proto-oncogene adjacent to the mouse mammary tumor virus long terminal repeat

(Tsukamoto et al., 1988). This construct, when added to the mouse germ line, was shown to result in high level mammary gland expression of *Wnt-1* mRNA. Male and female mice developed hyperplastic mammary glands and ultimately mammary adenocarcinomas. Virtually all females develop carcinomas by 12 months while less than 20% of males developed this tumor by twelve months of age (Tsukamoto et al., 1988).

Following crossing of the *Wnt-1* transgenic and p53-deficient mice, twelve groups of mice (each group containing at least 16 animals) were monitored for tumor development. The parameters defining each group were sex, p53 genotype (p53+/+, p53+/-, p53-/-), and *Wnt-1* transgene status (present or absent). The mammary tumor incidence in the six categories of mice containing the *Wnt-1* transgene are shown in Tables 2A and 2B. The six groups without the *Wnt-1* transgene did not develop mammary tumors.

Table 2A. Mammary tumor incidence in p53-deficient and normal *Wnt-1* transgenic female mice

p53 Genotype	Number of animals	50% tumor incidence	100% tumor incidence	Mean tumors per mouse
p53+/+	16	22.5 weeks	40 weeks	1.17
p53+/-	32	23.0 weeks	41 weeks	1.17
p53-/-	16	11.5 weeks	15 weeks	1.28

Table 2B. Mammary tumor incidence in p53-deficient and normal *Wnt-1* transgenic male mice

p53 Genotype	Number of animals	Tumor incidence Six months	Tumor incidence Twelve months
p53+/+	21	10%	43%
p53+/-	22	20%	32%
p53-/-	12[a]	100%	

[a] Four of 16 *Wnt-1 TG* p53-/- males developed early lymphomas.

Note above that the *Wnt-1 TG* p53-/- females and males developed mammary adenocarcinomas much sooner than their *Wnt-1 TG* p53+/- and p53+/+ counterparts. The *Wnt-1*

TG p53+/- males and females did not develop tumors significantly faster than the *Wnt-1 TG* p53+/+ males and females. During tumor development, roughly half of the *Wnt-1 TG* p53+/- tumors lost their remaining wild type p53 allele, as measured by Southern blotting (data not shown). These tumors with p53 loss of heterozygosity (LOH) did not develop any sooner than those p53+/- tumors without LOH. Thus, only those animals completely lacking p53 (p53-/-) showed accelerated mammary tumor development under the influence of the *Wnt-1* transgene.

p53 LOSS AFFECTS THE HISTOPATHOLOGY OF MAMMARY ADENOCARCINOMAS

In the mammary cancer study described above, mammary tumors were recorded when the tumor reached a size of roughly 0.5 cm. When the tumor became 1.5-2.0 cm in diameter, the animal was sacrificed and histopathology performed on the tumor by standard methods. Analysis of 32 *Wnt-1 TG* p53 mammary adenocarcinomas revealed dramatic differences in the tumor histopathology which directly depended on the presence or absence of wild type p53 in the tumor. Histology of representative tumors of each p53 genotype is shown below in Fig. 1.

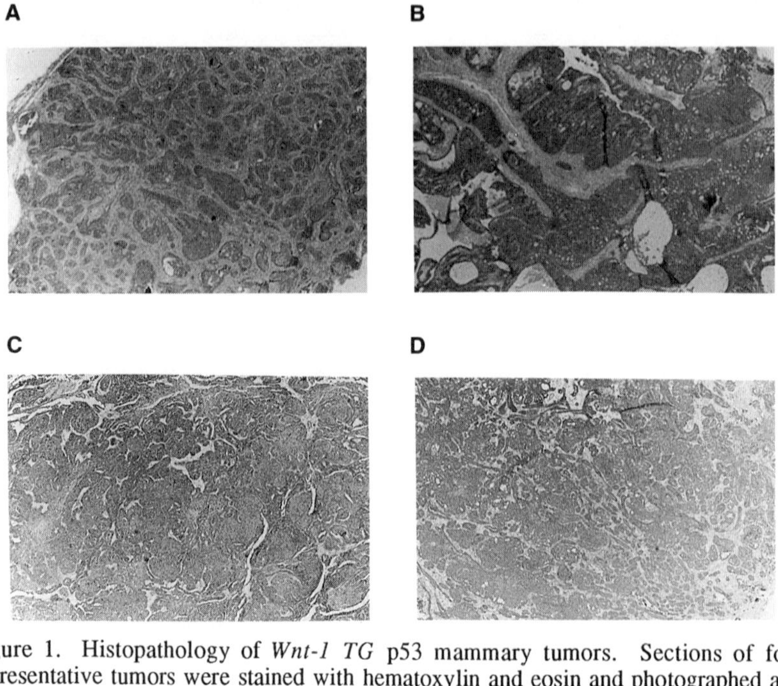

Figure 1. Histopathology of *Wnt-1 TG* p53 mammary tumors. Sections of four representative tumors were stained with hematoxylin and eosin and photographed at a magnification of 50X. (A) *Wnt-1 TG* p53+/+ tumor; (B) *Wnt-1 TG* p53+/- (no LOH) tumor; (C) *Wnt-1 TG* p53+/- (LOH) tumor; (D) *Wnt-1 TG* p53-/- tumor.

In most of those tumors which retained wild type p53 (p53+/+ and p53+/- without LOH), the tumor cells appeared more organized, with considerable stromal involvement or fibrosis. In contrast, tumors missing p53 (p53-/- or p53+/- with LOH) had much less stromal fibrosis. These tumor cells were also more anaplastic in appearance and had more mitotic figures. Table 3 shows the compilation of 32 *Wnt-1 TG* p53 female tumors analyzed by histopathology for a fibrotic or non-fibrotic appearance and their p53 genotypes.

Table 3. Histopathology of female *Wnt-1 TG* p53 tumors

p53 Genotype	With Fibrosis	Without Fibrosis
p53+/+	8 (73%)	3 (27%)
p53+/- (no LOH)	6 (75%)	2 (25%)
p53+/- (LOH)	1 (14%)	6 (86%)
p53-/-	0 (0%)	6 (100%)

Note above the strong correlation between the presence of functional wild type p53 and presence of fibrosis. The p53+/- (no LOH) tumors are believed to retain wild type p53, since the p53 cDNAs of four representative p53+/- (no LOH) tumors were sequenced and found to be wild type (data not shown). These results suggest that mammary tumorigenesis pathways in this model may be fundamentally different depending on the presence or absence of wild type p53.

EFFECTS OF p53 LOSS ON GENOMIC STABILITY IN A MAMMARY CANCER MODEL

The relatively early development of mammary tumors in the *Wnt-1 TG* p53 mice provided us with a useful model for exploring the genetic and biological effects of the presence and absence of p53 in tumor progression in a single tissue. One effect of p53 loss in tissue culture cells appears to be increased genetic instability as measured by abnormal chromosome numbers and susceptibility to gene amplification in the presence of certain drugs (Livingstone et al., 1992; Yin et al., 1992). However, we wanted to extend these observations and determine whether loss of p53 confers genetic instability in the context of an *in vivo* tumor model.

In our first set of experiments, we made cytogenetic preparations from the mammary tumor cells of p53+/+, p53+/-, and p53-/- *Wnt-1* mice to determine whether loss of p53 conferred chromosomal instability. Metaphase preparations were made according to standard procedures on tumor cells isolated 24-48 hours previously from intact tumors (Aldaz et al., 1992). The chromosome numbers of 25-50 metaphases for 15 *Wnt-1* tumors of different p53 genotypes were determined. The results of these chromosome counts are summarized in Fig. 2.

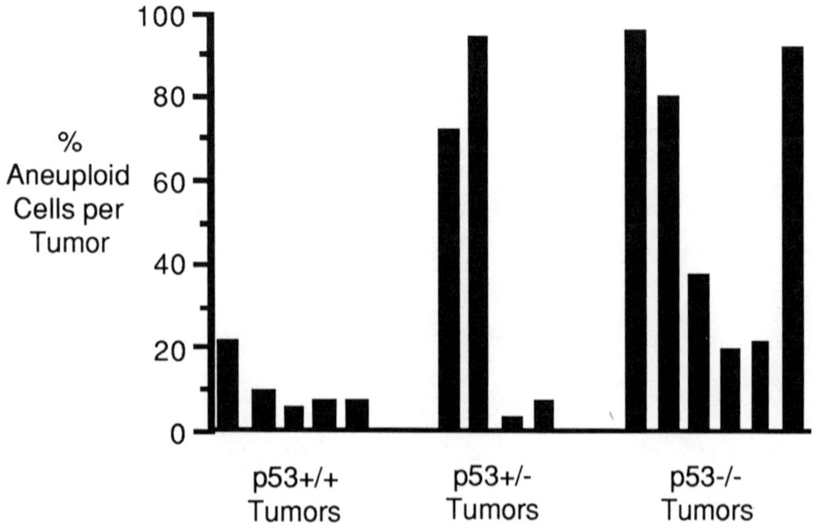

Figure. 2. Summary of cytogenetic studies in *Wnt-1 TG* p53 mice. Each tumor is represented by a bar indicating the percentage of examined cells that had chromosome numbers other than 40. The p53 genotype of each group is indicated below the graph.

Note that the great majority of cells from all of the *Wnt-1 TG* p53+/+ mammary tumors retained an apparent diploid karyotype, while several of the *Wnt-1 TG* p53-/- tumors had a high percentage of aneuploid cells. Interestingly, some of the *Wnt-1 TG* p53-/- tumors were primarily diploid in karyotype, indicating that p53 loss by itself was insufficient to confer genomic instability. The *Wnt-1 TG* p53+/- tumors displayed two patterns: one of high aneuploidy and one of apparent diploidy. When the status of the remaining wild type p53 allele in these tumors was assayed by Southern blot hybridization, both aneuploid tumors had lost the wild type allele, while in the diploid tumors, one tumor had retained the wild type allele and the second had partial loss of heterozygosity (data not shown).

The aneuploid cells in the individual *Wnt-1 TG* p53+/- and Wnt-1 p53-/- tumors tended to be heterogeneous in chromosome number. Typical tumors had high numbers of cells in the hypotetraploid range. Other tumors had a high percentage of cells missing a single chromosome (data not shown). Taken, together, these cytogenetic experiments support the concept, previously established by *in vitro* studies, that loss of p53 predisposes a developing tumor cell to chromosomal instability *in vivo*.

We employed a second type of assay, comparative genomic hybridization (CGH), to measure genomic instability in the *Wnt-1 TG* p53 tumor model. CGH detects regions of increases and decreases in DNA copy number throughout the entire genome of a tumor cell (Kallioniemi et al., 1992). This procedure was applied to 25 of our *Wnt-1 TG* p53 tumor DNAs and some of the results are shown in Table 4 and Fig. 3. First of all, the total number of chromosomal abnormalities in each tumor was partially dependent on the p53 genotype of the animal in which the tumor arose. Only two of six *Wnt-1 TG* p53+/+ tumors and two of four *Wnt-1 TG* p53+/- (no LOH) tumors exhibited chromosomal regions with DNA copy number gains or losses (Table 4). In contrast, all eight *Wnt-1 TG* p53+/- (LOH) and seven *Wnt-1 TG* p53-/- tumors displayed at least one chromosomal abnormality and many showed multiple changes in DNA copy number. As shown in Table 4, the average number of chromosomal changes per tumor was greatest in the *Wnt-1 TG* p53+/- (LOH) tumors, with an average of 4.2 abnormalities/tumor compared to 1.7 abnormalities per tumor for the *Wnt-1 TG* p53-/- tumors.

Table 4. Summary of CGH Abnormalities in the *Wnt-1 TG* p53 tumors

p53 Genotype	Tumors with Chromosome Abnormalities	Average Number of Chromosome Abnormalities per Tumor
p53+/+	2/6	0.3
p53+/- (no LOH)	2/4	1.0
p53+/- (LOH)	8/8	4.2
p53-/-	7/7	1.7

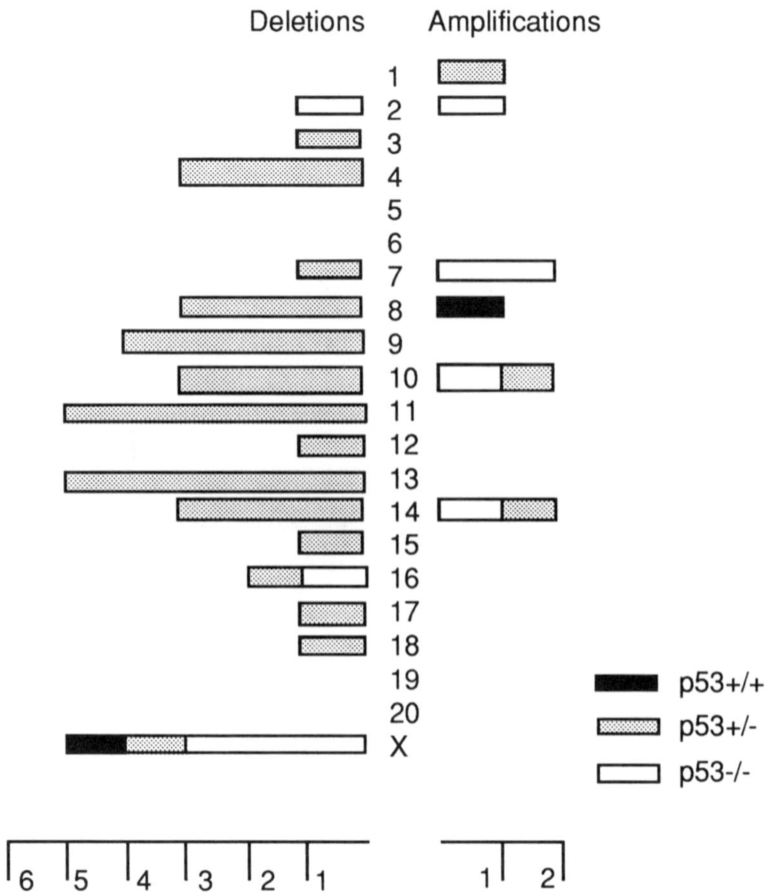

Figure 3. Chromosomal pattern of CGH DNA copy number gains and losses in the *Wnt-1 TG* p53 mammary tumors. CGH data from 25 *Wnt-1 TG* p53 tumors are compiled in this figure according to chromosome (listed in the middle column). The scale at the bottom indicates the number of tumors observed with a copy number gain or loss at a given chromosome. The p53 genotype of a tumor is indicated by black filling (p53+/+), shaded filling (p53+/-), or no filling (p53-/-).

The chromosomal abnormalities that were observed were both DNA copy number losses and gains, with losses predominating. Many of the copy number losses encompassed entire chromosomes or most of a chromosome. The pattern of chromosomal DNA gains and losses was at least partially non-random, with particular chromosomes displaying more frequent copy number gains and losses than others. These losses and gains are shown in Fig. 3. Note that DNA copy number losses were observed in at least four different tumors for chromosomes 9, 11, 13, and X. DNA copy number gains were observed at least twice on chromosomes 7, 10, and 14. Interestingly, in a *Wnt-1 TG* p53-/- tumor with evidence of DNA copy number gains on chromosome 7, we were able to demonstrate by Southern blot hybridization amplification (6-8 copies) of the *int-2/FGF3* gene (data not shown). This gene also was shown to be greatly increased in mRNA expression in this tumor. Since *int-2/FGF-3* has previously been activated in some mouse mammary carcinomas (Peters et al., 1986), this result not only validates the power of the CGH technique, it confirms the probable cooperation of *int-2/FGF-3* and *Wnt-1* in the generation of this tumor.

Chromosome 11 losses were usually associated with LOH of the wild type p53 allele in *Wnt-1 TG* p53+/- tumors, consistent with the location of the p53 gene on mouse chromosome 11. Fig. 3 also suggests that certain chromosomal losses tended to be associated with a particular p53 genotype. For example, the *Wnt-1 TG* p53+/- tumors showed losses in chromosomes 9 and 13, which were not observed in the *Wnt-1 TG* p53+/+ and *Wnt-1 TG* p53-/- tumors. In addition, half of the *Wnt-1 TG* p53-/- chromosomal abnormalities were increases in DNA copy number, whereas less than 10% of the chromosome alterations in the p53+/- tumors were increases in DNA copy number (Fig. 3). The CGH results confirm the cytogenetic data and support the hypothesis that loss of p53 results in increased genomic instability at the chromosomal and subchromosomal level.

DISCUSSION

This study represents our attempts to determine the effects of the presence or absence of p53 on tumor progression in a single targeted tissue. The results indicate that loss of p53 does have dramatic effects on both biological and genetic aspects of mammary tumor progression in our model. *Wnt-1* transgenic mice missing p53 (p53-/-) display (1) accelerated tumor development compared to *Wnt-1 TG* p53+/+ and *Wnt-1 TG* p53+/- mice; (2) altered tumor histopathology compared to p53+/+ mice; and (3) increased genomic instability compared to *Wnt-1 TG* p53+/+ mice. The *Wnt-1 TG* p53+/- mice, while not developing tumors any sooner than Wnt-1 p53+/+ mice, do exhibit altered mammary tumor histopathology (more anaplastic, less fibrotic) similar to the tumors of the *Wnt-1 TG* p53-/- mice when the remaining p53 wild type allele is lost. Surprisingly, the *Wnt-1 TG* p53+/- tumors with loss of the wild type allele display even more genomic instability (as measured by CGH) than *Wnt-1 TG* p53-/- tumors.

These *in vivo* tumorigenesis experiments extend previous *in vitro* studies which indicated that loss of p53 confers genomic instability. However, the existence of *Wnt-1 TG* p53-/- tumors with diploid karyotypes suggests that p53 loss predisposes a tumor cell to genomic instability rather than induces it directly. Evidence exists that p53 is a cell cycle checkpoint protein both at G1 and mitosis (Kastan et al., 1992; Livingstone et al., 1992; Yin et al., 1992; Cross et al., 1995). Cells which lose the p53-mediated mitotic spindle checkpoints may be likely to leave mitosis and enter G1 before completing chromosome segregation. Cross et al. (1995) have shown that the loss of the p53 mitotic checkpoint often results in tetraploid and octaploid cells *in vitro* and *in vivo*. Such results are consistent with our observations of hypotetraploidy in many of the *Wnt-1 TG* p53 mammary tumors.

Despite the correlation between loss of p53 and increased genomic instability in our model, it appears that increased genomic instability *per se* is not necessarily correlated with accelerated tumorigenesis. The tumors with the most chromosomal abnormalities, the *Wnt-1 TG* p53+/- (LOH) tumors, do not develop any sooner than *Wnt-1 TG* p53+/+ tumors, which show the least chromosomal instability. We hypothesize that chromosomal gains and losses which do occur may be selected for during tumor progression, but do not represent the key rate limiting events which determine the initial tumor formation.

One mechanism by which loss of p53 may confer accelerated tumorigenesis is through loss of p53-mediated apoptosis. Loss of p53 in other murine tumor models has been shown to result in decreased apoptosis of tumor cells and this has been correlated with increased rate and aggressiveness of tumor growth (Lowe et al., 1994; Symonds et al., 1994). Loss of p53-mediated apoptosis could explain the earlier appearance of the *Wnt-1 TG* p53-/- mammary tumors. However, why didn't the p53+/- (LOH) tumors show even slightly increased rates of tumor development over *Wnt-1 TG* p53+/+ tumors? One explanation is that loss of the remaining wild type allele is a relatively late event in tumor development, so that p53-mediated apoptosis is not lost in this type of tumor until it is too late to affect the time to overt tumor appearance. A second possibility is that p53 wild type allele loss does occur relatively early but that loss of p53-mediated apoptosis is not a rate limiting step to tumor formation in this particular model and that other mechanisms are crucial. Further experiments are currently underway to test both possibilities.

REFERENCES

Aldaz CM, Chen A, Gollahon LS, Russo J, Zappler K (1992): Nonrandom abnormalities involving chromosome 1 and Harvey-ras-1 alleles in rat mammary tumor progression. Cancer Res 52:4791-4798.

Clarke AR, Purdie CA, Harrison DJ, Morris RG, Bird CC, Hooper ML, Wyllie AH (1993): Thymocyte apoptosis induced by p53-dependent and independent pathways. Nature 352:849-852.

Cross SM, Sanchez CA, Morgan CA, Schimke MK, Ramel S, Idzerda RL, Raskind WH, Reid BJ (1995): A p53-dependent mouse spindle checkpoint. Science 267: 1353-1356.

Donehower LA, Harvey M, Slagle BL, McArthur MJ, Montgomery CA, Butel JS, Bradley A (1992): Mice deficient for p53 are developmentally normal but susceptible to spontaneous tumours. Nature 356: 215-221.

Finlay CA, Hinds PW, Levine AJ (1989): The p53 proto-oncogene can act as a suppressor of transformation. Cell 57: 1083-1093.

Greenblatt MS, Bennett WP, Hollstein M, Harris CC (1994): Mutations in the p53 tumor suppressor gene: clues to cancer etiology and molecular pathogenesis. Cancer Res 54: 4855-4878.

Harvey M, McArthur MJ, Montgomery CA, Butel JS, Bradley A, Donehower LA (1993): Spontaneous and carcinogen-induced tumorigenesis in p53-deficient mice. Nature Genet 5: 225-229.

Kallioniemi A, Kallioniemi O-P, Sudar D, Rutovitz D, Gray JW, Waldman F, Pinkel D (1992): Comparative genomic hybridization for molecular cytogenetic analysis of solid tumors. Science 258: 818-821.

Kastan MB, Zhan Q, El-Deiry WS, Carrier F, Jacks T, Walsh WV, Plunkett BS, Vogelstein B, Fornace AJ Jr (1992): A mammalian cell cycle checkpoint pathway utilizing p53 and GADD45 is defective in ataxia-telangiectiasia. Cell 71: 587-597.

Livingstone LR, White A, Sprouse J, Livanos E, Jacks T, Tlsty T (1992): Altered cell cycle arrest and gene amplification potential accompany loss of wild-type p53. Cell 70: 923-935.

Lowe SW, Schmitt EM, Smith SW, Osborne BA, Jacks T (1993a): p53 is required for radiation-induced apoptosis in mouse thymocytes. Nature 362: 847-849.

Lowe SW, Ruley HE, Jacks T, Housman DE (1993b): p53-dependent apoptosis modulates the cytotoxicity of anticancer agents. Cell 74: 957-967.

Lowe SW, Bodis S, McClatchey A, Remington L, Ruley HE, Fisher DE, Housman DE, Jacks T (1994): p53 status and the efficacy of cancer therapy *in vivo*. Science 266: 807-810.

Malkin D, Li FP, Strong LC, Fraumeni JF Jr, Nelson CE, Kim DH, Kassel J, Gryka MA, Bischoff FZ, Tainsky MA, Friend SH (1990): Germ line p53 mutations in a familial syndrome of breast cancer, sarcomas, and other neoplasms. Science 250: 1233-1238.

Srivastava S, Zou Z, Pirollo K, Blattner W, Chang EH (1990): Germ-line transmission of a mutated p53 gene in a cancer prone family with Li-Fraumeni syndrome. Nature 348: 747-749.

Symonds H, Krall L, Remington L, Saenz-Robles M, Lowe S, Jacks T, Van Dyke T (1994): p53-dependent apoptosis suppresses tumor growth and progression *in vivo*. Cell 78: 703-711.

Tsukamoto AS, Grosschedl R, Guman RC, Parslow T, and Varmus HE (1988): Expression of the *int*-1 gene in transgenic mice is associated with mammary gland hyperplasia and adenocarcinomas in male and female mice. Cell 55: 619-625.

Yin H, Tainsky MA, Bischoff FZ, Strong LC, Wahl GM (1992): Wild-type p53 restores cell cycle control and inhibits gene amplification in cells with mutant p53 alleles. Cell 70: 937-948.

Yonish-Rouach E, Resnitzky D, Lotem J, Sachs L, Kimchi A, Oren M. (1991): Wild-type p53 induces apoptosis of myeloid leukemic cells that is inhibited by interleukin-6. Nature 352: 345-347.

Genetics and Cancer Susceptibility:
Implications for Risk Assessment, pages 13–22

GENETIC SUSCEPTIBILITY TO *IN VIVO* AND *IN VITRO* CHEMICAL TRANSFORMATION

Cheryl Walker

Department of Carcinogenesis, Univeristy of Texas M.D. Anderson Cancer Center, Science Park - Research Division, Smithville, Texas 78957

INTRODUCTION

Germline transmission of a tumor suppressor gene mutation constitutes a well described form of cancer susceptibility that predisposes to the development of many types of spontaneous tumors in both rodents and humans. Loss or inactivation of the second, normal allele of the defective tumor suppressor gene as a somatic event results in the development of tumors in such predisposed individuals. This 2 event or "2-hit" mechanism for tumor suppressor gene inactivation in tumors was first hypothesized by Knudson for retinoblastoma (Knudson, 1971), and subsequently has been shown to be a general paradigm for the role of tumor suppressor genes in both hereditary and nonhereditary tumors (Weinberg, 1991; Bishop, 1991; Marshall, 1991).

The participation of tumor suppressor genes in carcinogen-induced tumors is less well described than for spontaneous tumors. In certains types of human cancer, such as hepatocellular carcinoma associated with aflatoxin and hepatitis exposure, it is clear that carcinogen inactivation of a tumor suppressor gene, in this case aflatoxin-induced mutation in the p53 tumor suppressor gene, plays a critical role in tumor development (Puisieux, 1991; Hsu, 1991; Greenblatt, 1994). As described in the accompanying chapter by Groopman et al, this is perhaps the clearest example to date of a tumor suppressor gene which is targeted by a known human carcinogen.

For experimental carcinogenesis, studies in animal cancer susceptibility models in which germline tumor suppressor gene alterations exist naturally or are created via knockout mutations can be used to address questions related to tumor suppressor gene inactivation by chemical carcinogens. Such animal models in which the intrinsic genetic defect is well defined offer the opportunity to dissect the process of tumor development within a defined system to elucidate the fundamental principals underlying cancer susceptibility. Animal models are amenable to intervention at all stages of neoplastic development, allowing investigators to study even the earliest events in this process. In addition, both normal and neoplastic cells and tissue can be readily accessed from donor animals for biochemical and molecular analysis. Because of the facility with which tumor development can be manipulated in animals, opportunities are also available for testing therapeutic approaches for various types of cancer and for identifying chemopreventative agents.

For genetic studies, well-defined animal models can be used to identify the genes responsible for cancer susceptibility. Human populations are generally heterogeneous, making it difficult to identify genes responsible for inherited cancer susceptibility if they have a low penetrance, cause a small increase in relative risk, or are involved in multilocus susceptibility. Using animal models, directed matings can be used in which the parental genotypes are known to dissect the genetic basis of cancer susceptibility. Such defined crosses also present an opportunity to generate linkage data that can be used to localize (and possibly identify) specific genes responsible for cancer susceptibility. Working with intact animals also has an advantage over in *vitro* studies, as in the whole animal, tumor development proceeds in the presence of other organ systems, such as the endocrine and immune systems, which can effect the process of tumor development. These interactions between the product of a susceptibility gene and specific organ systems, which might be required to confer the susceptible phenotype, can be studied only in the whole animal.

Both physiological and experimentally derived animal models of genetic susceptibility to cancer are available. Genetic susceptibility can be broadly grouped into one of two classes of physiologic animal models of tumorigenesis: (1) those for which the susceptibility gene itself is the target for tumor development and (2) those in which modifer genes are responsible for tumor susceptibility. Experimentally derived animal models may also be grouped into two classes. So called "knockout" animals are murine models in which the function of a specific gene has been ablated. In these animals, one or both copies of a tumor suppressor gene have been inactivated, resulting in an increased susceptibility for tumor development. Alternatively, transgenic animals, in which a specific gene such as an activated oncogene has been introduced into the germline, have also been developed that exhibit an increased susceptibility for tumor development.

One naturally occuring animal model which can be utilized in these types of studies is the Eker rat hereditary cancer model (Eker, 1961). In this model, rats that inherit a mutation in the Tuberous sclerosis gene (Tsc-2) develop spontaneous tumors of the kidney, uterus and spleen (Everitt, et al., 1992). The mutation results from an intronic insertion in the Tsc-2 gene, altering transcription and inactivating the mutated allele (Yeung, et al., 1994; Kobayashi, et al., 1995) Spontaneous tumors of the kidney develop in 100% of predisposed animals by 12-14 months of age, and uterine leiomyoma and splenic hemangiosarcoma also are observed with a high frequency (>60%) in these animals. Tumors develop in carrier rats as a result of a somatic mutation in in the remaining normal allele, consistent with Knudson's 2-hit hypothesis (Yeung, et al., 1995).

Renal cell carcinoma (RCC) in rats closely resembles that of man in many ways. Because of the many similarities between rat and human RCC, the rat appears to be particularly well suited for studies on mechanisms of carcinogenesis of kidney epithelial cells. However, spontaneous RCC in rats is very rare, occurring with a frequency of >0.5% (Barrett and Huff, 1991; Solleveld and Boorman, 1986). Histologically, RCC are similar in the two species (Hard, 1976). Tumors and tumor-derived cell lines from both rat and human RCC express transforming growth factor alpha (Walker, et al., 1991; Derynck, et al., 1987; Mydlo, et al., 1989; Gommela, et al., 1989; Petrides, et al., 1990). Activation of *ras* oncogenes appears to be an infrequent event in tumors of both species (Nagata, et al., 1990; Nanus, et al., 1990; Fujita, et al., 1988; Recio, et al., 1991).

The kidney is a target organ for many environmental carcinogens including lead, chloroform, trihalomethanes, components of unleaded gasoline and a number of other compounds, many of which have tested positive in the NTP rodent bioassays (Mehlman, 1984; Hamilton, 1975; Hiasa and Ito, 1987; Kluwe, et al., 1984; Barrett and Huff, 1991; MacFarland, 1982; IARC, 1980; NCI, 1976). In the rat, 2-year carcinogenicity bioassay data indicate that the kidney is the second most common site for tumor development, with liver being the primary site (Barrett and Huff, 1991). RCC arise from epithelial cells of the renal tubule (Richie and Skinner, 1981) and these tumors make up the largest proportion of primary kidney cancers in man, comprising ~ 85% of all renal tumors (Richie and Skinner, 1981), accounting for ~ 2% of the cancer deaths each year. The percentage of human renal cell carcinomas that may be the result of exposure to chemical carcinogens in the environment and the role of tumor suppressor genes in carcinogen induced RCC is unknown. The Eker rat model in which animals are susceptible to RCC and for which the normal allele of the Tsc-2 gene can be a target for spontaneous tumor development is well suited for dissecting the role of tumor suppressor genes as determinants of susceptibility to chemical carcinogenesis in the kidney.

TISSUE-SPECIFIC FACTORS MODULATE SUSCEPTIBILITY TO CHEMICAL CARCINOGENESIS

Several types of renal neoplasms exist and have been well described in the rat. In adult animals, renal mesenchymal tumors, arising from stromal cells of the kidney, and RCC, arising from tubular epithelial cells, are the most common. These tumors have distinct cell types of origin (mesenchymal and epithelial cells respectively) and are easily discriminated from each other histologically (Hard, 1976; Thoenes, et al. ,1986). Both these neoplasms can be induced by the renal carcinogen dimethylnitrosoamine (DMN) and the ability of this carcinogen to induce these tumors in rats has been well described by Hard (1986). Because the Eker mutation is carried in the germline, both renal epithelial and mesenchymal cells inherit the defective Tsc-2 allele, and thus at the genetic level are equally predisposed toward tumor development. However, the fact that only RCC and not renal mesenchymal tumors are observed as spontaneous tumors in these rats would suggest that other, tissue-specific factors, modulate the risk of tumor development in these genetically predisposed cells.

To test this hypothesis, rats carrying the Eker mutation were exposed to a single 30 mg/kg dose of the renal carcinogen DMN. As a control, rats that lacked this mutation were also exposed to the same dose, and the incidence of RCC and renal mesenchymal tumors in the 2 groups was determined at 14 months of age (Walker, et al., 1992). As shown in Figure1, while untreated carrier animals developed RCC spontaneously, the number of these tumors in the DMN treated animals was greatly increased. Relative to noncarrier rats that were exposed to DMN, the multiplicity of RCC in rats carrying the Eker mutation (after subtracting the background of spontaneous tumors) was > 70-fold higher than rats carrying 2 wild type alleles of this gene. Thus the presence of the Eker mutation in the Tsc-2 gene acted as a determinent of susceptibility to tumor development in the renal epithelial cells for both spontaneous and carcinogen-induced tumors.

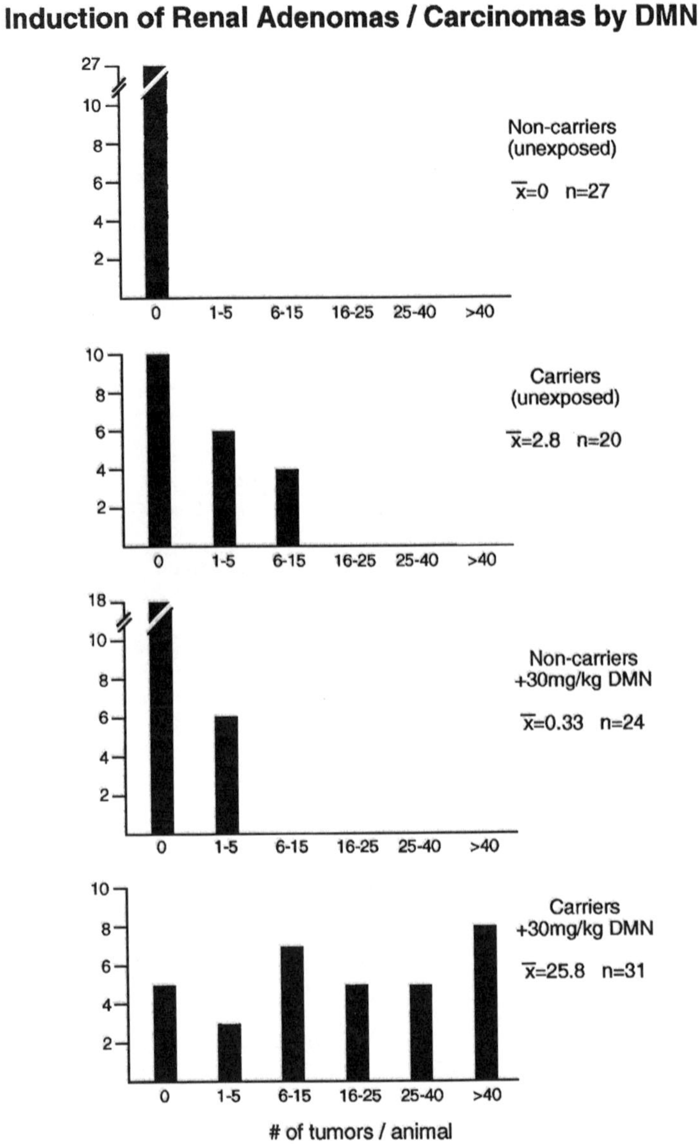

Figure 1. Tumor multiplicity is shown for (from top to bottom) spontaneous RCC in wild-type animals and rats carrying the Eker mutation and DMN-induced RCC in wild-type rats and gene carriers.
n = number of rats/group
$\overline{x}$ = mean number of tumors/animal

The incidence of renal mesenchymal tumors in control wild-type rats and rats carrying the Eker mutation was also determined (Figure 2). In both wild-type and carrier animals, DMN was a potent renal carcinogen for mesenchymal tumors. However, there was no difference in tumor multiplicity or incidence between rats carrying the mutant or wild-type allele of the Tsc-2 gene. Thus, in renal mesenchymal cells, the presence of the Eker mutation was modulated by other factors so that increased susceptibility to tumor development conveyed by the presence of this mutation did not manifest itself in this cell type. The nature of this tissue-specificity is not clear at this time, but does not appear to be accounted for by a trivial explanation such as lack of expression of this gene in mesenchymal cells. The Tsc-2 gene is ubiquitously expressed (Yeung, et al., 1995), and thus presumably plays some role in cellular physiology in a variety of cell types, including renal mesenchymal cells. This type of tissue-specificity for germline alterations has been noted for virtually all other tumor suppressor genes as tumors develop in only a subset of cells and tissues in which the altered gene is present. This is particularly interesting for genes such as RB and p53, which have critical and generalized functions in cell cycle control, presumably even in cells in which mutations in these genes do not predispose to tumor development.

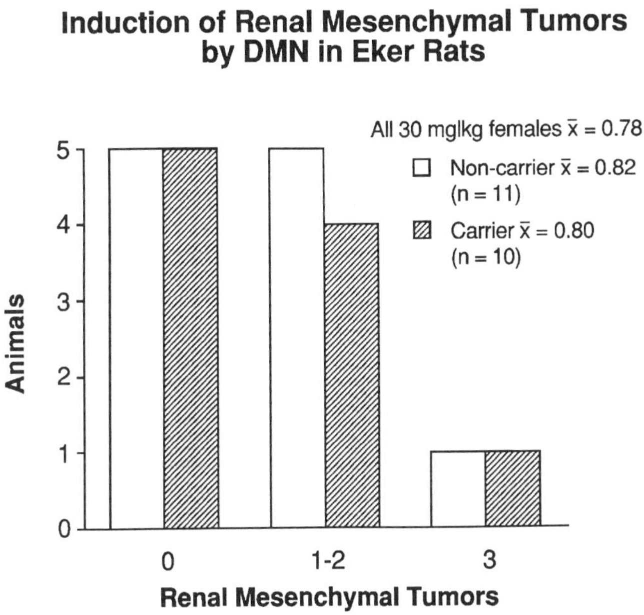

Figure 2. Multiplilcity of DMN-induced renal mesenchymal tumors in non-carrier (open bars) and carrier (hatched bars) rats.

TUMOR SUPPRESSOR GENES AS DETERMINANTS OF CELL TRANSFORMATION *IN VITRO*

Tumor development *in vivo* is a multistage process, involving many genes and alterations in numerous biological processes. Loss of function of tumor suppressor genes is permissive for tumor cell growth and the restraint mechanisms which are relieved following this loss of function appear to be quite varied. They can act at many different physiological levels from cell cycle checkpoint control in individual cells to regulating systemic biological functions such as angiogenesis. In contrast to studies of tumor growth *in vivo*, in which the entire spectrum of alterations required for tumor development can participate, *in vitro* studies of cell transformation by chemical carcinogens are generally more limited, often focusing on a particular window during the transformation process or quantitating the emergance of specific transformed characteristics. Thus studying susceptibility to cell transformation by tumor suppressor genes *in vitro* is problematic, due to both a lack of understanding of the relationship of various *in vitro* transformed characteristics to events occuring *in vivo* during tumor development and constrainsts on the nature of the transformed phenotypes amenable for study within any given in vitro transformation assay, which may or may not correspond to the mode of action of the particular tumor suppressor gene of interest.

To determine whether the presence of a tumor suppressor gene alteration can confer susceptibility to transformation *in vitro* as well as *in vivo*, experiments were performed to transform rat kidney epithelial (RKE) cells *in vitro* and quantitate cell transformation in cells which carried the Eker mutation in the Tsc-2 gene verses normal cells with 2 wild-type copies of this gene. Using an *in vitro* RKE transformation assay developed in our laboratory (Walker and Ginsler, 1992), proximal tubule cells derived from known Eker rat cariers (+/Ek) and non-carriers (+/+) were exposed to the carcinogen N-methyl-N'-nitro-N-nitrosoguanidine (MNNG). The percent transformation frequency following MNNG treatment was 7.5-fold higher in cells dervied from carrier animals when compared to cells from non-carrier animals (Horesovsky, et al., 1994). This increased susceptibility to transformation due to inheritance of the Eker mutation is consistent with a predisposition resulting from inactivation of a tumor suppressor gene.

Transformation of cells both in vitro and in vivo is a multistage process, and cells derived from animals carrying the Eker mutation can be thought to have inherited the first alteration in this process. In a two-hit model in which wild-type cells are exposed to a carcinogen for example, two relevant genetic alterations occurring at relatively low frequencies (10^{-4} to 10^{-5}) must be induced in the same cell lineage for cells to become transformed. Two such events would occurr in the same cell lineage only infrequently. In the case of cells carrying a germ-line susceptibility mutation, all cells have inherited the first relevant alteration and can be thought of as "primed" for transformation. Thus the effective target cell population is the entire cell culture, rather than the rare cell in which the first genetic alteration has been induced by the carcinogen, resulting in increased carcinogen-induced transformation frequencies in cells carrying the Eker mutation relative to non-carrier cells. Although it is not known how many events are required to transform cells in the RKE assay, subsequent events, such as inactivation of the remaining normal allele of this susceptibility locus by an agent such as MNNG, could result in a preneoplastic phenotype characterized by enchanced ability to grow *in vitro*. This enhanced growth potential would be recognized in the RKE assay as a transformed colony.

It was somewhat surprising that the difference in transformation was not higher between carrier and non-carrier cells, since the exposure of male carrier rats to DMN resulted in a 70-fold increase in renal tumors between carriers and non-carriers. This difference may be a result of the artificial environment involved with in vitro culture of primary cells. The environment of the kidny epithelial cell *in vivo* is likely to be markedly different from the environment encountered *in vitro*. The lowered transformation frequency *in vitro* may be a reflection of the absence of other factors that may participate in the transformation process *in vivo*.

Although cells carrying the Eker mutation would be predicted to be more susceptible to transformation, because the RKE assay measures a very early and specific transformed phenotype (enhanced growth potential *in vitro*), we could not know a priori whether inheritance of the Eker susceptibility mutation would result in increased susceptibility to transformation detectable in our assay. The fact that the mutation did predispose to the development of the very earliest transformants would be consistent with this genetic alteration playing a role in altered regulation of cell growth. It would also further suggest that the Eker susceptibility mutation influences the initial stages of cell transformation and tumor development. We do not know whether differences exist between MNNG transformed cells that carry the Eker mutation and non-carrier cells transformed by MNNG for other transformed phenotypes, such as tumorigenic potential *in vivo* or anchorage independent growth, but the establishment of cell lines from carrier and non-carrier transformants may prove a useful tool for addressing this question.

CONCLUSIONS

As our knowledge of the biology of tumor suppressor genes has grown, so has our understanding of the different biological levels at which these genes function. Clearly tumor suppressor genes can act as determinants of interindividual susceptibility to cancer, but it is also clear that there are constrainsts on the action of these genes. Tissue-specific factors can modulate the influence of tumor suppressor genes and it will be necessary in the future to characterize cancer risk for specific organs and tissues, not just at the level germline genetic alterations present in the individual. In addition, tumor suppressor genes can modulate the transformation of cells *in vitro* as well as *in vivo*. This may open new avenues for investigating the mechanism of action of these genes as well as provide opportunities for identifying cellular factors that modulate the influence of tumor suppressor genes on cell growth and transformation.

ACKNOWLEDGEMENTS

Several individuals have contributed to the work described in this chapter including Drs. Jeffery Everitt, Tom Goldsworthy, Doug Wolf and Greg Horesovsky. Technical assistance was provided by Wendy Stewart and Julie Ginsler, Michelle Gardiner was responsible for editorial assistance in the preparation of this manuscript and support for a portion of this work was obtained from a grant from the National Institutes of Health CA63613.

REFERENCES

Barrett JC and Huff J (1991): Cellular and molecular mechanisms of chemically induced renal carcinogenesis. Renal Failure 13:211-225.

Bishop JM (1991): Molecular themes in oncogenesis. Cell 64:235-248.

Derynck R, Goeddell DV, Ullrich A, Gutterman JU, Williams RD, Bringman TS, Berger WH (1987): Synthesis of messenger RNAs for transforming growth factors α and β and the epidermal growth factor receptor for human tumors. Cancer Res 47:707-712.

Eker R, and Mossige J (1961): A dominant gene for renal adenomas in the rat. Nature 189:858-859.

Everitt J, Goldsworth T, Wolf D, and Walker C (1992): Hereditary renal cell carcinoma in the Eker rat: A rodent familial cancer syndrome. J Urology 148:1932-1936.

Fujita J, Kraus MH, Onoue H, Srivastava SK, Ebi Y, Kitamura Y, Rhim JS (1988): Activated H-*ras* oncogenes in human kidney tumors. Cancer Res 48:5251-5255.

Gomella LG, Sargent ER, Wade TP, Anglard P, Linehan WM, Kasid A (1989): Expression of transforming growth factor α in normal human adult kidney and enhanced expression of transforming growth factors α and $\beta1$ in renal cell carcinoma. Cancer Res 49:6972-6975.

Greenblatt MS, Bennett WP, Hollstein M, and Harris CC (1994): Mutations in the *p53* tumor suppressor gene: clues to cancer etiology and molecular pathogenesis. Cancer Res 54:4855-4878.

Hamilton JM (1975): Renal carcinogenesis. Adv Cancer Res 22:1-66.

Hard GC (1976): Tumors of the kidney, renal pelvis and ureter. In Turusov VS (ed.): "Pathology of tumours in Laboratory Animals-Tumorus of the Rat." IARC Scientific Publications, Kyon, Vol. 6, No. 1, Part 2, pp. 73-102.

Hard GC (1986): Experimental models for the sequential analysis of chemically-induced renal carcinogenesis. Toxicol Pathol 14:112.

Hiasa Y and Ito N (1987): Experimental induction of renal tumors. Crit Rev Toxicol 17:279-343.

Horesovsky G, Ginsler J, Everitt J, and Walker C (1994): Increased susceptibility to in vitro transformation of cells carrying the Eker tumor susceptibility mutation. Carcinogenesis 15:2183-2187.

Hsu LC, Metcalf RA, Sun T, Welsh JA, Wang NJ, and Harris CC (1991): Mutational hotspot in the p53 gene in human hepatocellular carcinomas. Nature 350:427-431.

IARC (1980): "Monograph on the Evaluation of the Carcinogenic Risk of Chemicals to Humans". IARC, Lyon, Vol. 23, pp. 1-210.

Kluwe WM, Abdo KM and Huff J (1984): Chronic kidney disease and organic chemical exposures: evaluations of causal relationships in humans and experimental animals. Fundam Appl Toxicol 4:889-901.

Knudson AG (1971): Mutation and cancer: statistical study of retinoblastoma. PNAS USA 68:820-823.

Kobayashi T, Hirayama Y, Kobayashi E, Kubo Y, and Hino O (1995): A germline insertion in the tuberous sclerosis (*Tsc2*) gene gives rise to the Eker rat model of dominantly inherited cancer. Nature Genetics 9:70-74.

MacFarland HN (1982): "Chronic gasoline toxicity". In MacFarland HN, Holdsworth CE, MacGregor JA, Call RW and Kane N. (eds). The Toxicology of Petroleum Hydrocarbons. American Petroleum Institute.

Marshall CJ (1991): Tumor suppressor genes. Cell 64:313-326.

Mehlman MA (1984): "Renal Effects of Petroleum Hydrocarbons". Princeton Scientific. Princeton, NY Vol. VIII.

Mydlo JH, Michaeli J, Cordon-Cardo C, Goldenberg AS, Heston WDW, Fair WR (1989): Expression of transforming growth factor α and epidermal growth factor receptor messenger RNA in neoplastic and nonneoplastic human kidney tissue. Cancer Res 49:3407-3411.

Nagata Y, Abe M, Kobayashi K, Saiki S, Kotake T, Yoshikawa K, Yeda R, Nakayama E, Shiku H (1990): Point mutations of c-*ras* genes in human bladder cancer and kidney cancer. Jpn J Cancer Res 81:22-27.

Nanus DN, Mentle IR, Motzer RJ, Bander MH, Albino AP (1990): Infrequent ras oncogene point mutations in renal cell carcinoma. J Urol 143:175-178.

National Cancer Institute (1976) Carcinogenesis bioassay of chloroform. NCI, Bethesda, MD, Nat. Tech. Info. Service no. PB264018/AS.

Petrides PE, Bock S, Bovens J, Hofmann R, Jakse G (1990): Modulation of pro-epidermal growth factor, protransforming growth factor α and epidermal growth factor receptor gene expression in human renal carcinomas. Cancer Res 50:3934-3939.

Puisieux A, Lim S, Groopman J, and Ozturk M (1991): Selective targeting of p*53* gene mutational hotspots in human cancers by etiologically defined carcinogens. Cancer Res 51:6185-6189.

Recio L, Lane SC, Ginsler J, and Walker C (1991): Analysis of *ras* DNA sequences in rat renal cell carcinoma. Mol Carcinogenesis 4:350-353.

Richie JP and Skinner DG (1981): Renal neoplasia. In Brenner BM and Rector, FC (eds), The Kidney. W.B. Saunders, Philadelphia, Vol. II. pp. 2109-2134.

Solleveld HA and Boorman GA (1986): Spontaneous renal lesions in five rat strains. Toxicol Pathol 14:168-174.

Thoenes W, Storkel ST, and Rumpelt HJ (1986): Histopathology and classification of renal cell tumors. Path Res Pract 181:125.

Walker C and Ginsler J (1992): Development of a quantitative *in vitro* transformation assay for kidney epithelial cells. Carcinogenesis 13:25-32.

Walker C and Ginsler J (1992): Development of a quantitative in vitro transformation assay for rat kidney epithelial cells. Carcinogenesis 13:25-32.

Walker C, Everitt J, Freed JJ, Knudson AG, Whiteley LO (1991): Altered expression of transforming growth factor-a in hereditary rat renal cell carcinoma. Cancer Res 51:2973-2978.

Walker C, Goldsworthy TL, Wolf DC, and Everitt J (1992): Predisposition to renal cell carcinoma due to alteration of a cancer susceptibility gene. Science 255:1693-1695.

Weinberg RA (1991): Tumor suppressor genes. Science 254:1138-1146.

Yeung RS, Xiao G-H, Everitt JI, Jin F, and Walker CL (1995): Allelic loss at the tuberous sclerosis 2 locus in spontaneous tumors of the Eker rat. Mol Carcinogenesis, in press.

Yeung RS, Xiao G-H, Jin F, Lee W-C, Testa JR, and Knudson AG (1994): Predisposition to renal carcinoma in the Eker rat is determined by germ-line mutation of the tuberous sclerosis 2 (*TSC2*) gene. Proc Natl Acad Sci 91:11413-11416.

Genetics and Cancer Susceptibility:
Implications for Risk Assessment, pages 23–32

Tlag1, A NOVEL MURINE TUMOR SUSCEPTIBILITY GENE THAT REGULATES MNU-INDUCED THYMIC LYMPHOMA DEVELOPMENT

Ellen R. Richie, Joe M. Angel and Eugene M. Rinchik

Department of Carcinogenesis, University of Texas, M.D. Anderson Cancer Center, Science Park-Research Division, Smithville, TX 78957 (ERR, JMA)
Biology Division, Oak Ridge National Laboratory, Oak Ridge, TN 37831 (Present address: Sarah Lawrence College, Bronxville, NY 10708) (EMR)

ETIOLOGY OF SPONTANEOUS VERSUS CARCINOGEN-INDUCED THYMIC LYMPHOMA DEVELOPMENT

There is abundant evidence that genetic susceptibility to spontaneous and experimentally induced cancer is a complex phenomenon under multigenic control. Studies with inbred mice and recombinant congenic strains have facilitated the mapping of various genes that contribute to a predisposition for development of liver, lung or colon tumors (1,2). Genetic susceptibility also plays a crucial role in the development of hematopoietic neoplasms. It has been recognized for many years that inbred mouse strains are differentially susceptible to development of spontaneous thymic lymphoma. In fact, certain strains, such as AKR/J and C58/J, have been the subject of numerous investigations due to their characteristically high incidence (>90%) of spontaneous thymic lymphoma, which occurs between six and twelve months of age (3). Spontaneous thymic lymphomas develop as a result of somatic proviral integrations of a unique class of endogenous recombinant murine leukemia viruses (MuLVs), referred to as mink cell focus forming (MCF) viruses (4-6). Although non-viral genes have been reported to confer a degree of susceptibility to spontaneous lymphomagenesis (7), it is clear that inheritance of appropriate endogenous retroviral loci is a prerequisite for the high incidence of spontaneous lymphoma (3-6). The mechanism(s) by which proviral integration induces lymphoma development is not yet completely understood; however, activation of cellular oncogenes by integration of MCF proviral sequences is thought to play a key role in MuLV-mediated lymphomagenesis (8).

In contrast, proviral integrations are not required for development of thymic lymphomas induced by the direct-acting carcinogen N-methyl-N-nitrosourea (MNU). In this case, non-viral background genes are responsible for the differential susceptibility of various inbred mouse strains to MNU-induced lymphomagenesis. Figure 1 shows that in comparison to other inbred strains, AKR /J and DBA/2J mice develop an exceptionally high incidence of MNU-induced thymic lymphoma after a relatively short latency. Other laboratories also have reported that AKR mice are highly susceptible to MNU-induced lymphomagenesis (9,10). Initially, we speculated that MNU treatment indirectly resulted in the early emergence of MCF viruses thereby accelerating lymphoma development. However, subsequent analysis of DNA from MNU-induced lymphomas revealed that, unlike spontaneous lymphomas, MNU-induced tumors do not contain MCF proviral integrations (11). Furthermore, tumor incidence studies in AKR/J mice congenic for the b allele of the *Fv-1* locus supported the notion that distinct mechanisms are involved in the generation of spontaneous and MNU-induced thymic lymphomas. The b allele of the *Fv-1* locus restricts integration and replication of N-tropic MuLVs, the type of endogenous viruses present in AKR/J mice. Whereas conventional AKR/J mice have an $Fv\text{-}1^n$ genotype and a high incidence of spontaneous lymphoma characterized by numerous MCF proviruses, congenic AKR.Fv-1^b mice have a low incidence of spontaneous lymphoma due to the genetic restriction imposed on proviral integration (12). Interestingly, AKR and AKR.Fv-1^b mice develop MNU-induced lymphomas with similar incidence and latency. As expected, somatically acquired MuLV proviral sequences were not detected in lymphomas from AKR.Fv-1^b mice. These findings demonstrate that proviral integration does not contribute to the relative susceptibility of AKR mice to develop a high incidence of early appearing MNU-induced lymphomas (13). Consistent with this conclusion, we find that C58/J and HRS/J mice are relatively resistant to MNU-induced lymphoma development even though these strains, like AKR/J, have a high incidence of endogenous MuLV-induced spontaneous lymphoma.

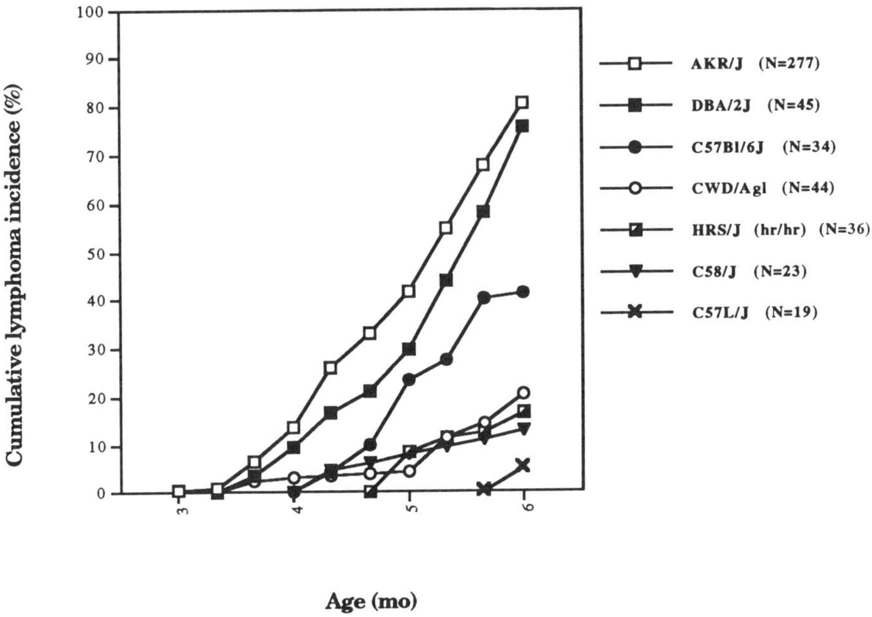

Figure 1. Differential susceptibility of various mouse strains to MNU-induced lymphoma development.

LOCALIZATION TO CHROMOSOME 7 OF A TUMOR SUSCEPTIBILITY GENE (*Tlag1*) THAT REGULATES MNU-INDUCED THYMIC LYMPHOMA DEVELOPMENT

Since non-viral genes apparently contribute to the predisposition of AKR/J mice to develop MNU-induced thymic lymphoma, we established genetic crosses between highly susceptible AKR/J mice and relatively resistant C57L mice as a first approach towards the identification of chromosomal regions responsible for genetic susceptibility. Mice were injected i.p. with a single dose of 75 mg/kg of MNU. The study was restricted to males because we observed that gender influences the progression of MNU-induced lymphomas (14). Experiments were terminated after the mice reached six months of age to avoid inclusion of spontaneous lymphomas in the analysis. The tumor incidence in parental strains as well as in (AKR x C57L)F_1, (AKR x C57L)F_2, AKR x (AKR x C57L)F_1 and (AKR x C57L)F_1 x AKR backcross progeny is shown in Figure 2. (By convention, the female parent is listed first when designating a cross).

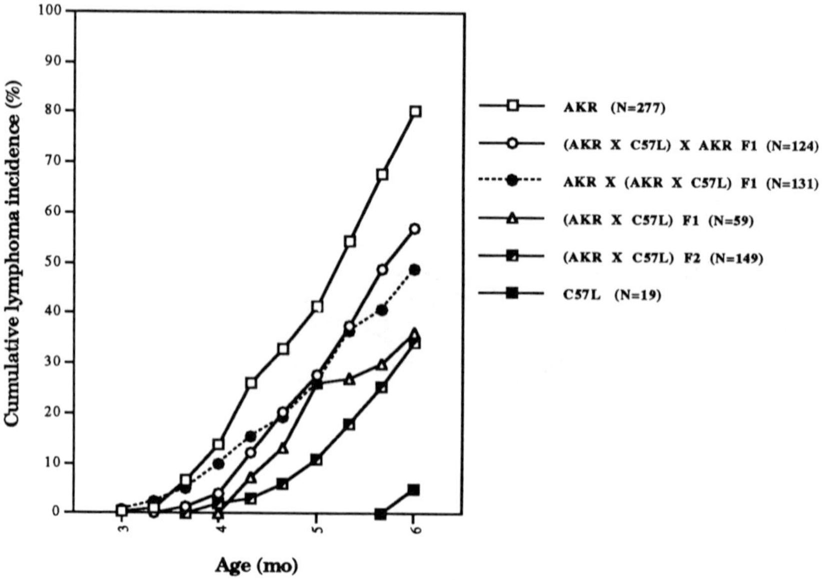

Figure 2. MNU-induced lymphoma incidence in crosses between AKR/J and C57L/J mice.

Approximately 80% of AKR/J mice developed MNU-induced lymphoma by six months of age. In contrast, only one lymphoma was observed in the C57L/J strain during the same interval. The tumor incidence in the various genetic crosses suggested that tumor susceptibility is under multigenic control. A fortuitous link between tumor susceptibility and coat color, demonstrated that one of these genes is linked to the albino locus (*c*) located on chromosome 7. In the (AKR x C57L)F_2 cross, we found that nonalbino mice have a significantly lower incidence of MNU-induced lymphoma than do albino mice (15). Since albino mice have a *c/c* genotype, whereas nonalbino mice are either *C/c* or *C/C* , these data indicate that homozygous inheritance of AKR/J alleles at a chromosome 7 locus confers enhanced susceptiblility to MNU-induced lymphoma. Restriction fragment length polymorphism analysis of the β-globin locus, located approximately 6 cM distal to *c*, provided verification of a chromosome 7 linkage. The data in Figure 3 show that F_2 mice that inherit two copies of the C57L β-globin allele (*Hbb*^{s}) are relatively resistant to tumor formation compared to mice that inherit two copies of the AKR/J β-globin allele (*Hbb*^{d}) (P<0.01). The tumor incidence of *Hbb*$^{s/d}$ heterozygotes is intermediate between the homozygous groups. Although not statistically significant, the data from heterozygous mice suggest either a gene dosage or an imprinting effect.

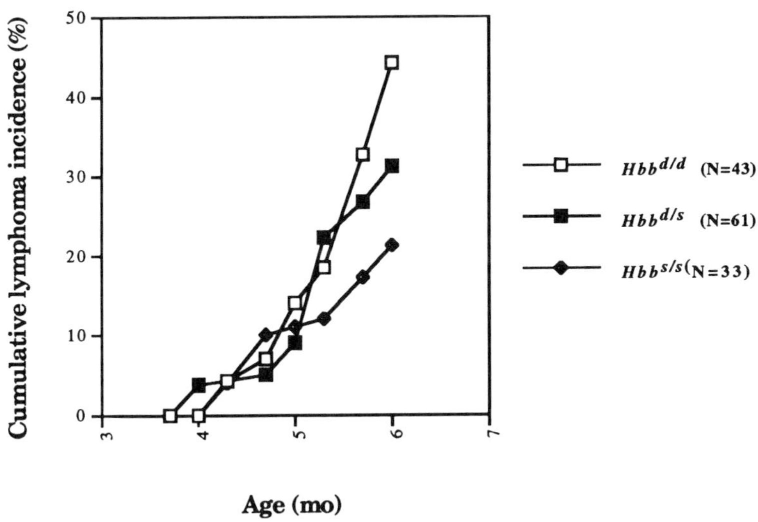

Figure 3. MNU-induced lymphoma incidence in (AKR x C57L)F_2 mice typed for homozygosity or heterozygosity at the *Hbb* locus.

Our initial observations were substantiated in AKR x (AKR x C57L)F_1 backcross progeny (16). Comparison of tumor incidence in backcross mice homozygous or heterozygous for additional polymorphic loci on chromosome 7 demonstrated that there is a stronger association between homozygous inheritance of AKR alleles and tumor incidence within the *c* to *Hbb* interval than outside this region. Because the tumor susceptibility gene apparently retards lymphoma development in the C57L/J strain, we have designated this locus as T-lymphoma attenuation gene 1 (*Tlag1*). Figure 4 shows a chromosome 7 map with the location of the polymorphic loci analyzed and the approximate position of *Tlag1*.

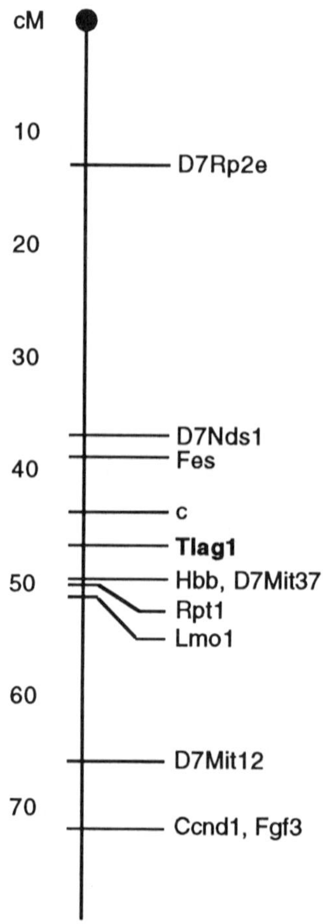

Figure 4. Locus map of murine chromosome 7. Locus symbols are given to the right of the chromosome and estimated map distances in centimorgans from the centromere are given at the left of the chromosome.

UTILIZATION OF ALBINO DELETION MUTANTS TO CONFIRM THE ASSIGNMENT OF *Tlag1* TO THE *c-Hbb* INTERVAL ON CHROMOSOME 7

In addition to conventional mapping studies, another approach we have taken to localize *Tlag1* involves complementation analyses in crosses between AKR/J mice and mice that carry overlapping radiation-induced interstitial deletions of the *c* locus on chromosome 7 (17). Since homozygosity for many of these deletions is lethal, the deleted chromosome is maintained in a hemizygous state opposite the chinchilla allele (c^{ch}) of the *c* locus. We are in the process of crossing male heterozygous deletion mutants with AKR/J females. The two types of F_1 progeny are easily distinguished by coat color. The albino progeny inherit an AKR/J chromosome 7 (*c*) opposite a deletion-containing chromosome 7, whereas the light chinchilla progeny inherit an AKR chromosome 7 opposite a nondeleted chromosome 7 containing the c^{ch} mutation. If the tumor susceptibility gene is located within the deletion, one would predict that lymphomagenesis would be accelerated in the albino compared to the light chinchilla progeny. To test this prediction and confirm the results of our F_2 and backcross analyses, we have assessed MNU-induced lymphoma development in albino and chinchilla males from a cross between AKR (*c/c*) females and hemizygous males carrying the c^{26DVT} deletion (c^{ch}/c^{26DVT}). The c^{26DVT}deletion spans a 6-11 cM region that includes the *c* locus and extends to a point just proximal to the *Hbb* locus. Figure 5 shows that progression of MNU-induced lymphoma in the albino progeny is similar to that of the AKR/J parental strain. In contrast, tumor development is delayed in the chinchilla progeny. These data confirm once again the notion that a gene which influences MNU-induced lymphoma development is localized within the *c* to *Hbb* interval on chromosome 7. We propose that the AKR/J strain contains a germline defect at the *Tlag1* locus resulting in enhanced susceptibility to development of a high incidence of early appearing MNU-induced lymphomas. Current efforts are directed towards utilizing a series of chromosome 7 deletion mutants to more precisely localize and clone the *Tlag1* gene.

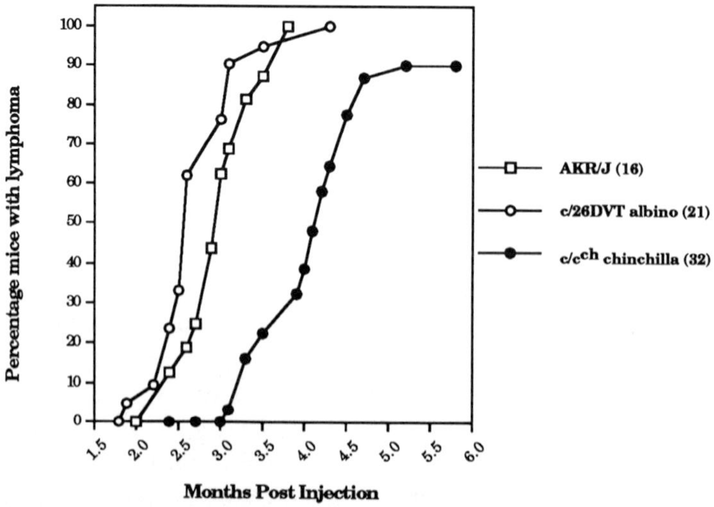

Figure 5. MNU-induced lymphoma incidence in (AKR x c^{ch}/c^{26DVT})F_1 albino and chinchilla progeny.

ACKNOWLEDGEMENTS

This work was supported by National Institutes of Health/National Cancer Institute grant CA37912, American Cancer Society grant ACS CN103, and the Bruce McMillan, Jr. Foundation.

REFERENCES

1. Demant P (1992): Genetic resolution of susceptibility to cancer-new perspectives. Seminars in Cancer Biology 3:159-166
2. Drinkwater NR and Bennet LM (1991): Genetic control of carcinogenesis in experimental animals. In Ito N and Sugano H (eds): "Modification of Tumor Development in Rodents." Prog Exp Res Basel Karger, vol 33, pp1-20
3. Gross L (1970): "Oncogenic Viruses" (2nd ed.). New York: Pergamon Press.
4. Chattopadhyay SK, Cloyd MW, Linemeyer DL, Lander MR, Rands E, Lowy DR (1982): Cellular origin and role of mink cell focus-forming viruses in murine thymic lymphomas. Nature (London), 295:25-31.

5. Herr W, Gilbert, W (1984): Free and integrated recombinant murine leukemia virus DNAs appear in preleukemic thymuses of AKR/J mice. J Virol. 50:51-62
6. Hartley JW, Wolford NK, Old LJ, Rowe WP (1977): A new class of murine leukemia virus associated with development of spontaneous lymphomas. Proc Natl Acad Sci USA 74:789-792
7. Chen S, Lilly F (1982): Suppression of spontaneous lymphoma by previously undiscovered dominant genes in crosses of high and low-incidence mouse strains. Virology 118:76-85
8. Corcoran LM, Adams JM, Dunn AR, Cory S (1984): Murine T lymphomas in which the cellular myc oncogene has been activated by retroviral insertion. Cell 37:113-122
9. Frei JV (1980): Methylnitrosourea induction of thymomas in AKR mice requires one or two "hits" only. Carcinogenesis 1:721-723
10. Warren W, Lawley PD, Gardner G, Harris G, Ball JK, Cooper CS (1987): Induction of thymomas by N-methyl-N-nitrosourea in AKR mice: interaction between the chemical carcinogen and endogenous murine leukaemia viruses. Carcinogenesis 8:163-172
11. Richie ER, Angel JM, McEntire B (1988): N-methyl-N-nitrosourea induced T-lymphomas of AKR/J mice contain somatically acquired ecotropic-like murine leukemia proviruses. Virology 164:211-219
12. Jolicoeur P, Rassart E (1980): Effect of *Fv-1* gene product on synthesis of linear and supercoiled viral DNA in cells infected with murine leukemia virus. J Virol 33:183-195
13. Richie ER, Angel JM, Cloyd MW (1991): Influence of murine leukemia proviral integrations on development of N-methyl-N-nitrosurea-induced thymic lymphomas in AKR mice. J Virol 65:5751-5756
14. Romach E, Moore J, Rummel S, Richie E (1994): Influence of sex and carcinogen treatment protocol on tumor latency and frequency of *K-ras* mutations in N-methyl-N-nitrosurea-induced lymphomas. Carcinogenesis 15:2275-2280
15. Angel JM, Morizot DC, Richie ER (1989): Genetics of N-methyl-N-nitrosourea induction of thymic lymphomas in AKR/J mice:assignment of a susceptibility gene to mouse chromosome 7. J Natl Cancer Inst 81:1652-1655
16. Angel JM, Morizot DC, Richie ER (1993): Localization of a novel chromosome 7 locus that suppresses development of N-methyl-N-

nitrosurea-induced thymic lymphomas. Mol Carcinog 7:151-156
17. Rinchik EM, Russell LB (1990): Germ-line deletion mutations in the mouse: tools for intensive functional and physical mapping of regions of the mammalian genome. In Davies K, Tilghman S (eds): "Genome Analysis Volume 1: Genetic and Physical Mapping" New York: Cold Spring Harbor Laboratory Press, pp.121-158

Genetics and Cancer Susceptibility:
Implications for Risk Assessment, pages 33–45

GENETIC ANALYSIS OF MULTISTAGE HEPATOCARCINOGENESIS

Therese M. Poole, Teresa A. Chiaverotti, Reynaldo A. Carabeo, and Norman R. Drinkwater

McArdle Laboratory for Cancer Research, University of Wisconsin Medical School, 1400 University Avenue, Madison, WI 53706

INTRODUCTION

Studies that began in the 1940s of skin tumor induction in mouse skin have provided the paradigm for multistage carcinogenesis (Boutwell, 1964; Berenblum and Shubik, 1947a,b). Treatment of mice with a limiting dose of chemical carcinogen followed by repetitive treatment with a non-carcinogenic, promoting agent resulted in the efficient induction of benign papillomas, while neither treatment alone was sufficient to yield skin tumors. In this model, the carcinogen-induced, initiating event for tumor development is irreversible; the activities of the promoting agent are largely reversible and result in the clonal expansion of the initiated cell (Boutwell, 1989).

The complexity of the promotion phase of carcinogenesis was indicated by the observation that chronic application of certain chemicals could promote the clonal growth of preneoplastic cells provided that these cells had previously received a single treatment with a promoting agent (Slaga, *et al.* 1980a,b). These growth-stimulating agents were termed "second-stage promoters" and appeared to act by increasing the rate of proliferation of preneoplastic cells (Slaga, *et al.* 1980b; Drinkwater, 1990). Based on these results, promotion was divided into two distinct stages, conversion, in which initiated cells become responsive to promotional stimuli, and propagation, which is the clonal expansion of a preneoplastic cell (Boutwell, 1964). Thus, complete promoters affect both conversion and propagation while second-stage promoting agents only increase the rate of propagation.

Multistage carcinogenesis in the liver has also been studied experimentally in mice and rats and the results of these studies are generally consistent with the skin model. Several initiation-promotion regimens have been utilized in rats to identify histological and biochemical changes associated with specific stages of carcinogenesis (rev. in Pitot, 1991). We have pursued a genetic approach to understanding the regulation of multistage hepatocarcinogenesis. Inbred mouse strains vary widely in their susceptibilities to spontaneous and chemically-induced hepatocarcinogenesis (Drinkwater and Bennett, 1991). Susceptible and resistant strains may differ by up to 100-fold in their relative risk for liver cancer development. We have compared several inbred strains for a variety of phenotypes associated with hepatocarcinogenesis and have determined the chromosomal locations of specific genes that determine their susceptibility to liver tumor induction. Our results demonstrate that hepatocarcinogenesis is under the control of several genes that act at different stages.

STRAIN VARIATION IN THE ROLE OF *HRAS1* ACTIVATION IN INITIATION

Initiation of carcinogenesis results from the induction of a mutation in a critical, cellular target gene. Genetic control of initiation could be mediated at several points, including carcinogen metabolism, the formation and repair of premutagenic DNA lesions, and the fixation of initiating mutations. However, the evidence to date indicates that regulation at these levels does not adequately explain the observed variation among inbred strains in susceptibility to hepatocarcinogenesis (Drinkwater and Ginsler, 1986). Recent studies demonstrate that the phenotypic effect of specific initiating events does depend on the genetic background of the host.

There is good evidence that mutational activation of the *Hras1* gene represents one pathway for initiation of hepatocarcinogenesis. Thus, a substantial fraction of spontaneous and chemically-induced liver tumors from $B6C3F_1$ mice contained mutant *Hras1* genes and the type of mutation present in the tumor depended on the nature of the carcinogen (Wiseman, *et al.*, 1986; Stowers, *et al.*, 1988). It has also been shown that these mutations are present in the earliest identifiable preneoplastic lesions (Buchmann, *et al.*, 1991). However, studies by Buchmann *et al.* (1991) and Dragani *et al.* (1991) demonstrated that, while preneoplastic lesions or liver tumors induced in C3H/HeJ or B6C3F1 mice had a high incidence of *Hras1* activating mutations, few lesions induced in genetically resistant C57BL/6J, BALB/c, or (C57BL/6 x BALB/c)F_1 hybrid mice carried mutant *Hras1* genes. One interpretation of these results is that the efficiency of promotion of the *Hras1*-initiated cells depends on the susceptibility phenotype of the animal (Buchmann, *et al.* 1991; Dragani, *et al.* 1991). This relationship is thought to be manifested through the preferential promotion of *Hras1*-initiated hepatocytes in the susceptible animal.

We have investigated this apparent correlation by comparing the frequencies of *Hras1* mutations in liver tumors from ten different inbred strains of mice with differing susceptibilities to hepatocarcinogenesis. Male mice of each strain were injected at twelve days of age with 0.1 μmol/g body weight of N,N-diethylnitrosamine (DEN). Sensitive and resistant strains were sacrificed at 32 and 50 weeks of age, respectively. At least two tumors were collected from each animal and analyzed for point mutations in codon 61 of *Hras1* using a polymerase chain reaction (PCR)-based assay (Lee and Drinkwater, 1995). Our data indicate that there is no significant correlation between the susceptibility phenotype and frequency of *Hras1* mutations in liver tumors. In our experiment, three of the five sensitive strains, CBA/J, C3H/HeJ (C3H), and C57BR/cdJ (BR) yielded frequencies of 11%, 25%, and 23%, respectively, values higher than for the resistant strains, C57BL/6J (B6) (4%), A/J (0%), AKR/J (4%), BALB/cByJ (0%), and SWR/J (0%) (Table 1). Two sensitive strains, SM/J and DBA/2J (D2) were exceptional, yielding frequencies of 0% and 4%, respectively. We have also compared the frequencies of *Hras1* activation and susceptibilities of recombinant inbred mouse strains derived from sensitive C3H and resistant B6 mice and observed that the two phenotypes were uncorrelated (Lee and Drinkwater, 1995). These results indicate that the phenotypes of susceptibility and *Hras1* mutant frequency are genetically distinct. We are currently attempting to determine the genetic basis for the prevalence of *Hras1* mutations in liver tumors.

Table 1: Analysis of frequency of mutations in codon 61 of *Hras1* in liver tumors of male mice treated with diethylnitrosamine (DEN)[a]

Inbred Strain	No. of animals	Mean tumor multiplicity (s.d.)	*Hras1* mutants/ tumors tested (%)
CBA/J	19	135 (55)	3/28 (11)
SM/J	28	82 (37)	0/91 (0)
C3H/HeJ	39	51 (50)	12/43 (28)
C57BR/cdJ	27	52 (32)	7/31 (23)
DBA/2J	24	29 (19)	1/26 (4)
SWR/J[b]	46	13 (12)	0/48 (0)
BALB/cByJ[b]	22	12 (9)	0/22 (0)
AKR/J[b]	23	7.7 (8.0)	1/29 (4)
C57BL/6J[b]	42	5.1 (12)	2/47 (4)
A/J[b]	42	4.8 (7.8)	0/19 (0)

[a] R. Carabeo, G.H. Lee, N. Drinkwater, unpublished.

[b] Denotes resistant animals sacrificed at 50 weeks of age.

COMPARISON OF INBRED STRAINS FOR RESPONSES TO PROMOTION OR INHIBITION OF HEPATOCARCINOGENESIS

A distinct advantage in studying multistage hepatocarcinogenesis is that early lesions that are the precursors of liver tumors can be readily identified and quantified (Moore, *et al.*, 1981; Pitot and Sirica, 1980). These preneoplastic foci are clonal growths of cells with altered histochemical staining properties; the number of foci per liver can be estimated by observing the number of foci in stained liver sections and extrapolating this value for the entire liver, and the growth rate of foci can be approximated by determining the rate of change in focus size over time (Moore, *et al.*, 1981). In order to discern the effect of genetic background on the induction and the proliferation of preneoplastic cells, we have studied the growth kinetics of these early lesions in mouse liver.

We have analyzed the number and the growth rate of hepatic foci deficient in glucose-6-phosphatase (G6Pase) expression in four inbred strains of mice with varying susceptibilities to chemically-induced hepatocarcinogenesis, C3H, D2, BR and B6. C3H males are the most sensitive of the listed strains, with tumor multiplicities that are approximately 50-80 fold higher than those in relatively resistant B6 male mice (Drinkwater and Ginsler, 1986). When treated perinatally, D2 males are about 70% as sensitive as the C3H males (20-fold more susceptible than B6 males) (Bennett, *et al.*, 1992; Lee, *et al.*, 1995) and BR males are intermediate in sensitivity with tumor multiplicities that are 10-15 fold higher than that in B6 males (Kemp and Drinkwater, 1989).

Table 2. Growth rate and number of glucose-6-phosphate-deficient hepatic foci in inbred mice.

Strain	Apparent doubling time (weeks)	Number of Foci per Liver[b]
MALES		
C3H/HeJ	2.0 (0.1)[c]	580 (310)[c]
C57BL/6J	3.5 (0.5)[d]	110 (150)[d]
C57BR/cdJ	3.3 (0.8)[d]	680 (410)[d]
DBA/2J	2.4 (0.4)[c]	170 (60)[c]
FEMALES		
C3H/HeJ	6.0 (0.7)[e]	299 (143)[e]
C57BL/6J	10.2 (2.3)[d]	226 (137)[d]
C57BR/cdJ	4.6 (2.1)[d]	160 (130)[d]

[a]Apparent doubling time (standard deviation), measured by regression of the change in the number of cells per focus over time.

[b]Values are mean (standard deviation) for foci at 24 weeks of age.

[c]Data from Bennett (1993).

[d]Data from Poole and Drinkwater (1993, 1994).

[e]Data are from Hanigan, *et al.*, (1990).

Male mice from each of these strains were treated at 12 days of age with DEN (0.05 μmol/g body weight) and groups of mice were sacrificed at various times between 12 weeks to 32 weeks of age. At the time of sacrifice, frozen liver sections were stained for G6Pase. For each of the two growth parameters, each phenotype in the studied strains fell into two groups, high growth rate (or focus number) and low growth rate (or focus number). However, the two phenotypes were independent of each other and among the four strains, all four of the possible combinations of phenotypes were observed (Table 2). In C3H males, foci are numerous and grow at a rapid rate; in D2 males, there are few foci but they grow at a high rate; in BR males, the number of foci is high but their rate of growth is low; and in B6 males, there are few foci that grow slowly (Hanigan, *et al.*, 1988; Bennett, *et al.*, 1992; Poole, *et al.*, 1994). Since the number of foci and their rate of growth are not correlated, we conclude that the mechanisms affecting these two phenotypes are distinct. We propose that the number of foci and the growth rate of foci each measures the two separate stages in promotion, conversion and propagation, respectively. Therefore, foci in C3H males have high conversion and propagation rates while those in D2 mice have a low conversion rate but a high propagation rate. Lesions in BR mice convert at a high frequency but proliferate relatively slowly and those in B6 males, have low rates of both conversion and propagation.

Hormonal Influence

Males of all inbred mouse strains are more sensitive to hepatocarcinogenesis than females (Kemp and Drinkwater, 1989), in part because androgens and ovarian hormones have opposite effects on the development and growth of preneoplastic lesions. These hormonal effects are most obvious when the tumor multiplicities of intact and gonadectomized animals are compared (Vesselinovitch, *et al.*, 1980, Vesselinovitch, 1990). We have compared tumor development in intact and gonadectomized male and female C3H, B6 and BR mice that were treated perinatally with DEN (Poole and Drinkwater, 1995). For all strains, castrated males developed 70-90% fewer tumors than intact controls, indicating that testosterone promotes tumor development. In B6 and C3H females, ovariectomy resulted in an 8-fold increase in the number of liver tumors, indicating that, in these strains, ovarian hormones inhibit the development of liver tumors. The BR strain was unusual in that ovariectomized BR females developed only 25 percent more tumors than intact controls, suggesting that the pathway that normally inhibits hepatocarcinogenesis in females is lacking in this strain.

We have shown that tumor multiplicity is not correlated with circulating levels of testosterone or with the relative affinity or abundance of androgen receptor present in hepatic cytosol (Kemp and Drinkwater, 1989). We have also demonstrated that BR and B6 females do not differ in the abundance or binding properties of hepatic estrogen receptors (Poole and Drinkwater, 1995). Studies of hepatocarcinogenesis in *Tfm* (*Testicular feminization*) mutant mice, which lack functional androgen receptors, demonstrated that the mechanism by which testosterone promotes liver tumor development is indirect (Kemp, *et al.*, 1989). Heterozygous female mice, which are mosaic for the expression of this X-linked gene, were treated perinatally with carcinogen, ovariectomized, treated chronically with testosterone, and tumors from these animals were analyzed for their androgen receptor content. The fraction of tumors containing functional receptors was equal to that lacking receptor activity, demonstrating that promotion by testosterone is indirect or non-cell autonomous (Kemp, *et al.*, 1989).

Analysis of the development of preneoplastic hepatic foci has allowed us to determine the role of sex hormones in the stages of promotion. We have shown that preneoplastic foci in B6 and C3H females grow at similar rates, whereas in BR females the net growth rate is 2-fold higher (Table 2). Because the foci in BR males and females grow at a similar rate we conclude that the focus growth rate in BR mice is testosterone independent. Because BR males have many more foci than BR females we believe that the conversion stage is promoted by testosterone. Testosterone may also stimulate conversion in C3H males, as this strain also develops a large number of preneoplastic foci. Preneoplastic foci in B6 and C3H females grow at a similar rate, which is half the rate seen in BR females. Thus, we believe that ovarian hormones suppress the growth of preneoplastic foci in B6 and C3H females; but that this inhibitory pathway is not active in BR mice.

Influence of Partial Hepatectomy

Partial hepatectomy (PH) or chemical injury to the liver of the mouse or rat induces the remainder of the liver to undergo several rounds of mitosis resulting in regeneration to its original mass (Harkness, 1957; Buchner, 1963). Studies in both species indicate that the growth stimulus provided by a partial hepatectomy may act as a promoter of hepatocarcinogenesis (Bartsch, *et al.*, 1988; Hanigan, *et al.*, 1990).

We have shown that preneoplastic hepatic lesions in B6 and C3H mice differ in their responses to partial hepatectomy. In these studies, partial hepatectomy four weeks after treatment of preweanling mice with the carcinogen, N-ethyl-N-nitrosourea (ENU), resulted in a 16-fold increase in the risk of liver tumor induction in B6 male mice, but not C3H male mice, relative to controls (Hanigan, *et al.*, 1990). We compared the number and growth rate of hepatic foci in ENU-treated intact and partially hepatectomized C3H and B6 male mice. We observed that the growth rate of the foci in unoperated C3H males was similar to that in partially hepatectomized C3H males. However, in partially hepatectomized B6 males, the growth rate of lesions was much higher than that in the unoperated controls, and was similar to that in the C3H males (Hanigan, *et al.*, 1990). In contrast, the number of foci in each of the strains was proportional to the fraction of the liver that remained following the surgery, suggesting that PH does not influence the process of preneoplastic focus formation. Thus, the increased risk for tumor development was a consequence of an increase in the growth rate of preneoplastic foci in the livers of B6 mice to the same level as that observed in C3H mice. We have also shown that the DNA labeling index of both normal and preneoplastic hepatocytes is higher in C3H mice compared to B6 mice (Hanigan, *et al.*, 1988) and that the C3H hepatocytes respond more rapidly to the proliferative stimulus of PH (Bennett, *et al.*, 1995), indicating that genetic factors increase the proliferation rate of all hepatocytes in the sensitive C3H males.

With the above data in mind, we have hypothesized that C3H hepatocytes are primed for growth such that, following conversion, propagation occurs without additional genetic or epigenetic changes whereas in B6 males an additional growth stimulus following the formation of the focus is required for the high rate of growth (Bennett, *et al.*, 1995). Conversely, it is possible that a growth inhibitor is present in B6 males but not in C3H males and that partial hepatectomy can overcome the resulting growth suppression in B6 male mice.

GENETIC MAPPING OF LOCI THAT CONTROL SUSCEPTIBILITY TO HEPATOCARCINOGENESIS

In order to understand the genetic basis for the differences among inbred strains in the promotion stages of carcinogenesis, we have used linkage analysis in crosses between sensitive and resistant strains to map the genes that affect the susceptibility of inbred mice to hepatocarcinogenesis. Mice from backcross and intercross populations were assayed for their tumor susceptibility and DNA from each mouse was genotyped at many marker loci (Lee, *et al.*, 1995; Dietrich, *et al.*, 1992; Lander and Botstein, 1989). The next sections describe some of the genes affecting murine hepatocarcinogenesis that have been identified in this manner.

Hcs

Tumor multiplicity in C3H male mice is 50 times higher than that in B6 males (Drinkwater and Ginsler, 1986). Twelve-day-old male mice from B6C3F$_1$ X B6 backcross and F$_2$ intercross populations were treated with DEN (0.2 μmol/g body weight) and tumor multiplicity was determined at 32 weeks of age. DNA markers in the distal region of chromosome 1 correlated well with susceptibility (Table 3) having a LOD score of 5.9 (i.e., it is nearly 1 million times more likely that a sensitivity gene is located in this region than that one is located in another part of the genome) (Bennett, 1993). This locus accounts for approximately 60% of the variance in sensitivity, slightly less than the 85% originally suggested for the magnitude of the effect of the major C3H susceptibility gene (Drinkwater and Ginsler, 1986). However, Dragani and coworkers have reported the identification of 6 additional *Hcs* genes in crosses between C3H and A/J or *Mus spretus* mice (Gariboldi, *et al.*, 1993; Manenti, *et al*, 1994). These results indicate that the genetics of tumor susceptibility in C3H mice is complex.

Table 3. Loci segregating with liver tumor susceptibility in backcross and intercross mice treated with DEN.

Locus	DNA Marker[a]	Chromosome	LOD score
Hcs[b]	*D1Mit15*	1	5.9
Hcr1[c]	*D4Mit9*	4	5.6
Hcr2	*D10Mit15*	10	4.3
Hcf1[d]	*D17NDS2*	17	15.8
Hcf2	*D1Mit10*	1	6.2

[a]Dietrich et al., 1992.
[b]Data taken from Bennett (1993).
[c]Data taken from Lee, *et al.* (1995)
[d]Data taken from Poole, *et al.* (1994).

By combining the information from the biological and genetic experiments, we hypothesize that the major *Hcs* gene is involved in the conversion stage of promotion. While hepatic foci in C3H males have high rates of both conversion and propagation, the data from partial hepatectomy experiments indicates that preneoplastic foci in C3H males are more readily responsive to growth stimuli than are the foci in B6 males. This observation indicates that the product of the *Hcs* gene may be involved in priming a preneoplastic hepatocyte for any proliferation stimulus to which it may be exposed. The analysis of tumor development in B6↔C3H chimeric mice demonstrated that the *Hcs* gene appears to be acting in a cell autonomous manner (Lee, *et al.*, 1991). A high proportion of tumors in C3H males harbor mutated *Hras1* genes (Buchmann, *et al.*, 1991; Carabeo, *et al.*, 1994), but whether the *Hcs* gene product cooperates in any way with the ras protein is unknown at this point.

Hcr

Male D2 mice are about 70% as sensitive as C3H males when chemically treated as preweanlings but are resistant to spontaneous liver tumor induction (Bennett, *et al.*, 1992). In order to identify genes affecting chemically-induced tumor induction, male B6D2F_1 X B6 backcross and F_2 intercross mice were treated as preweanlings with DEN (0.05 µmol/g body weight), analyzed for tumor development at 32 weeks of age, and genotyped for DNA markers spanning the mouse genome. Linkage analysis revealed that two loci segregated with susceptibility (Lee, *et al.*, 1995). Unexpectedly, the DBA alleles of these two genes confer a decrease in tumor multiplicity. These loci have been designated *Hcr* for "*Hepatocarcinogen resistance.*" *Hcr1* and *Hcr2* been mapped to chromosomes 4 (LOD = 5.6) and 10 (LOD = 4.3), respectively (Table 3). No chromosomal regions were identified in which the D2 alleles correlated with sensitivity which may indicate that many genes, each with a small effect, contribute to the sensitivity of D2 mice to chemically induced hepatocarcinogenesis (Lee, *et al.*, 1995). This hypothesis is supported by the observation that several recombinant inbred lines between D2 and B6 show a higher tumor multiplicity than the sensitive D2 mice (Lee, *et al.*, 1995).

At least one of the *Hcr* gene products appears to exert its effects at the stage of conversion. This hypothesis is based on the fact the hepatic foci in D2 males have a high rate of proliferation but a low rate of conversion. The *Hcr* genes serve to reduce the number of tumors that form, so it is highly likely that they do so by suppressing the conversion process. The high rate of proliferation seen in the hepatic foci in D2 males is likely the result of the combined action of many sensitivity genes, each with small effects (Lee, *et al.*, 1995).

Hcf

Male BR mice are approximately 10 times more sensitive that B6 males but BR females are 40 times more sensitive than B6 females (Kemp and Drinkwater, 1989). In order to determine the genetic basis for the difference in sensitivity between these two strains, backcross and intercross mice were treated with DEN (0.1 µmol/g body weight) at 12 days of age. Tumor multiplicity was determined in males at 32 weeks and in females at 50 weeks of age. In both sexes, two genes could account for a majority of the difference in sensitivity between these two strains (Table 3) (Poole, *et al.*, 1993, 1994). These two loci, *Hcf1* and *Hcf2* (*Hepatocarcinogenesis in females*) are located on chromosomes 17 (LOD = 15.8) and 1 (LOD = 6.2), respectively, and interact synergistically in females and additively in males. Together, the genes account for a 12-fold difference in tumor multiplicity in females and a nearly 6-fold difference in the males.

Because the BR strain is unusual in that females are sensitive to liver tumor induction, it was surprising to find no female-specific sensitivity genes. We speculate that the *Hcf1* gene, which strongly influences tumor development in females, functions either to counteract the suppression by ovarian hormones on the growth of preneoplastic cells or to independently increase the propagation rate of converted hepatocytes. This hypothesis is supported by the observation that hepatic foci in BR females grow at a significantly higher rate than those in B6 and C3H females (Poole, *et al.*, 1993; Poole and Drinkwater, submitted for publication).

One would predict that genes identified in crosses between BR and B6 would affect the rate of focus formation and not the rate of proliferation because preneoplastic foci grow at similar rates in the two strains while the foci are more numerous in BR males than in B6 males (Poole and Drinkwater, submitted for publication). Thus, *Hcf2* is likely to affect conversion because of its larger effect on the formation of tumors in BR males compared to the BR females. Interestingly, *Hcf2* and *Hcs* are both located on chromosome 1. It is tempting to speculate that they identify the same gene since both appear to affect the conversion stage of promotion. In addition, both BR and C3H mice have high incidences of *Hras1* activation in liver tumors, providing a possible pathway for tumor formation (Carabeo, *et al.*, 1994). At this point, however, it must be stressed that these observations are only correlations and do not prove that the two genes are identical.

CONCLUSIONS

We have presented a model for murine multistage hepatocarcinogenesis that dissects the process of promotion into stages of conversion and propagation. Figure 1 outlines these stages and indicates potential sites of hormonal action and genetic influences. Initiation is an irreversible step involving heritable genetic alterations, often activating oncogenes such as *Hras1*. We do not believe that genetic differences in the rate of initiation account for the strain differences in hepatocarcinogen sensitivity. Rather, we show that differences in the rates of conversion and growth of preneoplastic foci can explain the wide variation seen between inbred strains. Conversion is the transition from a single initiated cell to a preneoplastic cell primed to respond to growth stimuli. Males of all strains develop more tumors than females, in part because testosterone stimulates conversion. C3H and BR males have the highest rates of conversion, suggesting that genetic background affects this step. We have identified susceptibility loci, *Hcs* and *Hcf2*, on chromosome 1 in C3H and BR mice, respectively, and speculate that these loci encode a determinant that stimulates conversion. The hepatocarcinogen resistance loci, *Hcr1* and *Hcr2*, identified in D2 mice may act as negative regulators of conversion since these loci act to reduce tumor number.

Genetic modifiers also influence the propagation stage in which clonal expansion of preneoplastic cells occurs. Preneoplastic foci in C3H and B6 males have faster doubling times than in females. We believe this sex difference is a consequence of inhibition of the growth of preneoplastic foci by ovarian hormones. The BR strain is an exception in that this inhibitory pathway does not appear to function. We have shown that preneoplastic foci in C3H and D2 males have faster doubling times than foci in B6 and BR males. Both preneoplastic foci and resting hepatocytes have a higher ^{3}H-thymidine labelling index in C3H males relative to B6 mice, indicating that genetic factors define the rate of proliferation. Since foci in D2 males grow at a rapid rate, we predict that D2 males would also have a high ^{3}H-thymidine labelling index. Our model predicts that genetic factors regulating the rate of proliferation also determine a strain's response to PH.

If this hypothesis is correct, there should be an increase in tumor number in BR mice following PH, but not in D2 mice.

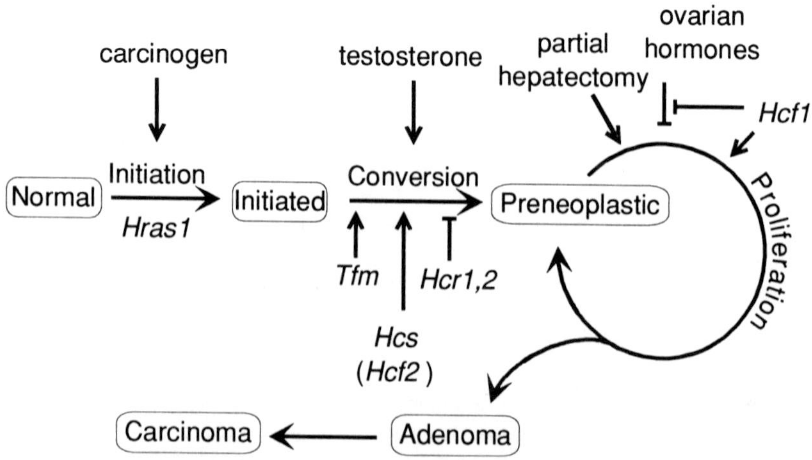

Figure 1. Genetic interactions in multistage hepatocarcinogenesis.

Experiments are in progress to test specific predictions of our model. We are analyzing the number of foci and kinetics of growth in intact and gonadectomized animals to characterize the effects of testosterone and ovarian hormones. In addition, we plan to examine the response of D2 and BR mice to PH. Our data indicate that genetic modifiers influence the frequency of tumors harboring activating mutations in *Hras1*, though we have not determined at what stage these genes act. We are analyzing segregating crosses to identify loci that effect the outgrowth of *Hras1* initiated cells. While the model detailed above is still speculative, the molecular characterization of the susceptibility genes identified in these studies will allow us to better define the stages of hepatocarcinogenesis.

ACKNOWLEDGEMENTS

We are grateful to our past colleagues, Drs. Marie Hanigan, Chris Kemp, Gang-Hong Lee, and Michelle Bennett, who were responsible for much of the work described above. This work was supported by grants CA22484, CA09135, and CA07175 from the National Cancer Institute. Reynaldo Carabeo is a Howard Hughes Medical Institute Predoctoral fellow.

REFERENCES

Bartsch H, Preat V, Aitio A, Cabral JRP, Roberfroid M (1988): Partial hepatectomy of rats ten weeks before carcinogen administration can enhance liver carcinogenesis: preliminary observations. Carcinogenesis 9:2315-2317.

Bennett LM, Winkler ML, Drinkwater NR (1992): Analysis of the genetic basis for the high susceptibility of DBA/2 mice to liver tumor induction by N,N-diethylnitrosamine Proc Am Assoc Cancer Res 33:164.

Bennett LM, Farnham PJ, Drinkwater NR (1995): Strain-dependent differences in DNA synthesis and gene expression in the regenerating livers of C57BL/6J and C3H/HeJ mice. Mol Carcinogenesis *in press*.

Bennett LM (1993): The genetics of hepatocarcinogenesis in inbred strains of mice. Ph.D. thesis. University of Wisconsin, Madison, WI.

Berenblum I, Shubik P (1947a): The role of croton oil applications associated with a single painting of a carcinogen, in tumour indiction in the mouse's skin. Brit J Cancer 1:379-383.

Berenblum I, Shubik P (1947b): A new quantitative approach to the study of stages of chemical carcinogenesis in the mouse's skin. Brit J Cancer. 1:383-391.

Boutwell RK (1964): Some biological aspects of skin carcinogenesis. Progress in Experimental Tumor Research 4:207-250.

Boutwell RK (1989): Model systems for defining initiation, promotion, and progression of skin neoplasms. In: Skin carcinogenesis: Mechanisms and Human Relevance. New York, Alan R. Liss, Inc. pp. 3-15.

Buchmann A, Bauer-Hofmann R, Mahr J, Drinkwater NR, Luz A, Schwartz M (1991): Mutational activation of the *c-Ha-ras* gene in liver tumors of different rodent strains: Correlation with susceptibility to hepatocarcinogenesis. Proc Natl Acad Sci USA 88:911-915.

Buchner NLR (1963): Regeneration of mammalian liver. Int Rev Cytol 15:245-300.

Carabeo R, Lee G-H, Drinkwater NR (1994): Correlation between frequency of Harvey *ras* mutational activation in codon 61 and susceptibility to hepatocarcinogenesis. Proc Am Assoc Cancer Res 35:152.

Dietrich W, Katz H, Lincoln SE, Shin H-S, Friedman J, Dracopoli NC, Lander ES (1992): A genetic map of the mouse suitable for typing intraspecific crosses. Genetics 131:423-447.

Dragani TA, Manenti G, Colombo BM, Falvella FS, Gariboldi M, Pierotti MA, Della Porta G (1991): Incidence of mutations at codon 61 of the *Ha-ras* gene in liver tumors of mice genetically susceptible and resistant to hepatocarcinogenesis. Oncogene 6: 333-338.

Drinkwater NR (1990): Experimental models and biological mechanisms for tumor promotion. Cancer Cells 2:8-14.

Drinkwater NR, Bennett LM (1991) Genetic control of carcinogenesis in experimental animals. In Ito N (ed): "Modification of Tumor Development in Rodents." Basel: S. Karger A. G, pp. 1 - 20.

Drinkwater NR, Ginsler JJ (1986): Genetic control of hepatocarcinogenesis in C57BL/6J and C3H/HeJ inbred mice. Carcinogenesis 7:1701-1707.

Festing MFW (1979): "Inbred Strains in Biomedical Research". New York: Oxford University Press.

Gariboldi M, Manenti G, Canzian F, Falvella FS, Pierotti MA, Della Porta G, Binelli G, Dragani TA (1993): Chromosome mapping of murine susceptibility loci to liver carcinogenesis. Cancer Res 53:209-211.

Hanigan MH, Winkler ML, Drinkwater NR (1990): Partial hepatectomy is a promoter of hepatocarcinogenesis in C57BL/6J male mice but not in C3H/HeJ male mice. Carcinogenesis 11:589-594.

Hanigan MH, Kemp CJ, Ginsler JJ, Drinkwater NR (1988): Rapid growth of preneoplastic lesions in hepatocarcinogen-sensitive C3H/HeJ male mice relative to C57BL/6J male mice. Carcinogenesis 9:885-890.

Harkness RD (1957): Regeneration of liver. Brit Med Bull 13:87-93.

Kemp CJ, Leary CN, Drinkwater NR (1989): Promotion of murine hepatocarcinogenesis by testosterone is androgen receptor-dependent but not cell autonomous. Proc Natl Acad Sc. USA 86:7505-7509.

Kemp C.J, Drinkwater NR (1989): Genetic variation in liver tumor susceptibility, plasma testosterone levels, and androgen receptor binding in sex inbred strains of mice. Cancer Res 49:5044-5047.

Lander ES, Botstein D (1989): Mapping mendelian factors underlying quantitative traits using RFLP linkage maps. Genetics 121:185-199.

Lee G-H, Nomura K, Kanda H, Kusakabe M, Yoshiki A, Sakakura T, Kitagawa T (1991): Strain specific sensitivity to diethylnitrosamine-induced carcinogenesis is maintained in hepatocytes of C3H/HeN↔C57BL/6N chimeric mice. Cancer Res 49:403-409.

Lee G-H, Bennett LM, Carabeo RA, Drinkwater NR (1995): Identification of hepatocarcinogen-resistance genes in DBA/2 mice. Genetics 139:387-395.

Lee G-H, Drinkwater NR (1995): Hepatocarcinogenesis in BXH recombinant inbred strains of mice: Analysis of diverse phenotypic effects of the *Hcs* (*Hepatocarcinogen sensitivity*) loci. Mol Carcinogenesis *in press.*

Manenti G, Binelli G, Gariboldi M, Canzian F, DeGregorio L, Falvella FS, Dragani TA, Pierotti MA (1994): Multiple loci affect genetic predisposition to hepatocarcinogenesis in mice. Genomics 23:118-124.

Moore MR, Drinkwater NR, Miller EC, Miller JA, Pitot HC (1981): Quantitative analysis of the time-dependent development of glucose-6-phosphatase-deficient foci in the livers of mice treated neonatally with diethylnitrosamine. Cancer Res 41:1585-1593.

Pitot HC, Sirica A (1980): The stages of initiation and promotion in hepatocarcinogenesis. Biochem Biophys Acta 605:191-215.

Pitot HC (1991): Characterization of the stage of promotion in hepatocarcinogenesis in the rat. In: Sudilovsky O (ed.) "Boundaries between promotion and progression during carcinogenesis." New York. Plenum Press, pp. 3-18.

Poole TM, Drinkwater NR (1995) Progress in Clinical and Biological Research *in press.*

Poole TM, Winkler ML, Kaehler DA, Drinkwater NR (1994): Two loci account for the sensitivity of male C57BR/cdJ mice to heptocarcinogenesis. Proc Am Assoc Cancer Res 35:122.

Poole TM, Winkler ML, Kaehler DA, Drinkwater NR (1993): C57BR/cdJ mice are genetically insensitive to inhibition of hepatocarcinogenesis by ovarian hormones. Proc Am Assoc. Cancer Res 34:255.

Slaga TJ, Fischer SM, Nelson K, Gleason GL (1980a): Studies on the mechanism of skin tumor promotion: evidence for several stages in promotion. Proc Natl Acad Sci USA 77:3659-3663.

Slaga TJ, Klein-Szanto AJP, Fischer SM, Weeks CE, Nelson K, Major S (1980b): Studies on the mechanism of action of anti-tumor-promoting agents: their specificity in two-stage promotion. Proc Natl Acad Sci USA 77:2251-2254.

Stowers SJ, Wiseman RW, Ward JM, Miller EC, Miller JA, Anderson MW, Eva A (1988): Detection of activated proto-oncogenes in N-nitrosodiethylamine-induced liver tumors: a comparison between B6C3F1 mice and Fischer 344 rats. Carcinogenesis 9:271-276.

Vesselinovitch SD (1990): Perinatal mouse liver carcinogenesis as a sensitive carcinogenesis model and the role of the sex hormonal environment in tumor development. In: Slaga T and Becker F (eds.), "Mouse Liver Carcinogenesis: Mechanisms and Species Comparisons." New York: Alan R. Liss, pp. 53-68.

Vesselinovitch SD, Itze L, Mihailovich N, Rao KVN (1980): Modifying role of partial hepatectomy and gonadectomy in ethylnitrosourea-induced hepatocarcinogenesis. Cancer Res 40:1538-1542.

Wiseman RW, Stowers SJ, Miller EC, Anderson MW, Miller JA (1986): Activating mutations of the c-Ha-*ras* protooncogene in chemically induced hepatomas of the male $B6C3F_1$ mouse. Proc Natl Acad Sci USA 83:5825-5829.

Genetics and Cancer Susceptibility:
Implications for Risk Assessment, pages 47–55

GENETIC SUSCEPTIBILITY TO TUMOR PROGRESSION IN MOUSE SKIN CARCINOGENESIS

Mariana C. Stern and Claudio J. Conti

Department of Carcinogenesis, University of Texas, M.D. Anderson Cancer Center, Science Park-Research Division, Smithville, Texas 78957

THE MOUSE SKIN MODEL

The mouse skin is one of the most widely used models for chemical carcinogenesis. Epidermal neoplasia can be induced in this organ by two different protocols, i.e., complete carcinogenesis and two stage carcinogenesis. In the first protocol, a large dose, or more commonly, multiple applications of a genotoxic carcinogen [e.g., Benzo(a)pyrene (BP) or 9,10-Dimethyl-1,2-benzantracene (DMBA)] is used to induce tumors on the back of susceptible mice. In the two stage protocols subcarcinogenic doses of a carcinogen (i.e., BP, DMBA) are followed by multiple applications of a non-carcinogenic but epidermal hyperplasiogenic agent [e.g., 12-0-tetradecanoylphorbol-13-acetate (TPA) Benzoyl peroxide (BzPo)] (Slaga, 1984, 1989; Yuspa, 1985; DiGiovanni, 1991; Conti, 1994).

The two-stage protocol has been the protocol of choice to study different aspects of chemical carcinogenesis including the genetic susceptibility to carcinogens. In this model three stages can be defined: 1) Initiation: the result of the application of a subcarcinogenic dose of a genotoxic carcinogen. It is believed to be genetic, irreversible and cumulative. In the case of initiation with DMBA the nature of the genetic damage appears to be a mutation in codon 61 of the H-ras gene. From the pathobiology point of view, the initiation is silent, i.e., the initiated skin behaves as a normal skin unless it is challenged with tumor promoters or wounding. 2) Promotion: the result of the action of tumor promoters on the initiated skin. Since most tumor promoters are not genotoxic, this stage of carcinogenesis has been presumed to be epigenetic. The endpoint of the promotion is the formation of papillomas which are exophytic noninvasive lesions consisting of hyperplastic epidermis folded over a core of stroma. 3) Progression: an ambiguous term that has been used with different meanings in different models. In the mouse skin model it is normally referred to as the conversion of papillomas to SCC. In the two stage protocol most, if not all the carcinomas derive from preexisting papillomas. This is not the case with the complete carcinogenesis protocol where a number of carcinomas appear *de novo* or from flat premalignant lesions (Slaga, 1984; 1989; Yuspa, 1985; DiGiovanni, 1991; Conti, 1994; Klein-Szanto, 1989).

GENETIC SUSCEPTIBILITY IN THE MOUSE SKIN MODEL

The genetic susceptibility to chemical carcinogens has been studied in this model for over 30 years. Early work by Boutwell and collaborators (1964) showed that the response of the skin to chemical carcinogens is strongly influenced by the genetic background of the host. Slaga (1984) rated the relative susceptibility of several mouse stocks and strains for complete carcinogenesis(SENCAR > CD1 > C57Bl/6J ≥ Balb/c ≥ ICR/Ha Swiss > C3H) and two stage carcinogenesis (SENCAR>DBA/2>CD-1 > C3H > BALB/c > C57BL/6J). Although this ranking is not absolute, particularly when different carcinogens are used, the differences between the extremes is dramatic; for example C57BL/6J animals can be almost totally refractory to two stage protocols using phorbol ester tumor promoters while in SENCAR mice relatively low doses of initiators and promoters induce more than 20 papillomas per mouse (Slaga, 1984).

Although the existence of genetic differences in the susceptibility of mouse skin to chemical carcinogenesis has been clearly documented, the mechanisms involved in this susceptibility are not fully understood. Early studies have focused on differences in the metabolism of carcinogens and DNA binding as a possible source of variability among species (reviewed by Yuspa, 1985; Naito and DiGiovanni, 1989). However, studies carried out by DiGiovanni and collaborators showed that although some differences among strains can be attributed to initiation, the major contribution to tumor susceptibility appears to be at the level of tumor promotion (Naito and DiGiovanni, 1989). Using a model with DBA/2, a strain susceptible to promotion with phorbol esters and C57BL/6J which is resistant, these investigators established that susceptibility to promotion in this model is inherited as an autosomal incomplete dominance and suggested that a minimum of two genes control the susceptibility to promotion (Naito, et al., 1988). Further studies by this group of investigators using recombinant inbred strains have better defined their genetic model postulating that a minimum of three loci, two dominant and one recessive, control sensitivity to tumor promotion (DiGiovanni, et al., 1992). These studies were carried out using TPA as promoter and therefore this genetic model may not necessarily be valid for other promoters because the susceptibility to promotion of different mouse strains has been shown to be largely dependent on the promotion agent (Reiners, et al., 1984). Nevertheless, DiGiovanni et al. (1991) has shown that at least one genetic locus controls a common pathway for susceptibility to different promoters.

ORIGIN OF SENCAR MICE AND DERIVED INBRED LINES

In the early 60's, Boutwell (1964) undertook a program of selective breeding for animals susceptible to skin tumor formation by a multistage protocol using DMBA as the initiation agent and croton oil as a promoter (Figure 1). He derived the STS (Skin Tumor Sensitive) mice from the Rockland stock by selecting animals with the earliest and most numerous tumors. The STS mice were subsequently outcrossed to outbred CD-1 mice to solve fertility problems, and further generations of selective breeding were performed. The result of these experiments was a mouse highly sensitive to two stage protocols, the SENCAR outbred stock. SENCAR was maintained as an outbred stock in Boutwell's laboratory and later on in Slaga's laboratory in the Oak Ridge National Laboratory. It is presently maintained as an outbred stock in the Frederick Animal Facility (NCI) (Environmental Health Perspectives, 1986).

The development of an inbred SENCAR strain was started in the Oak Ridge National Laboratory by Sue Fischer and Tom Slaga. They carried out 10 rounds of strict brother sister crosses followed by the selection of the more susceptible animals in each generation (similar to Boutwell's original experiment). This procedure was followed for 10 more generations of strict inbreeding without selection. The animals were later transferred to Science Park where the inbred nature of the strain was verified by skin transplant. The strain was registered as SSIN (SENCAR Sensitive Inbred) (Fischer, et al., 1987).

The susceptibility of SSIN to two-stage carcinogenesis protocols was characterized by Fischer et al (1987). SSIN mice initiated with DMBA showed higher sensitivity to tumor promotion by phorbol esters than the original outbred stock. A later study by DiGiovanni et al (1991) extended this observation, showing increased susceptibility of the SSIN in experiments with either DMBA or 1-Methyl-3- Nitro-1-Nitrosoguanidine (MNNG) as initiators and BzPo as a promoter. This study did not show increased sensitivity of the SSIN to promotion with Chrysarobin (DiGiovanni, 1991).

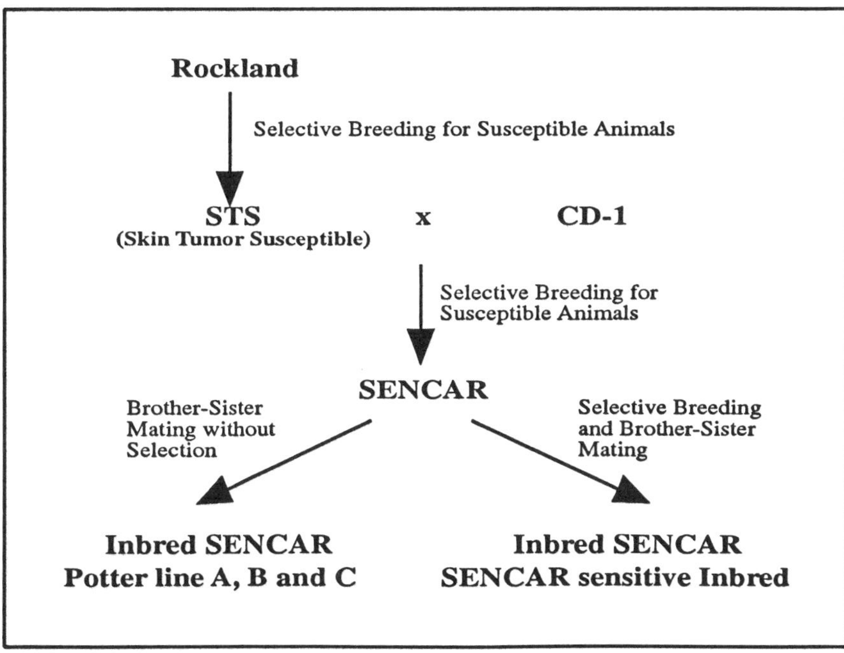

Figure 1. Diagram of the origin of the SENCAR stock and their derived inbred strains

Further characterization of the SSIN (Gimenez-Conti, et al, 1992) indicated that in spite of a high susceptibility to tumor promotion this strain did not develop malignant tumors. The lack of progression of SSIN papillomas was consistently shown at different doses of two different initiators (DMBA and MNNG) and two different promoters (TPA and BzPo). It was also observed that the expression of markers of premalignant progression (i.e., dysplasia, expression of keratin 13 and loss of keratin K1) was markedly suppressed in SSIN papillomas (Gimenez-Conti, et al., 1992). Since DMBA/TPA-induced papillomas in SENCAR mice exhibit a high incidence of H-ras mutations in codon 61, the presence of this genetic alteration was studied in SSIN papillomas. The majority of papillomas from SSIN presented H-ras mutations (although the frequency was lower than in the outbred SENCAR), suggesting that the lack of progression is probably not related to the putative initiation event in this model but rather to an independent genetic mechanism. In conclusion, the data from these experiments suggested that the putative gene(s) that confers susceptibility to tumor promotion were segregated from the gene(s) involved in tumor progression during the selection and inbreeding of the SENCAR mouse stock.

Independently of the studies carried out by the laboratories in Science Park, M. Potter (NCI, Bethesda, MD) developed three strains of inbred SENCAR. In this case, the strains were derived by inbreeding procedures without selection. Preliminary characterization of these mice was carried out by Hennings and Yuspa (Hennings, et al., 1993; 1994). The three strains, called A/pt, B/pt and C/pt showed high susceptibility to promotion and they developed carcinomas. Line B/pt was recently made available to our laboratory where we confirmed the high susceptibility to tumor promotion and also showed that the strain has a high incidence of carcinomas with a shorter latency time than the outbred SENCAR mice (Stern and Conti, unpublished results). It is presently unclear why the inbreeding in the SSIN strain has resulted in dissociation between promotion and progression while the strains developed by Potter maintain high susceptibility to both promotion and progression. It can be speculated that the selective breeding for tumor promotion put negative selection pressure on the tumor progression gene (or a tightly linked locus) but there is presently no evidence to support this hypothesis. Further, there are several alternative explanations, for example random segregation of the genes or selective pressure derived from experimental differences between the two laboratories involved in the inbreeding procedures.

SUSCEPTIBILITY TO PAPILLOMA PROGRESSION

The existence of different genetic mechanisms for controlling promotion and progression in the mouse skin carcinogenesis model has been suggested by early experiments carried out in our laboratory. Several years ago we used a mouse stock (obtained from Jackson Laboratory) that carries a constitutive chromosomal aberration. It was our intention to use this stock to investigate the role of chromosomal aberration in the progression of papillomas. Although high incidence and multiplicity of papillomas were obtained in this stock, no carcinomas were obtained (Trono and Conti, unpublished results). We also had a similar experience in a tumor experiment carried out on B6D2 F1 mice. This experiment (carried out to study allelic losses during tumor progression) produced a high number of papillomas as expected from the literature (Naito, et al, 1988), but again a small number of carcinomas was obtained over a very long latency period (over 2 years). Unfortunately, the purpose of those experiments was not to study promotion and progression, but to obtain tumors for cytogenetic and molecular analysis.

Consequently, data was not properly recorded (weekly follow-ups of the experiments with animals and tumor counting, histological examination of all the tumors and no-sampling or random sampling of animals) and thus the study was not adequate for publication. Although these early results from our laboratory were indicative of a differential genetic control of promotion and progression in the mouse skin model, it was not until we carried out the experiments with the SSIN mice that this phenomenon was fully apparent.

In order to characterize the dissociation between tumor promotion and progression observed in the SSIN mice, we designed an inter-strain breeding experiment using a DMBA/TPA protocol to study the susceptibility to tumor progression of F1 offsprings (Stern, et al., 1995). The strains used were SSIN, BALB/c (both of them known for their resistance to papilloma progression, and SENCAR. Both the SSIN x SENCAR and SENCAR x SSIN F1s showed a promotion sensitivity similar to that of the SSIN mice (Figure 2).

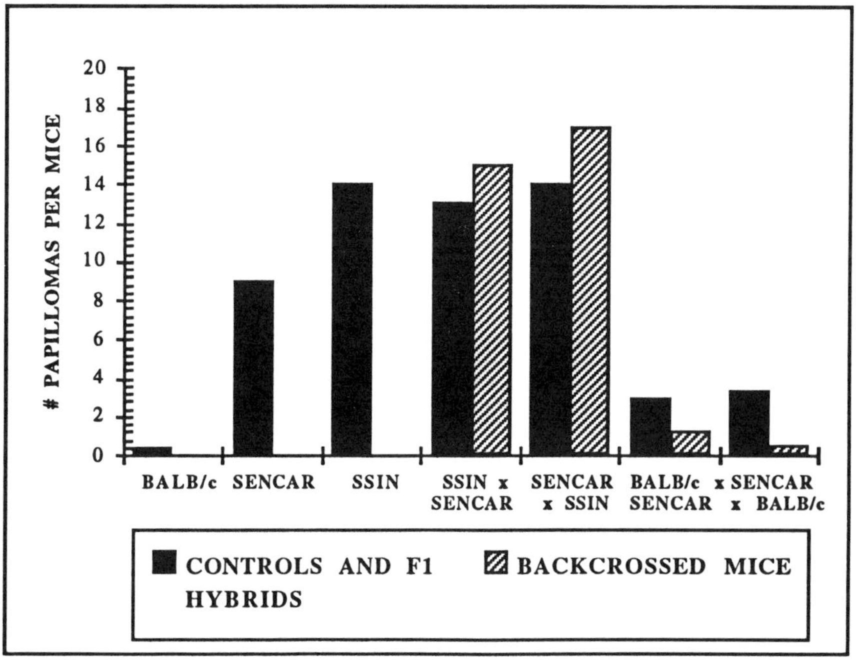

Figure 2.: Papilloma multiplicity in BALB/c, SENCAR, and SSIN control groups and F1 and Backcrossed hybrids.

This behavior was also seen in the SSIN x (SSIN x SENCAR), SSIN x (SENCAR x SSIN) backcrossed animals, suggesting that susceptibility to TPA promotion under these protocol conditions is inherited as a dominant trait. The BALB/c x SENCAR F1s showed an average response that was intermediate between the two parental strains/stock (Figure 2).

Regarding the papilloma progression, all F1s showed a cumulative number of SCCs similar to the SENCAR progenitor (Figure 3). We also investigated the previously described switch of keratin 1 to 13 as a marker of premalignant progression, which is significatively delayed in SSIN mice compared to SENCAR mice. The SSIN x SENCAR F1s expressed this switch in a way similar to the SENCAR mice.

Based on this evidence, we postulate that tumor progression in the mouse skin model (i.e., the ability of papillomas to progress to malignant tumors) is genetically regulated by modifier genes which are independent of the genes conferring susceptibility to tumor promotion.

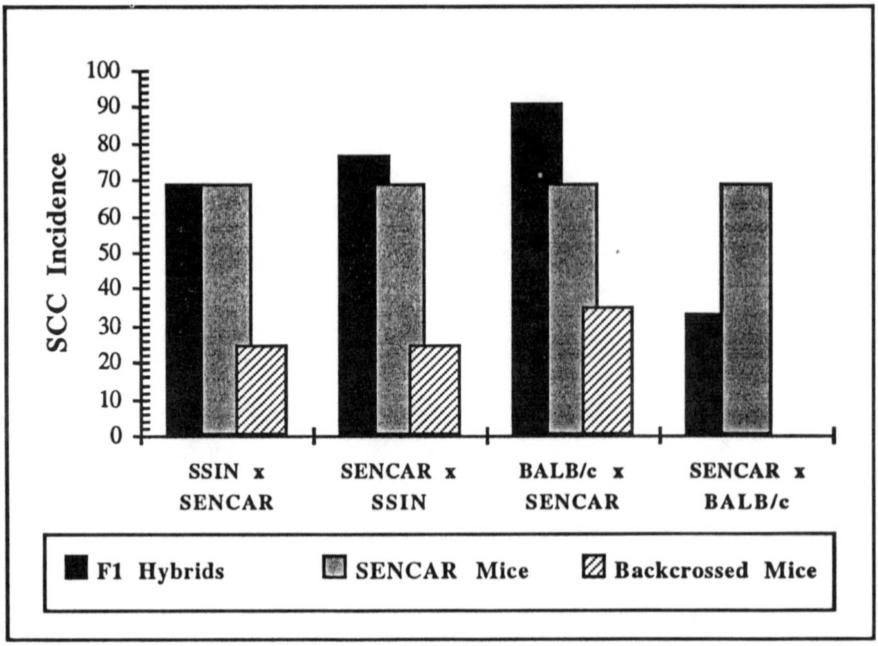

Figure 3. Squamous cell carcinoma incidence in SENCAR parental strain, F1 offsprings and Backcrossed hybrids

Recently Nagese et al (1995) have formulated a similar hypothesis. They have studied the susceptibility to chemical skin carcinogenesis on interspecies crosses between Mus spretus and susceptible strains of Mus musculus. Using this approach they have been able to identify three susceptibility loci, two on Chromosome 7 that seem to control the development of benign lesions and one in Chromosome 5 that affects early and late stages of tumor development. They concluded that benign and malignant tumors are largely under independent genetic control.

In order to formulate an accurate genetic model and to map the putative susceptibility genes controlling papilloma progression, we are presently carrying on a series of experiments using two SENCAR derived inbred lines, SSIN and SENCAR B/pt. The advantage of this model is that both inbred lines are highly susceptible to tumor promotion but in only one of them, SENCAR B/pt, do papillomas progress to squamous cell carcinomas. Therefore, these strains are excellent tools for performing mapping studies. Preliminary results from our laboratory indicate the existence of several polymorphic markers among these two strains. Preliminary results have shown that F1 hybrids between SSIN and SENCAR B/pt are highly susceptible to tumor progression, confirming our hypothesis that progression susceptibility is inherited as a dominant trait.

ACKNOWLEDGMENTS

The author wishes to thank Yolanda C. Valderrama for her secretarial assistance, Sharon Stockman for her editoria! expertise, Donna Schutz, Dale Weiss and Jimi Lynn Rosborough for their assistance in the breeding and animal experiments, and the Histology Department for the processing of samples. This work was supported by grants CA42157, CA52157 and CA57596.

REFERENCES

Boutwell RK (1964): Some biological aspects of skin carcinogenesis. Prog Exp Tumor Res 4:207-250.

Conti CJ (1994): The mouse skin as a model for chemical carcinogenesis. In Sundberg, JP (ed): "Handbook of mouse mutations with skin and hair abnormalities." Boca Raton: CRC press, pp 39-46.

DiGiovanni J (1991): Multistage carcinogenesis in mouse skin. Pharmac Ther 54:63-128.

DiGiovanni J, Walker SC, Beltrán L, Naito M, Eastin WC (1991): Evidence for a common genetic pathway controlling susceptibility to mouse skin tumor promotion by diverse classes of promoting agents. Cancer Res 51:1398-1405.

DiGiovanni J, Imamoto A, Naito M, Walker SE, Beltrán, L, Chenicek KJ, and Skow L (1992): Further genetic analyses of skin tumor promoter susceptibility using inbred and recombinant inbred mice. Carcinogenesis 13:525-531.

Environmental Health Perspectives. The SENCAR mouse in toxicology testing. Vol 68:3-203, 1986.

Fischer SM, O'Connel FJ, Conti CJ, Tacker KC, Fries JW, Patrick KE, Adams LM, Slaga TJ (1987): Characterization of an inbred strain of the SENCAR mouse that is highly sensitive to phorbol esters. Carcinogenesis 8:421-424.

Gimenez-Conti IB, Bianchi AB, Fischer SM, Reiners Jr JJ, Conti CJ, Slaga TJ (1992): Dissociation of sensitivities to tumor promotion and progression in outbred and inbred SENCAR mice. Cancer Res 52:3432-3435.

Hennings H, Krsmanpvic LS, Glick AB, Yuspa SH, Potter M (1993): Inbred mouse strains to study carcinoma development in mouse skin. 84th Annual meeting of the American Association for Cancer Research, Vol. 34, p 145.

Hennings H, Lowry DT, Yuspa SH, Mock BA, Potter M (1994): Skin carcinogenesis in the F1 hybrid of sensitive SENCAR A/Pt and resistant BALB/cAnPt mice. 85th Annual meeting of the American Association for Cancer Research, Vol. 35, p 121.

Klein-Szanto AJP (1989): Pathology of human and experimental skin tumors. In Conti CJ, Slaga TJ, Klein-Szanto AJP (eds): "Skin Tumors: Experimental and Clinical Aspects." New York: Raven Press, pp 19-53.

Nagase H, Bryson S, Cordell H, Kemp CJ, Fee F, Balmain A (1995) Distinct genetic loci control development of benign and malignant skin tumours in mice. Nature Genetics 10:424-429.

Naito M, Chenicek KJ, Naito Y, DiGiovanni J (1988): Susceptibility to phorbol ester skin tumor promotion in (C57BL/6 x DBA/2) F1 mice is inherited as an incomplete dominant trait: evidence for multi-locus involvement. Carcinogenesis 9:639-636.

Naito M, DiGiovanni J (1989): Genetic background and development of skin tumors. In Conti CJ, Slaga TJ, Klein-Szanto AJP (eds): "Skin Tumors: Experimental and Clinical Aspects." New York: Raven Press, pp 187-212.

Reiners JJ, Nesnow S, Slaga TJ (1984): Murine susceptibility to two stage skin carcinogenesis is influenced by the agent used for promotion. Carcinogenesis 5:301-307.

Slaga TJ (1984): Mechanisms involved in two-stage carcinogenesis in mouse skin. In Slaga TJ (ed): "Mechanisms of Tumor Promotion." Boca Raton, Florida: CRC Press, Vol. II, pp 1-16.

Slaga TJ (1989): Cellular and molecular mechanisms involved in multistage skin carcinogenesis. In Conti CJ, Slaga TJ., Klein-Szanto AJP (eds): "Carcinogenesis, A Comprehensive Survey." Skin Tumors: Experimental and Clinical Aspects." New York: Raven Press, Vol. 11, pp 1-18.

Stern MC, Gimenez-Conti IB, Conti CJ (1995): Genetic susceptibility to papilloma progression in SENCAR mice. Carcinogenesis 16:1947-1943.

Yuspa SH (1985): Cellular and molecular changes during chemical carcinogenesis in mouse skin cells. In Huberman E, Barr SH (eds.): "Carcinogenesis, The Role of Chemicals and Radiation in the Etiology of Cancer." New York: Raven Press, Vol. 10, pp. 210-210.

Genetics and Cancer Susceptibility:
Implications for Risk Assessment, pages 57–80

ONE DECADE OF COMPARATIVE MOLECULAR CARCINOGENESIS

Tamra L. Goodrow

Department of Pathology, Fox Chase Cancer Center, Philadelphia, PA 19111

Introduction

That the biological, physiological, and evolutionary processes in other mammals including rodents might be similar to those of humans was recognized more than two centuries ago. Indeed, animals have long been studied in an effort to understand human disease or alternatively to evaluate or assess the effects of various compounds administered on living beings. The reasons for using animal models and in studying comparative molecular carcinogenesis have changed little. They include: 1) to develop and compare animal models with human carcinogenesis to determine how well different animal models may recapitulate human disease, 2) to better understand the mechanisms underlying cell growth and cancer, 3) to define and evaluate the toxicity/carcinogenicity of different chemical agents, 4) to attempt to determine the etiological agents causing cancer, and 5) to provide information for use in extrapolation of cancer risk in animals to humans. Assessment of the similarity of the carcinogenic process in animal models as compared to that in humans is central for putting the other goals in perspective and thus is perhaps one of the most important questions that comparative molecular carcinogenesis seeks to address. Although the similarity of animal models to human disease must necessarily be defined at the histological, pathological, and biological levels, in addition to the molecular level, this discussion will be focused on the latter and will also be restricted to comparison of human carcinogenesis with rodent rather than other larger animal models of carcinogenesis.

Advantages and problems inherent in the study of comparative carcinogenesis

Rodent models have several advantages for the study of carcinogenesis. In rodents, opposed to humans, tumorigenesis may be easily studied temporally, as a sequence of events. This is partially due to the fact that the tumor latency period is much shorter for rodents than for humans. Animal models also allow study of this disease in a genetically defined and distinct population. The effects of multiple exposures to exogenous agents via the diet or environment may be experimentally limited and controlled. Furthermore, etiological agents (chemical carcinogens) may be defined and used, potentially allowing for study of different carcinogenesis pathways and for direct correlation of the identified genetic alterations with those predicted due to the given chemical exposure. In vitro correlates are also often more easily obtained. However, some of these same advantages also confound interpretation of results in relation to those obtained in humans since they are also the result of important differences between the rodent and human populations. Table 1 lists a summary of potential problems and confounding factors in the study of comparative molecular carcinogenesis. These are discussed in greater detail below.

Table 1. Problems inherent in comparative carcinogenesis

1) genetic diversity differences	
2) complexity of etiological factors	multiple:in humans limited: in rodents
3) complexity of modulating	genetic susceptibility factors
	environmental exposures endogenous factors (metabolism differences, hormones, immune system)
4) complexity of cancer	multiple genetic events multiple pathways
5) limited knowledge of genetic/epigenetic events involved	

The heterogeneity of the human population is not reflected in most laboratory rodent populations, even with outbred strains. This makes the study of different genetic susceptibility factors difficult. Nevertheless, both the use of transgenic mice and also some strains of rodents that are uniquely susceptible to certain forms of cancer are proving to be extremely valuable as potential models of the genetically susceptible human population. Furthermore, isolation of genes leading to such susceptibilities in rodents will also almost undoubtably lead to the identification and isolation of human homologues of these critical genes. The Eker rat, which is highly susceptible to kidney carcinogenesis is one such example of an animal susceptibility model (Eker, R and Mossige, J. 1961). The Eker rat is more susceptible to spontaneous and chemically induced renal carcinogenesis than other strains of rats (Walker et al., 1992). Recently, the gene responsible for this increased susceptibility, TSC2, has been determined to be the rat homologue of the human tuberous sclerosis gene II (Yeung et al., 1994). In addition, several mouse strains exhibit widely differing susceptibilities to chemically-induced liver or lung carcinogenesis and several studies are underway to identify the genes responsible for such different susceptibilities. Chromosomal regions have been described as possible locations for the susceptibility loci. Both the Eker rat model and mouse liver tumor susceptibility models are discussed in more detail in other chapters of this volume.

The etiological factors involved in human carcinogenesis are multiple and complex while those in rodents may be experimentally limited. During their lifetime, humans are exposed to thousands of agents via their environment, work place, or diet which may interact to contribute to carcinogenesis. These are virtually impossible to identify let alone imitate in rodent models. In addition, different species-specific viruses may contibute to tumorigenesis and may be very difficult to compare in human and rodent models. Lastly, the required amount of carcinogen used in many animal models of carcinogenesis is often considerably higher than that to which the human population is exposed. Furthermore, use of high doses of chemicals may dictate or alter the carcinogenic pathways making them difficult to compare with humans.

Another confounding factor in comparative carcinogenesis is that carcinogenesis is a highly complex process that is thought to result from several different alterations in multiple target genes. One example of this has been described in the colon, where at least 4-5 different genetic changes appear to be necessary for the development of the fully malignant lesions. These include loss of the specific chromosomal regions 5q and 18q which harbor the APC, MCC and DCC tumor suppressor genes, mutations in the K-ras gene, and loss or mutation of the p53 tumor suppressor gene (reviewed in Fearon, 1992). Moreover, cancer may arise via many different pathways, depending often upon the organ, cell of origin, or etiological agents. These pathways may also in turn depend upon other modulating factors mentioned above such as genetic susceptibility of the host, environmental exposures, or the presence of viruses.

The final problem is that there is only limited knowledge of the genetic and/or epigenetic events involved in carcinogenesis. Alterations in only a handful, though increasing number of gene families have been widely identified in human or rodent tumors. These are generally grouped into 2 different classes: the oncogenes and the tumor suppressor genes. Tables 2 and 3 list the putative onco- and suppressor genes and the human tumors in which they have been implicated. Other classes of genes recently postulated to play a role in cancer or susceptibility to cancer are the DNA repair enzymes, drug metabolizing enzymes, and genes involved in cell cycle control. The isolation of genes has proceeded at a more rapid pace as the number of experimental approaches has broadened. As more genes are isolated and examined, the gaps in the tumorigenesis pathways are being filled in allowing increasingly more critical and detailed comparisons of carcinogenesis in rodents and man. Some examples of the scope of genetic alterations in comparative molecular studies are described below.

Table 2. Oncogenes implicated in carcinogenesis[1,2]

gene	types of human tumors
abl	chronic myelogenous leukemia, acute lymphocytic leukemia
erb B1	squamous cell carcinoma, astrocytoma
erb B2/neu	breast, ovary, stomach
met	Burkitts lymphoma,lung, breast, cervix
myc (family)	(L-) lung, (N-) neuroblastoma, lung(SCLC), breast, Burkitt lymphoma, acute T cell leukemia, cervix
ras (family)	lung (adenocarcinomas), pancreas, bladder, colon, thyroid, melanoma, acute myelogenous and lympho-blastic leukemia
ret	thyroid
sis	astrocytoma
src	colon
trk	thyroid

[1]with genetic alterations found in at least 10% of primary tumors
[2] table modified from Bishop (1991)

Table 3. Tumor suppressor genes[1]

gene	chrom. loc.	type of cancers(human)	ref. for cloning of gene
APC	5q21	colon	Groden et al., 1991
BRCA	17q21	breast, ovarian	Miki et al., 1994
DCC	18q21	colon, endometrial, bladder	Fearon et al., 1990
MCC	5q21	colon	Kinzler et al., 1991
NF1	17q11.2	neurofibrosarcomas	Viskochil et al, 1990 Wallace et al., 1990
NF2	22q	neuromas, melanomas mesotheliomas, meningiomas	Trofatter et al., 1993
p16 (CDKN2)	9p21	esophagus, melanoma, mesotheliomas, lung HNSCCs[2], gliomas	Serrano et al., 1993
p53	17p13.1	breast, lung, SCCs, lymphomas, liver, pancreas osteosarcomas, leukemias, ovarian, esophagus, sarcoma bladder, brain	Harlow et al., 1985 Zakut-Houri et al., 1985
Rb	13q14	retinoblastoma, lung, colon, breast, prostate, sarcoma, osteosarcoma	Friend et al., 1986
VHL	3p25	kidney, CNS hemangioblastomas	Latif et al., 1993
WT1	11p13	Wilms	Call et al., 1990 Gessler et al., 1990

[1]with genetic alterations found at least approximately 10% in primary tumors

[2]squamous cell carcinomas of the head and neck

Examples of comparative studies of molecular carcinogenesis in various organs

The development of molecular techniques has allowed comparative carcinogenesis studies to be done at the molecular level on a large scale using primary tumor material from rodents and humans. This approach has been tremendously valuable in that it eliminates the artifacts potentially linked with using cell culture or other in vitro analyses. Tumors may be analyzed for abnormalities at the chromosomal level or at the DNA level for alterations such as gene loss, amplification, rearrangement, and mutation. Furthermore, both the type of altered genes and their specific alterations or mutations may be compared across species. Alterations in gene expression are also often examined. Tables 4, 5, 6, and 7 show examples of comparative molecular carcinogenesis in rodents vs. humans in liver, kidney, lung, and squamous cell tumorigenesis. The data in these tables is a compilation of results from several different laboratories. Only data on alterations in primary tumors or very short term cultures is included. While an attempt at completeness has been attempted, the references are not inclusive.

Conclusions

A number of observations may be drawn from examination of Tables 4-7. First, most genes found with alterations in some form of human cancer are also found to be altered in at least some type of rodent cancer. However, the combination of genetic alterations or genetic pathway can be similar or differ greatly for tumorigenesis in a given organ between rodents and humans. For example, examination of the alterations found in rodent vs human liver cancer (Table 4) indicate significant differences in the genetic pathways between mice and humans: ras mutations appear to play a large role in most chemically-induced and spontaneously occurring (susceptible strain) murine liver tumors while they play a minimal role in human hepatocarcinogenesis. The converse is true in the case of the p53 gene. We and others examined several different chemically-induced and spontaneous murine hepatocellular carcinomas (HCCs) and found no mutations in the hotspot regions of the p53 gene (Goodrow et al., 1992, Kress et al., 1992) while a relatively high proportion of p53 mutations are found in human HCCs from regions with population at risk for exposure to aflatoxins. In the rat, the extent to which ras and p53 are altered appears to be strongly chemical/model specific. This illustrates another important observation: that the genetic alterations found in most animal models are largely chemical-specific. In the case of adenocarcinoma of the lung, K-ras and p53 alterations appear to play a significant role in humans but the p53 gene appears to play a much more limited role in murine lung adenocarcinomas. Again, there appears to be some chemical specificity since a total of 35 spontaneous, DMBA, and DEN-induced lung murine adenocarcinomas exhibited no mutations in exons 5-8 of the p53 gene while 2/8 adenocarcinomas induced by 1,3-butadiene contained p53 mutations (Goodrow et al., 1992, Goodrow and Wiseman, unpublished results). In rats,

Table 4: Comparative molecular carcinogenesis of the liver

	mouse	rat	human
ras	60-80%[1] H-ras (susc. strains) 0% spontaneous (resistant strains) 0-100% H-ras all chemicals 8-25% K-ras 1,3 butadiene, tri-,tetrachloroethylene	spon. 8-100% K-ras aflatoxin 0-8% H, N, K-ras all chemicals 0% spontaneous	7-17% N-ras predominantly also H-, K-ras

refs: mouse: Reynolds et al., 1986, 1987, Fox et al., 1990, Goodrow et al., 1990, Buchmann et al., 1991, Dragani et al., 1991, Manam et al., 1992, Anna et al., 1994, Devereux et al., 1994 rat: Ishikawa et al., 1985, McMahon et al., 1986, Funato et al., 1987, Sinha et al., 1988, Watatani et al., 1989, Stowers et al., 1988, McMahon et al., 1990, Li et al., 1990, Li et al.,1991, Buchman et al., 1991, Soman and Wogan, 1993, Bitsch et al., 1993, Tokusashi et al., 1994, Ostermayr et al, 1991, Fujimoto et al., 1991, Sakai and Ogawa, 1990, human: Gu, J, 1988, Tsuda et al., 1989, Ogata et al., 1990, Tada et al., 1990.

	mouse	rat	human
p53	0% spontaneous DMBA, AAB, AAF DEN, phenobarbital	0% aflatoxin DEN, DMAAB, solt farber, perox. prolif., NMU 50% tamoxifen 30% choline deficient 82% aflatoxin (RFLPs)	50% Quidong 5%TaiwanChina 2% Xian 8% Shanghai 30% S. Africa 0-36% Japan

refs: mouse: Goodrow et al., 1992, Kress et al., 1992a, Rumsby et al., 1994, unpublished observations. rat: Lilleberg et al., 1992, Smith et al., 1993a, 1993b, Vancutsem et al., 1994, Tokusashi et al., 1994 human: Bressac et al., 1991, Hsu et al., 1991, Hosono et al., 1991, Murakami et al., 1991, Ozturk et al., 1991, Buetow et al., 1992, Scorcone et al., 1992, , Kress et al., 1992b, Volkmann et al., 1994.

[1] % is frequency of mutations/genetic alterations in primary solid tumors

Table 5. Comparative molecular carcinogenesis of the kidney

species	rat	human
ras	K-ras 44% DMN-OMe(mesenchymal) K-ras 75% DEN (mesenchymal) K-ras 100% ENU (nephroblastoma) K-ras 91% spon (nephroblastoma) 0% ras N-ethyl-Nhydroxyethyl-nitrosamine/n-nitrosomorpholine 0% ras renal cell carcinomas	H-ras 2-13%
references	rat: Peratoni et al., 1990, Sukamar et al, 1986, Ohgaki et al, 1991, Matsumoto et al.,1990, Recio et al., 1991 human: Fujita et al., 1988, Nanus et al., 1990, Nagata et al., 1990, Rochlitz et al., 1992	
p53	10% DMN-OMe (mesenenchymal) 0% nickel subsulfide 100% ENU (nephroblastoma)	5%
references	rat: Weghorst et al., 1994, Ohgaki et al., 1992. human: Strohmeyer et al., 1993, Suzuki et al., 1992	
LOH	Eker: 4,5,6	3p, 6q, 8p, 9pq, 14q17p
OTHER	overexp. TGF alpha Eker strain: TSC 2 gene mutations	overexp. TGF EGF receptor, c-myc VHL gene mutations
references	rat: Funaki et al., 1991, Walker et al., 1991, Yeung et al., 1994 human: Strohmeyer and Slamon, 1994, Thrash-Bingham et al., 1995,Gnarra et al., 1994,Shuin et al. 1994, Shuin et al., 1994.	

Table 6. Comparative studies of adenocarcinomas of the lung

	mouse	rat	human
ras	K- 10-43% spon. (resist. strains)	K- 40% spontaneous	K- 20-33%
		K- 75% tetranitromethane	N,H- rare
	K- 90-100% spon. (susc. strains)	K- 6% N-nitrosobis(2-oxopropyl) amine (BOP)	
	K- 22-100% all chemicals	K- 17% beryllium	
refs.	mouse: Belinsky et al, 1989, You et al., 1989, Goodrow et al., 1990, Candrian et al., 1991, Devereux et al., 1991, 1993, Manam et al., 1992, Re et al., 1992. rat: Stowers et al., 1987, Stegelmeier et al., 1991, Ohgaki et al., 1993, Nickell-Brady et al., 1994 human: Mitsudomi et al., 1991a, Reynolds et al., 1991, Rodenhuis et al., 1987, 1988, Slebos et al., 1990, Suzuki et al., 1990.		
p53	0% spon., DEN, DMBA, NNK	0% beryllium	35-55%
	7% $MeCl_2$		
	25% butadiene		
refs.	mouse: Goodrow et al., 1992, Hegi et al., 1993 rat: Nickell-Brady et al., 1994 human: Chiba et al., 1990, Miller et al., 1992, Suzuki et al., 1992, Kishimoto et al., 1992		
LOH	chr. 11, methylene chloride, 1,3-butadiene chr. 14, methylene chloride chr. 4, 1,3-butadiene		1, 3p, 9p, 17p, 11p, 13q
OTHER			20%-75% EGF receptor, Neu overexpression 20% mut. in Rb
refs.	mouse: Wiseman et al., 1994. humans: Weston et al., 1989, rev. in Pastorino et al., 1993.		

Table 7a. Comparative squamous cell carcinogenesis

	mouse skin	rat lung
ras	H61 90-100% DMBA/TPA H12 50-100% MNU, MNNG H13,61 25-40% 3MC H61 50% DMBA H61 56-78% promoters alone 0% X-ray H13 23% Benzo-a-pyrene H61 (H13) 90-100% methylbenzanthracene, fluoromethylbenz(a)anthracene	K- lung: 71% BOP K- lung: 75% TNM K- skin: 25% radiation
refs.	mouse: DiGiovanni et al., 1993, Brown et al., 1990, Jaffe and Bowden, 1989, Bonham et al., 1989, Pelling et al., 1987, 1988, rev. in Conti and Klein-Szanto, 1994 rat: Ohgaki et al., 1993, Stowers et al., 1989, Sawley et al., 1987	
p53	50% BaP 25%-50% DMBA/PMA 0% in papillomas 20-100%, UVB	nasal 45% formaldehyde
refs:	mouse: Ruggeri et al., 1991, 1993, Burns et al., 1991, Kanjilal et al., 1993, Kress et al., 1993c, Recio et al., 1992	
other	LOH at 7, 11 no Rb alterations trisomy at chrom. 6,7	
refs.	mouse: Bremner and Balmain, 1990, Bianchi et al., 1991, Ruggeri et al., 1991	

Table 7b. Comparative squamous cell carcinogenesis

	human skin	human lung SCC	human head and neck
ras	H-ras 20% K-ras 2%	K-ras 0-10%	H-ras 35% (India) H-ras 0-5% (Europe/USA) 22% LOH of ras allele
p53	47%	46-75%	23-58%
OTHER		75% LOH at Rb locus overexp. EGF R altered exp. RAR beta	15% LOH at Rb locus 73% LOH at APC locus 12.5% APC mutations 10% p16 mutations LOH at 3p, 5q, 7q, 8, 9p21-22, 9q, 11q, 13q14, 17p overexp: EGFR, c-myc amp:int-2, hst-1, cyclinD

refs. skin: Brash et al., 1991, Pierceall et al., 1991a, 1991b, Corominas et al., 1989, van der Schroeff et al., 1990
lung: included in references for Table 6 for NSCLCs
head and neck: Rumsby et al., 1990, Chang et al., 1991, Saranath et al., 1991, Sakai et al., 1992, Ah See et al., 1994, Carey et al., 1993, Grandis and Tweardy, 1993, Somers et al., 1992, Sakai and Tsuchida, 1992, Field et al., 1993, Zhang et al., 1994.

K-ras appears to be involved in lung tumorigenesis however mutations in p53 have not been detected.

In contrast, some animal tumor models of squamous cell carcinogenesis of the skin show a stronger target gene and mutation similarity with that found in human tumors of similar histology. As shown in Tables 7a and 7b, most tumor models producing murine skin SCCs exhibit alterations in the ras gene and p53 gene, while in humans, alterations in each of these genes are also observed in SCCs of the skin and/or head and neck. In rats, ras involvement is seen in SCCs of the esophagous, skin, and lung and p53 mutations are detected in esophageal and nasal SCCs.

In summary, definition and comparison of the complex molecular changes in human and rodent carcinogenesis shows that although etiological agents, exposures, and genetic susceptibilites may differ substantially, the critical genes involved in tumorigenesis are often common in rodents and humans. The multistep nature is also exhibited in animals and humans despite a much shorter latency period in animals. However, of equal importance is the observation that the specific pathways, genes, and mutations found in each animal model are largely organ, rodent strain, and/or chemical specific and thus may be either more or less similar to those identified in the correlate human tumors. This observation points to a strength rather than a weakness however, of using animal models since different pathways dependent upon organ, etiological agents, host susceptibility factors, and genetic differences are also likely to play a role in human tumorigenesis. Nevertheless, since in many cases the putative etiological agents are unknown in human tumors, this makes true comparison of genetic lesions of human tumors and animal tumors difficult. One way that this problem is beginning to be addressed is by new molecular epidemiological studies.

Molecular epidemiology

Information obtained from the rapidly evolving field of molecular epidemiology has proved tremendously valuable for the study of comparative molecular carcinogenesis and the study of carcinogenic mechanisms. Molecular epidemiology studies can correlate specific gene alterations and mutations with defined human environmental or dietary exposures and risk factors. Thus, the molecular lesions identified in human tumors with known exposures may be directly compared with those observed in animal tumorigenesis models induced by the same agents. These studies allow an optimal test, at the molecular level, of the similarity between the animal models and the human situation.

Molecular epidemiology studies are also important to comparative molecular carcinogenesis in that they enable further comparisons of the mutational targets, spectra, and frequency in human tumors with rodent tumors and with those predicted from the chemical/agent exposures. The results of such comparisons may contribute to the identification of etiological agents and form a basis for risk assessment. Table 8 lists some examples of comparisons facilitated by molecular epidemiology studies. These studies show both a close correlation between the lesions characterized in human and rodent tumors (induced by the same or similar etiological agents/exposures) and a good correlation between the specific molecular lesions identified and the predicted base changes due to adduct formation and or repair processes. For example, the mutations in the p53 gene in human SCCs from sunlight-exposed areas are similar to those found in UVB-induced mouse skin models: the p53 gene shows a high frequency of C to A transitions and several double mutations at dipyrimidine sites (Brash et al., 1991, Pierceall et al., 1991a, 1991b). These are completely consistent between mouse and human tumors and are also consistent with the mutations predicted from in vitro studies of UV radiation damage. Good correlations are also observed in the lesions identified in human and murine tumors induced by tobacco smoke and its components.

Transgenic mice and comparative molecular carcinogenesis

Transgenic mice strains represent other relatively new and valuable tools in comparative molecular carcinogenesis for several reasons. Many different transgenic mice have been created using cancer-related genes (Table 9). Each of these has tremendous potential value for the study and dissection of the effects of a single gene alteration on both spontaneously occuring and chemically-induced tumorigenesis. In addition, some transgenic mice models may be used as surrogate models for the susceptible human population. For example, the heterozygous mutant p53 mouse or the p53 knockout mouse may represent good models for individuals with the Li-Fraumeni syndrome. The use of these mice and other transgenics was the topic of another presentation and will be discussed in more detail in another chapter in this book.

Table 9. Examples of putative oncogenes or suppressor genes engineered into in transgenic mouse strains

bcl-2	EBV
erbB2/neu	lck
myc	papillomavirus
mutant p53	p53 knockout
pim-1	ras
Rb mutant	Rb + p53 mutants
SV40	TGF alpha

Transgenic technologies might also be applied in comparative molecular carcinogenesis to "engineer" or drive a carcinogenesis pathway in rodent tumors such that it better recapitulates a pathway observed in the correlate human tumors. For example, many chemically-induced non-transgenic mouse lung adenocarcinomas exhibit K-ras mutations but a very low frequency of p53 mutations (Goodrow et al., 1992). However, as indicated in Table 6, approximately 30-50% of human lung adenocarcinomas contain p53 mutations. This suggests that a mutant p53 transgenic mouse model might be a good surrogate model for comparison to human adenocarcinomas of the lung. We have examined spontaneously-occurring lung adenocarcinomas from transgenic mice heterozygous for a mutant p53 transgene containing a codon 135 (ala-val) mutation for ras mutations and found a high incidence of K-ras mutations (Goodrow, Shafarenko, and Wiseman, unpublished results). Thus, these tumors exhibit genetic alterations very similar to human lung adenocarcinomas. Further studies of these tumors might include analysis of other genetic changes often seen in human adenocarcinomas such as Rb alterations and/or examination of EGF receptor and neu expressison. Once such a model is characterized and developed, it may be easier to study other novel epigenetic and genetic alterations required to complement these changes for tumorigenesis. A further advantage of using transgenic mice is that the latency period for spontaneous and or chemically-induced tumor formation in many transgenic animals is decreased compared to their non-transgenic counterparts, making the bioassays potentially shorter, cheaper, and more practical to perform.

Summary

The field of comparative carcinogenesis has expanded greatly during the last decade. During this decade, the advent of molecular biology techniques allowed the isolation and identification of several oncogenes and tumor suppressor genes. Analysis of genetic alterations in these genes enabled the first dissection and comparison of carcinogenesis pathways in humans and rodents at the molecular level. The results showed that most of the oncogenes-/tumor suppressor genes found to be altered in humans were also altered in rodents. Even the molecular pathways involved in carcinogenesis appear to be similar in some organs. Unfortunately, there are still many unknown steps in the process of carcinogenesis. However, overall, the results still indicate that in spite of the differences between rodents and humans, the use and comparison of rodent models with human tumorigenesis is one of the best ways to 1) examine the mechanisms of carcinogenesis, 2) to identify potential carcinogenic compounds, and 3) to help determine potential carcinogenic risk for humans. The potential validity of the comparative carcinogenesis approach should become even more valuable as it becomes more fine-tuned due to the application of new approaches and the identification of new genes for study. The rapid pace of genomic mapping, the use of loss of heterozygosity studies, and the use of genetically susceptible populations (rodents and humans) has and will continue to allow the localization, isolation, and identification of new cancer genes. As each gene is analyzed in human and rodent tumors, the molecular pathway comparisons will become more accurate and detailed. This combined with molecular epidemiological and transgenic approaches will assure that the field of comparative carcinogenesis will continue to grow and be important in the next decade.

Acknowledgements

The author wishes to thank Dr. Steven Reynolds for his comments and critical review of this chapter.

References

Ah-See KW, Cooke TG, Pickford IR, Soutar D, Balmain A (1994): An allelotype of squamous carcinoma of the head and neck using microsatellite markers. Canc. Res. 54: 1617-1621.

Anna CH, Maronpot RR, Pereira MA, Foley JF, Malarkey DE, Anderson MW (1994): ras proto-oncogene activation in dichloroacetic acid-, trichloroethylene- and tetrachloroethylene-induced liver tumors in B6C3F1 mice. Carcinogenesis 15: 2255-2261.

Belinsky SA, Devereux TR, Maronpot RR, Stoner GD, Anderson MW (1989): Relationship between the formation of promutagenic adducts and the activation of the K-ras protooncogene in lung tumors from A/J mice treated with nitrosamines. Canc. Res. 49: 5305-5311.

Bianchi AB, Navone NM, Aldaz CM, Conti CJ (1991): Overlapping loss of heterozygosity by mitotic recombination on mouse chromosome 7F1-ter in skin carcinogenesis. PNAS 88: 7590-7594.

Bishop JM: (1991) Molecular themes in oncogenesis. Cell 64: 235-248.

Bitsch A, Roschlau H, Deubelbeiss C, Neumann HG (1993): The structure and function of the H-ras proto-oncogene are not altered in rat liver tumors initiated by 2-acetylaminofluorene, 2-acetylaminophenathrene and trans-4-acetylaminostilbene. Toxicol. Lett. 67:173-86.

Bonham K, Embry T, Gibson D, Jaffe DR, Roberts RA, Cress AE, Bowden GT (1989): Activation of the cellular Harvey ras gene in mouse skin tumors initiated with urethane. Molec. Carc. 2:34-39.

Brash DE, Rudolph JA, Simon JA, Lin A, McKenna GJ, Baden HP, Halperin AJ, Ponten J (1991): A role for sunlight in skin cancer: UV-induced p53 mutations in squamous cell carcinoma. PNAS 88: 10124-10128.

Bremner R and Balmain A (1990) Genetic changes inskin tumor progression correlation between presence of a mutatnt ras gene and loss of heterozygosity on mouse chromosome 7. Cell 61: 407-418.

Bressac B, Kew M, Wands J, Ozturk M (1991): Selective G to T mutations of p53 gene in hepatocellular carcinoma from southern Africa. Nature 350: 429-431.

Brown K, Buchmann A, Balmain A (1990): Carcinogen-induced mutations in the mouse c-Ha-ras gene provide evidence of multiple pathways for tumor progression. PNAS 87: 538-542.

Buchmann A, Bauer-Hofmann R, Mahr J, Drinkwater NR, Luz A, Schwartz M (1991): Mutational activation of the c-Ha-ras gene in liver tumors of different rodent strains: correlation with susceptibility to hepatocarcino-genesis. PNAS 1,88:911-915.

Buetow KH, Sheffield VC, Zhu M, Zhoe T, Shen F, Hino O, Smith M, McMahon Bj, Lanier AP, London WT, Redeker AG, Govindarajan S. (1992): Low frequency of p53 mutations observed in a diverse collection of primary hepatocellular carcinomas. PNAS 89: 9622-9626.

Burns PA, Kemp CJ, Gannon JV, Lane DP, Bremner R, Balmain A (1991): Loss of heterozygosity and mutational alterations of the p53 gene in skin tumours of interspecific hybrid mice. Oncogene 6: 2363-2369.

Call,KM, Glaser T., Ito CY, Buckler AJ, Pelletier J, Haber DA, Rose EA, Kral A, Yeger H, Lewis WH, Jones C, and Housman DE (1990): Isolation and characterization of a zinc finger polypeptide gene at the human chromosome 11 Wilms'tumor locus. Cell 60: 509-520.

Candrian U, You M, Goodrow T, Maronpot R, Reynolds SH, Anderson MW (1991): Activation of protooncogenes in spontaneously occurring non-liver tumors from C57BL/6 x C3H F1 mice. Canc. Res. 51: 1148-1153.

Carey TE, Worsham MJ, VanDyke DL (1993): Chromosomal biomarkers in the clonal evolution of head and neck squamous neoplasia. J. Cell. Biochem. 17F: 213-222.

Chang SE, Bhatia P, Johnson NW, Morgan PR, McCormick F, Young B, Hiorns L (1991): Ras mutations in United Kingdom examples of oral malignancies are infrequent. Int. J. Cancer 48: 409-412.

Chiba I, Takahashi T, Nau M, D'Amico D, Curiel D, Mitsudomi TDB, Carbone D, Piantadosi S, Koga H, Reissmann P, Slamon D, Holmes E, Minna J (1990): Mutations in the p53 gene are frequent in primary, resected non-small cell lung cancer. Oncogene 5: 1603-1610.

Conti CJ and Klein-Szanto AJP (1994): "Biochemistry and molecular biology of skin tumors" in Biochemical and molecular aspects of selected cancers, Vol. 2. Academic Press.

Corominas M, Kamino H, Leon J, Pellicer A (1989): Oncogene activation in human benign tumors of the skin(keratoacanthomas): is H-ras involved in differentiation as well as proliferation? PNAS 86: 6372-6376.

Devereux T, Anderson MW, Belinsky SA (1991): Role of ras protooncogene activation in the formation of spontaneous and nitrosamine-induced lung tumors in the resistant C3H mouse. Carcinogenesis 12: 299-303.

Devereux TR, Belinsky SA, Maronpot RR, White CM, Hegi ME, Patel AC, Foley JF, Greenwell A, Anderson MW (1993): Comparison of pulmonary O6 methylguanine DNA adduct levels and Ki-ras activation in lung tumors from resistant and susceptible mouse strains. Molec. Carc. 8: 177-185.

Devereux TR, White CM, Sills RC, Bucher JR, Maronpot RR, Anderson MW (1994): Low frequency of H-ras mutations in hepatocellular adenomas and carcinomas and in hepatoblastomas from B6C3F1 mice exposed to oxazepam in the diet. Carcinogenesis 15: 1083-1087.

DiGiovanni J, Beltran L, Rupp A, Harvey RG, Gill RD (1993): Further analysis of c-Ha-ras mutations in papillomas initiated by several polycyclic aromatic hydrocarbons and papillomas from uninitiated, promoter-treated skin in SENCAR mice. Molec. Carc. 8:272-279.

Dragani TA, Manenti G, Colombo BM, Falvella FS, Gariboldi M, Pierotti MA, Della Porta G (1991): Incidence of mutations at codon 61 of the Ha-ras gene in liver tumors of mice genetically susceptible and resistant to hepato carcinogenesis. Oncogene 6: 333-338.

Eker R and Mossige J (1961): A dominant gene for renal adenomas in the rat. Nature 189: 858-859.

Fearon ER (1992): Genetic alterations underlying colorectal tumorigenesis. Canc. Surv. 12: 119-136.

Fearon ER, Cho KR, Nigro JM, Kern SE, Simons JW, Ruppert JM, Hamilton SR, Preisinger AC, Thomas G, Kinzler KW, Vogelstein B (1990): Identifica tion of a chromosome 18q gene that is altered in colorectal cancers. Science 247: 49-56.

Field JK, Zlatko P, Pavelic ZP, Spandidos DA, Stambrook PJ, Jones AS, Gluckman JL (1993): The role of the p53 tumor suppressor gene in squamous cell carcinoma of the head and neck. Arch. Otolaryn. Head Neck Surg. 119: 1118-1122.

Fox TR, Schumann AM, Watanabe PG, Yano BL, Maher VM, McCormick JJ (1990): Mutational analysis of the H-ras oncogene in spontaneous C57BL/6 x C3H/He mouse liver tumors and tumors induced with genotoxic and non-genotoxic hepatocarcinogens. Canc. Res. 50: 4014-4019.

Friend SH, Bernards R, Rogelj S, Weinberg RA, Rapaport JM, Albert DM Dryha TP (1986): A human DNA segment with properties of the gene that predisposes to retinoblastoma and osteosarcoma. Nature 323: 643-646.

Fujimoto Y, Ishizaka Y, Tahira T, Sone H, Takahashi H, Enomoto K, Mori M, Sugimura T, Nagao M (1991): Possible involvement of c-myc but not ras genes in hepatocellular carcinomas developing after spontaneous hepatitis in LEC rats. Mol. Carc. 4: 269-74.

Fujita J, Kraus MH, Onoue H, Srivastava SK, Ebi Y, Kitamura, Rhim JS (1988): Activated H-ras oncogenes in human kidney tumors. Canc. Res. 48: 5251-5255.

Funato T, Yokota J, Sakamoto H, Kameya T, Fukushima S, Ito N, Terada M, Sugimura T (1987): Activation of N-ras gene in a rat hepatocellular carcinoma induced by dibutylnitrosamine and butylated hydroxytoluene. Gann 78:689-694.

Funaki K, Everitt J, Oshimura M, Freed JJ, Knudson AG, Walker C (1991): Hereditary renal cell carcinoma in the rat associated with non-random loss of chromosomes 5 and 6. Canc. Res. 51: 4415-4422.

Gessler M, Poustka A, Cavenee W, Neve RL, Orkin SH, Bruns GAP (1990): Homozygous deletion in Wilms'tumors of a zinc finger gene identified by chromosome junping. Nature 343: 774-778.

Gnarra JR, Tory K, Schmidt L, Wei MH, Li H, Latif F, Liu S, Chen F, Duh FM et al. (1994): Mutations of the VHL tumour suppressor gene in renal carcinoma. Nature Gene. 7: 85-90.

Goodrow T, Reynolds S, Maronpot R, Anderson M (1990): Activation of K-ras by codon 13 mutations in C57BL/6 x C3H F_1 mouse tumors induced by exposure to 1,3-butadiene. Canc. Res. 50: 4818-4823.

Goodrow TL, Storer RD, Leander KR, Prahalada SR, van Zwieten MJ, Bradley MO (1992): Murine p53 intron sequences 5-8 and their use in polymerase chain reaction/direct sequencing analysis of p53 mutations in CD-1 mouse liver and lung tumors. Molec. Carc. 5: 9-15.

Grandis JR and Tweardy DJ (1993): TGF alpha and EGFR in head and neck cancer. J. Cell. Biochem. 17F:188-191.

Groden J, Thliveris A, Samowitz W, Carlson M, Gelbert L, Albertsen H, Joslyn G, Stevens J, Spirio S, Robertson M, Sargeant L, Krapcho K, Wolff

E, Burt R, Hughes JP, Warrington J, McPherson J, Wasmuth J, LePaslier D, Abderrahim H, lCohen D, Leppert M, White R (1991): Identification and characterizationof the familial adenomatous polyposis coli gene. Cell 66: 589-600.

Gu J (1988): Molecular aspects of human hepatic carcinogenesis. Carcinogene sis 9: 697-703.

Harlow E, Williamson NM, Ralston R, Helfman DM, Adams TE (1985): Molecular cloning and in vitro expression of a cDNA clone for human cellular tumor antigen p53. Mol. Cell. Biol. 5:1601-1610.

Hegi ME, Soderkvist P, Foley JF, Schoonhoven R, Swenberg JA, Kari F, Maronpot R, Anderson MW, Wiseman RW (1993): Characterization of p53 mutations in methylene chloride-induced lung tumors from B6C3F1 mice. Carcinogenesis 14: 803-810.

Hosono S, Lee C-S, Chou M-J, Yang, C-S, Shih C (1991): Molecular analysis of the p53 alleles in primary hepatocellular carcinomas and cell lines. Oncogene 6: 237-243.

Hsu IC, Metcalf RA, Sun T, Welsh JA, Wang NJ, Harris CC (1991): Mutation al hotspot in the p53 gene in human hepatocellular carcinomas. Nature 350: 427-428.

Ishikawa F, Takaku F, Nagao M, Ochiai M, Hayashi K, Takayama S, Sugimura T (1985): Activated oncogenes in a rat hepatocellular carcinoma induced by 2-amino-3-methyl-imidazo{4,5-f}quinoline. Gann, 76:425-428.

Jaffe DR and Bowden GT (1989): Detection of distint transforming genes in X-ray induced tumors. Carcinogenesis 10: 2243-2247.

Kanjilal S, Pierceall WE, Cummings KK, Kripke ML, Ananthaswamy HN (1993): High frequency of p53 mutations in ultraviolet radiation-induced murine skin tumors: evidence for strand bias and tumor heterogeneity. Canc. Res. 53: 2961-2964.

Kinzler KW, Nilbert MC, Vogelstein B et al. (1991): Identification of a gene located at chromosome 5q21 that is mutated in colorectal cancers. Science 251: 1366-1370.

Kishimoto Y, Murakami Y, Shiraishi M, Hayashi K, Sekiya T (1992): Aberrations of the p53 tumor suppressor gene in human non-small cell carcinomas of the lung. Canc. Res. 52: 4799-4804.

Kress S, Konig J, Schweizer J, Lohrke H, Bauer-Hofmann R, Schwarz M (1992a): p53 mutations are absent from carcinogen-induced mouse liver tumors but occur in cell lines established from these tumors. Mol. Carc. 6: 148-158.

Kress S, Jahn U-R, Buchmann A, Bannasch P, Schwarz M (1992b): p53 mutations in human hepatocellular carcinomas from Germany. Canc. Res. 52: 3220-3223.

Kress S, Sutter C, Strickland PT, Mukhtar H, Schweizer J, Schwarz M (1992c): Carcinogen-specific mutational pattern in the p53 gene in ultraviolet B radiation-induced squamous cell carcinomas of mouse skin. Canc. Res. 52: 6400-6403.

Latif F, Tory K, Gnarra J, Yao et al., (1993): Identification of the von

Hippel-Lindau disease tumor suppressor gene. Science 260: 1317-1320.

Li H, Lee GH, Cui L, Liu J, Nomura K, Ohtake K Kitagawa T (1990): Absence of H-ras point mutation at codon 12 in N-methyl-N-nitrosourea-induced hepatocellular neoplasms in the rat. J. Can. Res. Clin. Oncol. 116: 331-335.

Li H, Lee GH, Liu K, Nomura K, Ohtake K, Kitagawa T (1991): Low frequency of ras activation in 2-acetylaminofluorene- and 3' -methyl-4-(dimethylamino)azobenzene-induced rat hepatocellular carcinomas. Canc. Lett. 56: 17-24.

Lilleberg SL, Cabonce MA, Raju NR, Wagner LM, Kier LD (1992): Alterations in the structural gene and the expression of p53 in rat liver tumors induced by Aflatoxin b_1. Molec. Carc. 6: 159-172.

Manam S, Storer RD, Prahalada S, Leander KR, Kraynak AR, Ledwith BJ, van Zwieten MJ, Bradley MO, Nichols WW (1992): Activation of the Ha-, Ki-, and N-ras genes in chemically induced liver tumors from CD-1 mice. Canc. Res. 52: 3347-3352.

Manam S, Storer RD, Prahalada S, Leander KR, Kraynak AR, Hammer meister CL, Joslyn DJ, Ledwith BJ, vanZwieten MJ, Bradley MO, Nichols WW. (1992): Activation of the Ki-ras gene in spontaneous and chemically induced lung tumors in CD-1 mice. Molec. Carc. 6: 68-75.

McMahon G, Hanson L, Lee J-J, Wogan GN (1986): Identification of an activated c-Ki-ras oncogene in rat liver tumors induced by aflatoxin B_1. PNAS 83: 9418-9422.

McMahon G, Davis EF, Huber J, Kim Y, Wogan GN (1990): Characterization of c-Ki-ras and N-ras oncogenes in aflatoxin B_1-induced rat liver tumors. PNAS 87: 1104-1108.

Miki Y, Swensen J, Shattuck-Eidens D, Futreal PA, Harshman K, Tavtigian S, Liu Q, Cochran C, Bennett LM, ding W, Bell R, Rosenthal J et al.(1994): A strong candidate for the breast and ovarian cancer susceptibility gene BRCA1. Science 266: 66-71.

Miller CW, Simon K, Aslo A, Kok K, Yokota J, Buys CH, Terada M, Koeffler HP (1992): P53 mutations in human lung tumors. Canc. Res. 52: 1695-1698.

Mitsudomi T, Steinberg SN, Oie HK, Mulshine JL, Phelps R, Viallet J, Pass H, Minna JD, Gadzar AF (1991): Ras gene mutations in non-small cell lung cancers are associated with shortened survival irrespective of treatment intent. Canc. Res. 51: 4999-5002.

Murakami Y, Hayashi K, Hirohashi S, Sekiya T (1991): Aberrations of the tumor suppressor p53 and retinoblastoma genes in human hepatocellular carcinomas. Canc. Res. 51: 5520-5525.

Nagata Y, Abe M, Kobayashi K, Saiki S, Kotake T, Yoshikawa K, Yeda R, Nakayama E, Shiku H (1990): Point mutations of c-ras genes in human bladder cancer and kidney cancer. Jpn. J. Canc. Res. 81: 22-27.

Nanus DM, Mentle IR, Motzer RJ, Bander NH, Albino AP (1990): Infrequent ras oncogene point mutations in renal cell carcinoma. J. Urol. 143:175-178.

Nickell-Brady C, Hahn FF, Linch GL, Belinsky SA (1994): Analysis of K-ras,

p53, and c-raf-1 mutations in beryllium-induced rat lung tumors. Carcino genesis 15: 257-262.
Ogata N, Kamimura T, Asakura H (1990): Point mutation, allelic loss and increased methylation of c-Ha-ras gene in human hepatocellular carcinoma. Hepatology 31: 31-37.
Ohgaki H, Kleihues P, Hard GC (1991): Ki-ras mutations in spontaneous and chemically induced renal tumors of the rat. Molec. Carc. 4: 455-459.
Ohgaki H, Hard GC, Hirota N, Maekawa A, Takahashi M, Kleihues P (1992): Selective mutation of codons 204 and 213 of the p53 gene in rat tumors induced by alkylating N-nitroso compounds. Canc. Res. 52: 2995-2998.
Ohgaki H, Furukawa F, Takahashi M, Kleihues P (1993): K-ras mutations are frequent in pulmonary squamous cell carcinomas but not in adenocarcinomas of WBN/Kob rats induced by N-nitrosobis (2-oxopropyl) amine. Carcino genesis 14: 1471-3.
Ostermayr R, Suchy B, Rabes HM. (1991): Carcinogen-induced liver tumours of Wistar rats: absence of activated ras genes and of N-rasC. J. Canc. Res. Clin. Oncol 117: 381-4.
Ozturk M, Bressac B, Kew M, Volkmann M, Bozcall S, Mura J, de la Monte S, Carson R, Blum H, et al.(1991): p53 mutation in hepatocellular carcinoma after aflatoxin exposure. Lancet 338: 1356-1359.
Pastorino U, Sozzi G, Miozzo M, Tagliabue E, Pilotti S, Pierotti MA (1993): J. Cell Biochem. Suppl 17F: 237-248.
Pelling JC, Fischer SM, Neades R, Strawhecker J, Schweickert L (1987): Elevated expression and point mutation of the Ha-ras proto-oncogene in mouse skin tumors promoted by benzoyl peroxide and other promoting agents. Carcinogenesis 8: 1481-1484.
Pelling JC, Neades R, Strawhecker J (1988): Epidermal papillomas and carcinomas induced in unititiated mouse skin by tumor promoters alone contain a point mutation in the 61st codon of the Ha-ras oncogene. Carcino genesis 9: 665-667.
Pierceall WE, Goldberg LH, Tainsky MA, Mukhopadhyay T, Ananthaswamy HN (1991a): Ras gene mutation and amplification in human non-melanoma skin cancers. Molec. Carc. 4: 196-202.
Pierceall WE, Mukhopadhyay T, Goldberg LH, Ananthaswamy HN (1991b): Mutations in the p53 tumor suppressor gene in human cutaneous squamous cell carcinomas. Molec. Carc. 4: 445-449.
Re FC, Manenti G, Borrello MG, Colombo MP, Fisher JH, Pierotti MA, Della Porta G, Dragani TA (1992): Multiple molecular alterations in mouse lung tumors. Molec. Carc. 5: 155-160.
Recio L, Lane SC, Ginsler G, Walker C (1991): Analysis of ras DNA sequences in rat renal cell carcinoma. Molec. Carc. 4: 350-353.
Recio L, Sisk S, Pluta L, Bermudez E, Gross EA, Chen Z, Morgan K, Walker C (1992): p53 mutations in formaldehyde-induced nasal squamous cell carcinomas in rats. Canc. Res. 52: 6113-6116.
Reynolds SH, Stowers SJ, Maronpot RR, Anderson MW, Aaronson SA (1986): Detection and identification of activated oncogenes in spontaneously

occurring benign and malignant hepatocellular tumors of the B6C3F1 mouse. PNAS 83: 33-37.
Reynolds SH, Stowers SJ, Patterson RM, Maronpot RR, AAronson SA, Anderson MW (1987): Activated oncogenes in B6C3F1 mouse liver tumors: Implications for risk assessment. Science 237: 1309-1316.
Reynolds SH, Anna CK, Brown KC, Wiest JS, Beattie EJ, Pero RW, Iglehart JD, Anderson MW (1991): Activated protooncogenes in human lung tumors from smokers. PNAS 88: 1085-1089.
Rochlitz CF, Peter S, Willroth G, deKant E, Lobeck H, Huhn D, Herrmann R (1992): Mutations in the ras protooncogenes are rare events in renal cell cancer. Eur. J. Cancer 28: 333-
Rodenhuis S, Vande Wetering ML, Mooi WJ, Evers SG, Van Zandwijk N, Bos JL (1987): Mutational activation of the K-ras oncogene. A possible pathogenic factor in adenocarcinoma of the lung. New Engl. J. Med. 317: 929-935.
Rodenhuis S, Slebos RJC, Boot AJM, Evers SG, Mooi WJ, Wagennan SS, Bodegom PC, Bos JL. (1988): Incidence and possible clinical significance of K-ras oncogene activation in adenocarcinoma of the human lung. Canc. REs. 48: 5738-5741.
Ruggeri B, Caamano, J, Goodrow T, DiRado M, Bianchi A, Trono D, Conti CJ, Klein-Szanto AJP (1991): Alterations of the p53 tumor suppressor gene during mouse skin tumor progression. Canc. Res. 51: 6615-6621.
Ruggeri B, DiRado M, Zhang SY, Bauer B, Goodrow T, Klein-Szanto AJP. (1993): Benzo-a-pyrene-induced skin tumors exhibit frequent and character istic G to T mutations in the p53 gene. PNAS 90: 1013-1017.
Rumsby G, Carter RL, Gusterson BA (1990): Low incidence of ras oncogene activation in human squamous cell carcinomas. Br. J. Cancer 61: 365-368.
Sakai E, Rikimaru K, Ueda M, Matsumoto Y, Ishii N, Enomoto S, Yamamoto H, Tsuchida N (1992): The p53 tumor suppressor gene and ras oncogene mutations in oral squamous cell carcinoma. Int. J. Cancer 52: 867-872.
Sakai E and Tsuchida N (1992): Most human squamous carcinomas in the oral cavity contain mutated p53 tumor-suppressor genes. Oncogene 7: 927-933.
Sakai H and Ogawa K (1990): Mutational activation of H-ras and K-ras is absent in N-nitroso-N-methylurea-induced liver tumors in rats. Gann 81: 437-439.
Saranath D, Chang SE, Bhoite LT, Panchal RG, Kerr IB, Mehta AR, Johnson NW, Deo MG (1991): High frequency mutation in codons 12 and 61 of H-ras oncogene in chewing tobacco-related human oral carcinoma in India. Br. J. Cancer. 63: 573-578.
Sawey MJ, Hood AT, Burns FJ, Garte SJ (1987): Activation of c-myc and c-K-ras oncogenes in primary rat tumors induced by ionizing radiation. Mol. Cell. Biol. 7: 932-935.
Scorsone KA, ZHou Y-Z, Butel JS, Slagle BL (1992): p53 mutations cluster at codon 249 in hepatitus B virus-positive hepatocellular carcinomas from China. Canc. Res. 52: 1635-1638.
Serrano M, Hannon GJ, Beach D (1993): A new regulatory motif in cell-cycle

control causing specific inhibition of cyclin D/CDK4. Nature 366: 704-707.

Shuin T, Kondo K, Torigoe S, Kishida T, Kubota Y, Hosaka M, Nagashima Y, Kitamura H, Latif F, Zbar B et al. (1994): Frequent somatic mutations and loss of heterozygosity of the von-Hippel-Lindau tumor suppressor gene in primary human renal cell carcinomas. Canc. Res. 11: 2852-2855.

Sinha S, Webber C, Marshall CJ, Knowles MA, Proctor A, Barrass NC, Neal GE (1988): Activation of ras oncogene in aflatoxin-induced rat liver carcinogenesis. PNAS 85: 3673-3677.

Slebos RJC, Kibbelaar RE, Dalesio O, Kooistra A, Stam J, Meyer CJ, Wagenaar SS, Vanderschueren RG, Van Zandwijk N, Mooi WF, Bos JL, Rodenhuis S (1990): K-ras oncogene activation as a prognostic marker in adenocarcinoma of the lung. New Engl. J. Med. 323: 561-565.

Smith ML, Yeleswarapu L, Locker J, Lombardi B (1993a): p53 mutation in hepatocellular carcinomas induced by a choline-devoid diet in male Fischer 344 rats. Carcinogenesis 14: 503-510.

Smith ML, Yeleswarapu L, Lombardi B, Shinozuka H (1993): Lack of mutations of the p53 tumor suppressor gene in hepatocellular carcinomas induced in rats by a peroxisome proliferator. Molec. Carc. 7: 89-93.

Somers KD, Merrick MA, Lopez ME, Incognito LS, Schechter GL, Casey G (1992): Frequent p53 mutations in head and neck cancer. Canc. Res. 52: 5997-6000.

Soman NR and Wogan GN (1993): Activation of the c-Ki-ras oncogene in aflatoxin B_1-induced hepatocellular carcinoma and adenoma in the rat: detection by denaturing gradient gel electrophoresis. PNAS 90: 2045-2049.

Stegelmeier BL, Gillett NA, Rebar AH, Kelly G (1991): The molecular progression of plutonium-239-induced rat lung carcinogenesis: Ki-ras expression and activation. Molec. Carc. 4:43-51.

Stowers SJ, Glover PL, Reynolds SH, Boone LR, Maronpot RR, Anderson MW (1987): Activation of the K-ras protooncogene in lung tumors from rats and mice chronically exposed to tetranitromethane. Canc. Res. 47: 3212-3219.

Stowers SJ, Wiseman RW, Ward Jm, Miller EC, Miller JA, Anderson MW, Eva A (1988): Detection of activated proto-oncogenes in N-nitrosodiethylamine-induced liver tumors: a comparison between B6C3F1 mice and Fischer 344 rats. Carcinogenesis 9: 271-276.

Strohmeyer TG, Imai Y, Fleischhacker M, Slamon DJ, Koeffler HP (1993): Study on p53 mutations and mdm-2 alterations in human renal cell carcino mas. J. Urol. 149: 460A, abstract 990.

Strohmeyer TG and Slamon DJ (1994): Proto-oncogenes and tumor suppressor genes in human urological malignancies. J. Urol. 151: 1479-1497.

Sukamar S, Peratoni A, Reed C, Rice JM, Wenk ML (1986): Activated K-ras and N-ras oncogenes in primary renal mesenchymal tumors induced in F344 rats by Methyl(meethoxymethyl)nitrosamine. Mol. Cell. Biol. 6: 2716-2720.

Suzuki H, Takahashi T, Kuroishi T, Suyama M, Ariyoshi Y, Ueda R (1992): P53 mutations in non-small cell lung cancer in Japan: Association between mutations and smoking. Canc. Res. 52: 734-736.

Suzuki Y, Orita M, Shiraishi M, Hayashi K, Sekiya T (1990): Detection of ras gene mutations in human lung cancers by single-strand conformation polymorphism analysis of polymerase chain reaction products. Oncogene 5: 1037-1043.

Suzuki Y, Tamura G, Satodate R, Fujioka T (1992): Infrequent mutation of p53 gene in human renal cell carcinoma dtected by polymerase chain reaction single strand conformation polymorphism analysis. Jap. J. Canc. Res. 83: 233-236.

Tada M, Omata M, Ohto M (1990): Analysis of ras gene mutations in human hepatic malignant tumors by polymerase chain reaction and direct sequenc ing. Canc. Res. 50: 1121-1124.

Thrash-Bingham C, Greenberg RE, Howard S, Bruzel A, Bremer M, Goll A, Salazar H, Freed JJ, Tartof KD (1995): PNAS in press.

Tokushashi Y, Fukuda I, Ogawa K. (1994): Absence of p53 mutations and various frequencies of K--ras exon 1 mutations in rat hepatic tumors induced by different carcinogens. Molec. Carc. 10: 45-51.

Trofatter JA et al. (1993): A novel moesin-, ezrin-, radixin-like gene is a candidate for the neurofibromatosis 2 tumor suppressor. Cell 72: 791-800.

Tsuda H, Hirohashi S, Shimosato Y, Ino Y, Yoshida T, Terada M (1989): Low incidence of point mutation of c-ki-ras and N-ras oncogenes in human hepatocellular carcinoma. Jpn. J Canc. Res 80: 196-199.

Vancutsem Pm, Lazarus P, Williams GM (1994): Frequent and specific mutations of the rat p53 gene in hepatocarcinomas induced by tamoxifen. Canc. Res. 15: 3864-3867.

van der Schroeff JG, Evers LM, Boot AJM, Bos JL (1990): Ras oncogene point mutations in basal cell carcinomas and squamous cell carcinomas of the human skin. J. Invest Dermatol. 94: 423-425.

Viskochil D, Buchberg AM, Xu Gl, Cawthon RM, Stevens J, Wolff RK, Culver M, Carey JC, Copeland NG, Jenkins NA, White R, O'Connell P (1990): Deletions and a translocation interrupt a cloned gene at the neurofi bromatosis type 1 locus. Cell 62: 187-192.

Volkmann M, Hofmann WJ, Muller M, Rath U, Otto G, Zentgraf H, Galle PR (1994): p53 overexpression is frequent in European hepatocellular carcinoma and largely independent of the codon 249 hot spot mutation. Oncogene 9: 195-204.

Walker C, Everitt J, Freed JJ, Knudson AG, Whiteley LO (1991): Altered expression of transforming growth factor alpha in hereditary rat renal cell carcinoma. Canc. Res. 51: 2973-2978.

Walker C, Goldsworthy TL, Wolf DC, Everitt J (1992): Predisposition to renal cell carcinoma due to alteration of a cancer susceptibility gene. Science 255: 1693-1696.

Wallace MR, Marchuk DA, Andersen LB, Letcher R, Odeh HM, Saulino AM, Fountain JW, Brereton A, Nicholson J, Mitchell Al, Brownstien BH, Collins FS (1990): Type 1 neurofibromatosis gene: identification of a large transcript disrupted in three NF1 patients. Science 249: 181-186.

Watatani M, Peratoni AO, Reed CD, Enomoto T, Wenk ML, Rice JM (1989):

Infrequent activation of K-ras, H-ras, and other oncogenes in hepatocellular neoplasms initiated by methyl(acetoxymethyl)nitrosamine, a methylating agent, and promoted by phenobarbital in F344 rats. Canc. Res. 49: 1103-1109.

Weghorst CM, Dragnev KH, Buzard GS, Thorne KL, Vandeborne GF, Vincent KA, Rice JM. (1994): Low incidence of point mutations detected in the p53 tumor suppressor gene from chemically induced rat renal mesenchy mal tumors. Canc. Res. 54: 215-219.

Weston A, Willey JC, Modali R, Sugimura H, McDowell EM, Resau J, Light B, Haugen A, Mann DL, Trump BF, Harris CC (1989): Differential DNA sequence deletions from chromosomes 3, 11, 13, and 17 in squamous cell carcinoma, large cell carcinoma, and adenocarcinoma of the human lung. PNAS 86: 5099-5103.

Wiseman RW, Cochran C, Dietrich W, Lander ES, Soderkvist P (1994): Allelotyping of butadiene-induced lung and mammary adenocarcinomas of B6C3F1 mice: frequent losses of heterozygosity in regions homologous to human tumor-suppressor genes. PNAS 91: 3759-3763.

Wiseman RW, Stowers SJ, Miller EC, Anderson MW, Miller JA (1986): Activating mutations of the c-Ha-ras protooncogene in chemically induced hepatomas of the male B6C3F1 mouse. PNAS 83: 5825-5829.

Yeung RS, Xiao GH, Jin F, Lee WC, Testa JR, Knudson AG (1994): Predisposition to renal carcinoma in the Eker rat is determined by germ-line mutation of the tuberous sclerosis (TSC2) gene. PNAS 91: 11413-11416.

You M, Candrian U, Maronpot RR, Stoner GD, Anderson MW (1989): Activation of the Ki-ras protooncogene in spontaneously occurring and chemically induced lung tumors of the strain A mouse. PNAS 86: 3070-3074.

Zakut-Houri R, Bienz-Todmor B, Givol D, Oren M (1985): Human p53 cellular tumor antigen: cDNA sequence and expression in COS cells. EMBO J. 4:1251-1255.

Zhang S-Y, Klein-Szanto AJP, Sauter ER, Shafarenko M, Mitsunaga S, Nabori T, Carson DA, Ridge JA, Goodrow TL (1994): Higher frequency of alterations in the p16/CDKN2 gene in squamous cell carcinoma cell lines than in primary tumors of the head and neck. Canc. Res. 54: 5050-5053.

Genetics and Cancer Susceptibility:
Implications for Risk Assessment, pages 81–108

VALIDATION ISSUES FOR THE USE OF TRANSGENIC MOUSE MUTATION ASSAYS IN RISK ASSESSMENT[1]

Nancy J. Gorelick

Miami Valley Labs, Procter & Gamble Company, Cincinnati, OH 45253-8707

INTRODUCTION

Regulatory agencies throughout the world have guidelines for genotoxicity testing to determine the safety of new chemicals, foods and drugs. In general, the acceptable sets of assays utilize bacterial systems and cell culture systems as well as rodents to predict the potential for carcinogenicity and/or heritable effects. Each of the regulatory guidelines includes assays which detect gene mutation and/or chromosome effects. The commonly used assays at this time include cytogenetic assays (*in vitro* and *in vivo* in rodent somatic tissue) and *in vitro* gene mutation assays. An *in vivo* somatic cell gene mutation assay in rodents has not been included because, until recently, one has not been available. There is significant interest in the possible use of the mutation assays in transgenic mice as part of regulatory test sets (U.S. FDA, 1993; Questions and Answers, 1993). Protocols for routine study designs and a complete evaluation of how well these assays predict potential carcinogenicity, however, are not yet complete. The progress to date in the evaluation of these assays is reviewed here. Because much of the transgenic mouse mutation data developed to date remains unpublished or has been presented only as meeting abstracts, a comprehensive review of the data generated is not possible.

---

[1]This manuscript has appeared in part in "Introduction: Update on Transgenic Mouse Mutation Assays. Workshop Proceedings from the 1994 Environmental Mutagen Society Meeting", by N.J. Gorelick, *Environmental and Molecular Mutagenesis*, and in "Overview of Mutation Assays in Transgenic Mice for Routine Testing" by N.J. Gorelick, *Environmental and Molecular Mutagenesis*, Copyright © (1995 John Wiley & Sons, Inc.). Reprinted by permission of Wiley-Liss, a division of John Wiley & Sons, Inc.

Furthermore, it is difficult to evaluate completely some of the studies reported. In this regard, let it be said at the outset that this report is not a comprehensive review of all transgenic mouse mutation data, with apologies to any colleagues whose data may have been omitted.

Mutation Assays in Transgenic Mice

Currently, two transgenic mouse mutation assays are commercially available. Both carry bacterial genes as mutational targets in a λ shuttle vector; one, called Muta™Mouse, carries the *lacZ* gene (Gossen et al., 1989) and the other, called Big Blue®, carries the *lacI* gene (Kohler et al., 1991a, 1991b; reviewed in Provost et al., 1993; Dycaico et al., 1994). In each case, multiple copies of the respective shuttle vector are integrated stably in a head-to-tail fashion in one chromosomal location (Gossen et al., 1989; Dycaico et al., 1994). Whereas each mouse can be treated by any route of administration with a potentially mutagenic agent, the λ shuttle vector technology permits excision of the mutational target from genomic DNA from any tissue for analysis in *E. coli*. Specifically, genomic DNA is exposed to λ packaging extract which excises individual transgenes and packages each as an infectious phage particle. *E. coli* cultures grown on agar plates are infected with the phage and, under standard conditions, each infection produces a plaque in the bacterial lawn containing ~ 10^5-10^6 phage particles of clonal origin. Plaques that contain mutant target genes are then identified by a color selection system. Wild type *lacZ* genes produce functional β-galactosidase, which cleaves the chromogenic substrate, 5-bromo-4-chloro-3-indolyl-β-D-galactopyranoside (X-gal), producing a blue plaque. On the other hand, mutants in *lacZ* do not produce functional β -galactosidase, do not cleave the chromogenic substrate, and produce a white or clear plaque. Mutants are thus scored as clear plaques on a background of blue plaques. Alternatively, *lacI* mutants are scored as blue plaques on a background of clear plaques. Wild type *lacI* genes encode proteins which repress the expression of the *lacZα* reporter gene and the production of functional β-galactosidase. X-gal is therefore not cleaved and clear plaques are produced. Mutant *lacI* genes encode proteins that do not repress the expression of the *lacZα* reporter gene and cells do produce functional β-galactosidase, resulting in the cleavage of X-gal and the production of blue plaques. Data from each system are expressed finally as mutant frequencies, the ratio of the observed number of mutant transgenes to the total number of transgenes sampled.

Mutation Studies to Date

To review the progress made to date in evaluating the transgenic mutation assays, data that have been published or presented previously are summarized here. Tissues in which a mutant frequency (MF) has been determined include skin, liver, spleen, splenic T-lymphocytes, lung, kidney, forestomach, urinary bladder, heart, brain, bone marrow and male germ cells. These include tissues in which chemically-induced tumors are commonly found as well as surrogate tissues that could be used for routine testing, such as bone marrow. Tissue-specific background MFs have been reported; MFs in various tissues from adult male transgenic mice are collected in Table 1. These data show that

Table 1. Tissue-Specific Spontaneous Background Mutant Frequencies

Tissue	Transgene, Strain[a]	MF[b] x 10^5 (No. mice)	Reference
Skin	*lacI*, C57BL/6	7.1 ± 2.1[c] (3)	Thompson et al., 1992
Liver	*lacI*, C57BL/6	4.1 ± 0.7 (10)	Rogers et al., 1993
Spleen (T-lymphocytes)	*lacI*, B6C3F1	3.5 ± 0.7 (8)	Walker et al., 1994
Lung	*lacI*, B6C3F1	6.6 ± 1.1 (4)	O'Kelly et al., 1994
Kidney	*lacI*, B6C3F1	5.4 ± 2.0 (4)	O'Kelly et al., 1994
Small Intestine	*lacI*, C57BL/6 x SWR	25[d] (5)	Tao et al., 1993b; Morrison and Ashby, 1994
Urinary Bladder	*lacI*, B6C3F1	2.7[d] (3)	Morrision and Ashby, 1994
Brain	*lacI*, B6C3F1	3.3 ± 0.4 (3)	Provost et al., 1993
Bone Marrow	*lacI*, B6C3F1	3.8 ± 0.1 (3)	Sisk et al., 1994a
Male Germ Cells	*lacI*, B6C3F1	0.6 ± 0.3 (8)	Provost et al., 1993
Skin	*lacZ*, CD2F1	2.8 ± 0.5 (7)	Myhr, 1991
Liver	*lacZ*, CD2F1	3.1 ± 1.0 (5)	Hoorn et al., 1993
Lung	*lacZ*, CD2F1	4.4 (5 pooled)	Recio et al., 1992
Brain	*lacZ*, CD2F1	0.1 (4 pooled)	Gossen et al., 1991
Bone Marrow	*lacZ*, CD2F1	4.1 ± 3.6 (7)	Hoorn et al., 1993
Testes	*lacZ*, CD2F1	0.6 (2 pooled)	Hoorn et al., 1993

[a] Data are from adult male mice. The *lacI* transgenic mice (Big Blue) are available with either of two genetic backgrounds, C57BL/6 or B6C3F1. The *lacZ* transgenic mice (MutaMouse) are BALB/c x DBA/2 mice.
[b] MF, mutant frequency; MFs in *lacI* or *lacZ* are reported.
[c] Avg ± SD
[d] Only the average was reported.

background MFs in most somatic tissues are similar whereas the background MF in germ cells is approximately an order of magnitude less and the background MF in small intestine is approximately an order of magnitude greater. The unusually high MF in the small intestine may be attributable to the high replication rate in the intestinal epithelium or, in part, to the small number of transgenes analyzed (Morrison and Ashby, 1994) and thus the uncertain nature of these data. Some of the classes of agents tested for mutagenicity in transgenic mice are listed in Table 2. These agents include mutagens and nonmutagens, as determined in *in vitro* tests, as well as rodent carcinogens and noncarcinogens. To date, at least 35 agents have been tested in at least one of the mouse strains. Finally, MF response depends on the number of exposures (e.g., Kohler et al., 1991b), the dosage (e.g., Mirsalis et al., 1993a), the expression time (e.g., Provost et al., 1993; Winegar et al., 1994) and the tissue (e.g., Hoorn et al., 1993; Provost et al., 1993). Reviews of different aspects of these data are available (Dycaico et al., 1994; Mirsalis et al., 1994; Morrison and Ashby, 1994).

Considerations for Routine Testing

There are multiple possible uses for the mutation assays in transgenic mice in terms of the genetic toxicity screening of chemical and physical agents. One use is to assess mutation induction in somatic cells as a follow-up *in vivo* mutagenicity test for positive results in *in vitro* gene mutation assays for predicting potential carcinogenicity. Another use is as a germ cell assay for assessing mutation induction in gonadal DNA to show interaction with gonadal DNA and to predict heritable effects, as a complement to or replacement for the specific locus tests currently in use. Mechanisms of mutagenesis can also be studied in the transgenic mice used for mutation assays (for examples, see Gorelick et al., 1995; Sisk et al., 1994a; Monroe and Mitchell, 1993). Finally, transgenic animals can be used to evaluate multiple endpoints, such as gene mutation, micronuclei, unscheduled DNA synthesis (UDS), DNA adducts, cell proliferation, metabolism and carcinogenicity. This could lead to a reduction in animal use for safety testing overall. Multiple endpoints have been combined in some studies reported to date. For example, Suzuki et al. (1993, 1994) measured gene mutation in liver and bone marrow as well as micronuclei in peripheral blood after treatment of MutaMouse™ with mitomycin C, diethylnitrosamine, ethylnitrosourea (ENU), or ethyl methane sulfonate. In *lacI* transgenic mice, UDS has been measured in liver after dimethylnitrosamine treatment (Ashby et al., 1993a; Tinwell et al., 1994b) and cell proliferation was determined in liver after treatment with phenobarbital, carbon tetrachloride, dimethylnitrosamine or partial hepatectomy (Mirsalis et al., 1993a). Steptozotocin-induced DNAdamage (comet assay) and mutation in *lacI* have been reported by Schmezer et al. (1994). ENU-induced micronuclei in peripheral blood and *lacI* mutation in various tissues have been measured (O'Kelly et al., 1994). The same endpoints were measured in ethylene oxide-treated *lacI* mice (Sisk et al., 1994b). Sofuni et al. have studied a number of different markers, including DNA adducts, micronuclei, cell proliferation and gene mutation in 2-amino-3,4-dimethylimidazo[4,5-*f*]quinoline (MeIQ)-treated *lacI* transgenic mice (Suzuki et al., 1995; Ushijima et al., 1995).

For an assay to be appropriate for use in the routine screening of new chemical and physical agents, it is necessary that the assay is validated and sufficient information about the assay is available to develop appropriate study designs. In the remainder of this discussion, I will review some of the validation and study design issues and the progress to address them.

Table 2. Classes of Agents Tested in the Transgenic Mouse Mutation Assays[a]

Class of Agent	Examples[a]	References
Alkylating Agents	Methyl nitrosourea	Provost et al., 1993
	DMN, MMS	Mirsalis et al., 1993b
	Ethyl nitrosourea	Kohler et al., 1991a,b; O'Kelly et al., 1994; Recio et al., 1992 Suzuki et al., 1993; Walker et al., 1994
Polycyclic Aromatic Hydrocarbons	Benzo[a]pyrene	Kohler et al., 1991b
	7,12-Dimethylbenzanthracene	Myhr, 1991; Thompson et al., 1992; Ashby et al., 1993b
Aromatic Amines	4-Acetylaminofluorene	Provost et al., 1994
	2-Acetylaminofluorene	Shephard et al., 1993; Gunz et al., 1993
Epoxides	Ethylene oxide	Sisk et al., 1994b
Antineoplastic Agents	Procarbazine, CP, Chlorambucil	Myhr, 1991
Radiation	Radon	Layton et al., 1994
	γ-rays	Winegar et al., 1994
"Nongenotoxic" liver carcinogens	Phenobarbital, carbon tetrachloride	Mirsalis et al., 1993a
	Di(2-ethylhexyl)phthalate	Gunz et al., 1993
	Methylclofenapate	Ashby et al., 1993a
Noncarcinogens	Acetone	Myhr, 1991
	Phosphate-buffered saline	Walker et al., 1994

[a] CP: cyclophosphamide, DMN: dimethylnitrosamine, MMS: methyl methanesulfonate

VALIDATION

Issues in Validation

Three aspects of the assay require validation. The first aspect is whether the assay techniques yield data that is reproducible within a laboratory and between laboratories. The second aspect is whether the test system measures what we are intending to measure. In other words, how closely does the transgene approximate an endogenous mammalian gene as a mutational target? It is also of interest to know if the transgenic mouse responds as the nontransgenic mice respond in terms of metabolism, DNA adduct formation, DNA repair, other genotoxicity endpoints, and spontaneous and agent-induced carcinogenesis. Finally, it is important to know if the assay is predictive of the endpoints of interest, namely, rodent carcinogenicity and heritable effects. Part of the difficulty in assessing the predictivity of the assay is to decide against which data base one should compare the responses in the transgenic assay. If mouse carcinogenicity tests are used, which chemicals are appropriate and which are most important among the genotoxins and nongenotoxins and among the carcinogens and noncarcinogens? Should one consider carcinogenicity assays in all mouse strains, including those that differ in susceptibility? Furthermore, which tissues (target and/or surrogate) should be the focus of the first effort and the total effort toward validation?

Progress in Validation

Some studies have been conducted to address the above issues and these studies are reviewed here. First of all, assay results are qualitatively reproducible. The spontaneous MF in liver from *lacI* transgenic mice has been determined in repeat experiments in one lab and in comparable experiments in multiple independent laboratories. Rogers et al. (1993) reported that the determination of MF was reproducible within a single lab using groups of 10 or 9 adult male mice for either the C57BL/6 or the B6C3F1 strains, respectively. In this study, two liver DNA samples were prepared independently from the same groups of mice and the DNA samples were analyzed independently. These data were analyzed by Piegorsch et al. (1994) for sources of variability and it was found that the largest contribution was from the variability between animals, which was significant. Similar inter-animal variability has been reported in data from other labs (Piegorsch et al., 1994; Carr and Gorelick, 1994). Comparison of the results of Rogers et al. with the adult male B6C3F1 liver MFs determined in two other labs shows the reproducibility of the results within the range of interanimal variability (Table 3) (Young et al., 1993; Carr and Gorelick, 1994). Results from independent studies in other labs are summarized elsewhere (Morrison and Ashby, 1994). Considering that nonoptimized protocols were used early on, the expected interanimal variability, and possible age effects, with the exception of the occasional outlier, the spontaneous MFs in liver from other labs are consistent with the findings reported here.

Table 3. Mutant Frequencies in Liver from *lacI* Transgenic Mice

Lab	Strain[a]	MF[b] x 10^5	Reference
Stratagene	C57BL/6	4.1 ± 0.7[c]	Rogers et al., 1993
	B6C3F1-study 1	4.3 ± 1.2	Rogers et al., 1993
	B6C3F1-study 2	4.1 ± 0.8	Rogers et al., 1993
Microbiological Associates	B6C3F1	4.2 ± 1.4	Young et al., 1993
Procter & Gamble	B6C3F1	4.4 ± 1.6	Carr and Gorelick, 1994

[a] Livers from adult (8-12 week old) male mice were analyzed in these studies.
[b] MF, mutant frequency
[c] Average ± sd; n=9 or 10; standard procedures were used in these studies (Rogers et al., 1993).

The reproducibility of MF determination in treated mice has not been determined in a single set of experiments, although there are multiple reports in the literature which follow similar study designs. For example, there are four MutaMouse™ studies (Gossen et al., 1989; Myhr, 1991; Recio et al., 1992; Hoorn et al., 1993; Suzuki et al., 1993) and four Big Blue® studies (Kohler et al., 1991b; Provost et al., 1992; Provost and Short, 1994; Walker et al., 1994) of ENU-induced mutagenesis. Many of these experiments unfortunately followed what are now, in hindsight, considered to be inadequate designs. In most cases, each treatment group consisted of only 2-3 mice. The small group sizes, in combination with the small numbers of plaque forming units (pfu) per animal, compromised the statistical analysis, as discussed elsewhere by Carr and Gorelick (1994, 1995), making it difficult to judge interlaboratory reproducibility based on these data. Future research requirements include well-designed interlaboratory comparisons of induced MFs. Thus, it is proposed that repeat experiments are conducted in each lab at least once during the validation process to define reliable detection limits and demonstrate reproducible MF determinations.

A second validation issue is the test system. Does the test system measure what we are intending to measure? More specifically, how closely does the transgene approximate an endogenous mammalian gene as a mutational target? These questions have been addressed experimentally in two kinds of studies. Both are comparisons of mutation in the transgene and in an endogenous gene. Tao et al. (1993a) showed that spontaneous and ENU-induced MFs at the *Dlb-1* locus are similar to the spontaneous and ENU-induced MFs in the *lacI* transgene, whereas X-ray induced-mutation, which is detected at the *Dlb-1* locus, is not detected in the transgene. The nature of the mutations recovered at either loci was not determined in this study, so it remains speculation that each locus may be differentially sensitive to the mutagenicity of the different types of DNA damage. It can be reasoned, however, that large deletions are not likely to be detected readily in the transgene (where the target and reporter genes as well as the phage genome must remain intact to be recovered) and that this limitation is the basis for the difference in X-ray-induced MFs in *lacI* and *Dlb-1*.

In a second type of study, we (Walker et al., 1994) have compared MFs and mutational spectra in the *lacI* transgene with the same in the endogenous *hprt* gene in splenic T-lymphocytes. ENU-induced MFs in the two genes are similar (average ± SEM: *lacI*, 8.0 ± 2.3; *hprt*, 5.4 ± 0.2) and the mutational spectra are similar as well. However, the ~10-fold higher background MF in the *lacI* gene (average ± SEM: *lacI*, 3.4 ± 0.4; *hprt*, 0.4 ± 0.03) makes it a somewhat less sensitive target for detecting increases in MF. There are several possible explanations for the differences in spontaneous MF in the transgene and in the *hprt* gene. Besides the differences in target sequence and protein function that could contribute to differences in the frequency of phenotypic detection of mutants, the differences in spontaneous MF could be due in part to the genomic location of each gene. For example, the position of the *hprt* gene itself can influence spontaneous mutagenesis (Lichtenauer-Kaligis et al., 1993a, 1993b). The methylation status of the various genes may also play a role in determining the spontaneous MF as methylation-dependent mutations appear to occur more frequently in the *lacI* transgene than in the endogenous *hprt* gene from untreated mice (Walker et al., 1994; Gorelick et al., 1993; Sisk et al., 1994b). It is likely that other endogenous genes would display a similar range of spontaneous MFs depending on these and other factors. The limitation in addressing this issue experimentally is that we can measure the spontaneous MF in only a few endogenous genes.

The question of whether the transgenic mouse lines respond as nontransgenic mice respond in terms of metabolism, DNA adduct formation, DNA repair, other genotoxicity endpoints, and spontaneous and agent-induced carcinogenesis has also been studied. The issue has been addressed in a few studies where chromosome damage (Suzuki et al., 1993, 1994; Sisk et al., 1994b; O'Kelly et al., 1994; D. Gibson et al., 1995), DNA adducts (Brown et al., 1994; Mirsalis et al., 1994), or UDS (Ashby et al., 1993a) as well as gene mutation have been determined. In all cases, the transgenic mouse responded as expected for a nontransgenic mouse with a similar genetic background.

The third validation issue is assay predictivity for carcinogenicity as well as for heritable effects. The carcinogenicity in rodents is known for many of the chemicals tested in the available transgenic mouse mutation assays and the predictivity of the two *lac* assays for carcinogenicity is described here.

There are a number of assumptions that should be noted for this assessment. Some of the data on which this analysis is based are available only in abstract form, not in peer-reviewed literature. In many cases, the raw MF data for individual mice are not reported and the conclusions of the authors are assumed to be fully supported by the raw data. Furthermore, it is still early in the evaluation of the mutation assays, and the choice of chemicals tested to date has been without deliberate attention to a balance of agents from different chemical or physical classes. Nonetheless, a number of chemical classes are represented, including carcinogens, noncarcinogens, *in vitro* mutagens and *in vitro* nonmutagens. Finally, it is not clear from all reports whether the mutation assays were conducted using standard methods for the assay or with the optimal study design; such parameters can significantly affect the results (e.g., Rogers et al., 1995). All the chemicals listed were tested in a tissue where tumors develop. Most of the chemicals were tested for carcinogenicity in the B6C3F1 or C57Bl mouse strains, although a positive carcinogenicity result in any strain was considered to prevail for purposes of classification (see discussion below). Here, mutagenicity is defined solely by the response in the *Salmonella*/microsome test. The 21 chemicals presented in the analysis of *lacI* data and the 12 chemicals presented in the analysis of the *lacZ* data were included because data from a rodent carcinogenicity study as well as results from the *Salmonella*/microsome test were available for comparison with the transgenic mouse mutation data (Tables 4 and 5). The breakout of carcinogenicity predictivity according to mutagenicity activity for both transgenic systems is presented in Table 6.

The most direct analysis of carcinogenicity predictivity would employ carcinogenicity data from the same mouse strains as used in the transgenic mutation assay. In this case, one would be able to conduct a predictivity analysis for the *lacI* system only, as carcinogenicity results are not available in Balb/c x DBA/2 mice for the compounds tested in the *lacZ* system. Such an analysis of the *lacI* system can be made based on a subgroup of chemicals listed in Table 4, including o-anisidine, 1,3-butadiene, 7,12-dimethylbenzanthracene, ethylene oxide, ethylnitrosourea, benzene and carbon tetrachloride. For these chemicals, which are all carcinogens, the transgenic mutation assay correctly identifies all but carbon tetrachloride, which is a nonmutagenic carcinogen that would not be expected to be positive. Thus, the assay performs very well in this analysis. Nonetheless, this is a small data base that is not reflective of a variety of chemicals.

It is useful to consider a larger data base that includes chemicals for which carcinogenicity data are available from any mouse strain, not just those strains that are genetically similar to the transgenic mouse mutation assay strains, although it is acknowledged that strain differences affect tumor outcome. This approach can be justified if transgenic mutation assays are to be used in routine screening by the fact that mutation induction is known to be a key step in carcinogenesis and mutation in many different systems is used to predict tumor outcome. In this light, it is appropriate to use the transgenic mutation assays for routine screening to predict the outcome of a bioassay in any mouse strain. Analyses of the *lacI* system and the *lacZ* system follow.

In the *lacI* system, all three of the noncarcinogens were negative and 12 of the 18 carcinogens were positive in the transgenic assay. Four of the six carcinogens that were negative in the transgenic mutation assay are nonmutagenic liver carcinogens, so the

Table 4. Chemicals Used in the Predictivity Analysis of the *lacI* Transgenic Mouse Mutation Assay for Carcinogenicity

Test Agent[a]	Carcinogenicity Strain[b]	Transgenic Tissue[c]	Transgenic Result	Transgenic Strain	Transgenic Reference
Mutagenic carcinogens					
2-Acetylaminofluorene[d,8,7]	B6C3F1, Balb/c	liver	+	C57Bl/6	Shephard et al., 1993
o-Anisidine[e,13,2]	B6C3F1	bladder	+	B6C3F1	Provost et al., 1994; Ashby et al., 1994
Benzo[a]pyrene[8,3]	Balb/c, Sencar	lung, spleen, liver	+	B6C3F1	Kohler et al., 1991a; Provost et al., 1994
1,3-Butadiene[4,4]	B6C3F1	bone marrow	+	B6C3F1	Sisk et al., 1994a
7,12-Dimethylbenzanthracene[8;14,18]	C57Bl/6, DBA/2	skin	+	C57Bl/6	Thompson et al., 1992
Dimethylnitrosamine[5,5]	C3H, Swiss	liver	+	B6C3F1, C57Bl/6	Mirsalis et al., 1993b; Tinwell et al., 1994a,b; Shephard et al., 1994[d]
Ethylene Oxide[4,1]	B6C3F1	lung, spleen	+	B6C3F1	Sisk et al., 1994b
Ethylnitrosourea[5,5]	B6C3F1	lung, kidney, spleen	+	B6C3F1	Kohler et al., 1991b; O'Kelly et al., 1994

MeCCNU[f,14;1,7]	Swiss	bone marrow	-	not reported	Ashby et al., 1993
Methylnitrosourea[5,5]	C3H	liver, lung, spleen	+	C57Bl/6	Kohler et al., 1991a; Shephard et al., 1994[d]
Phenobarbital[4,16;10,1]	C3H	liver	-	C57Bl/6, B6C3F1	Gunz et al., 1993[d]; Mirsalis et al., 1993a
Streptozotocin[5,5]	Swiss	kidney, liver	+	C57Bl/6	Schmezer et al., 1994
Nonmutagenic carcinogens					
Benzene[4,7]	B6C3F1	spleen	+	B6C3F1	Provost et al., 1994
Carbon Tetrachloride[4,7]	B6C3F1	liver	-	B6C3F1	Mirsalis et al., 1993a
Diethylhexylphthalate[d,9,9]	B6C3F1	liver	-	C57Bl/6	Gunz et al., 1993
Heptachlor[d,4;1,14]	B6C3F1	liver	-	C57Bl/6	Gunz et al., 1993
Methylclofenapate[15,17]	B6C3F1	liver	-	C57Bl/6	Lefevre et al., 1994
Urethane[d,e,14,6]	C3H, Balb/c	lung	+	C57Bl/6	Shephard et al., 1994
Mutagenic noncarcinogens					
4-Acetylaminofluorene[11,12]	not reported	liver	-	B6C3F1	Provost et al., 1994

Nonmutagenic noncarcinogens

Acetone	not reported	skin	-	C57Bl/6	Thompson et al., 1992
Phosphate-Buffered Saline	not reported	spleen	-	B6C3F1	Walker et al., 1994

[a] Mutagenicity is defined by the result in the *Salmonella*/microsome test and carcinogenicity is defined by the result in mouse bioassays. The first number or set of numbers following the chemical name indicates the reference for the *Salmonella* results. The second number or set of numbers following the chemical name indicates the reference for the carcinogenicity results. The references are coded as follows: 1- IARC, 1987b; 2- IARC, 1982; 3- IARC, 1983; 4- IARC, 1987a; 5- IARC, 1978; 6- IARC, 1974; 7- NTP, 1991; 8- Takehiko and Michiko, 1991; 9- Tennant et al., 1987; 10- Gold et al., 1993; 11- EPA (1988); 12- Nesnow et al. (1986); 13- Zeiger et al., 1990; 14- Registry of Toxic Effects of Chemical Substances (1993); 15- Lefevre et al., 1994; 16- Albertini and Gocke, 1992; 17- Stanley et al., 1994; 18- DiGiovanni et al., 1984.

[b] A relevant but not comprehensive list of strains in which the chemical was reported to be carcinogenic (references in footnote a).

[c] The first tissue listed for each chemical is a tumor target.

[d] Female mice were used in the transgenic studies; all other transgenic studies were conducted with male mice.

[e] The dose routes for the carcinogenicity studies and the transgenic studies were different.

[f] MeCCNU, 1-(2-chloroethyl)-3-(4-methylcyclohexyl)-1-nitrosourea.

Table 5. Chemicals Used in the Predictivity Analysis of the *lacZ* Transgenic Mouse Mutation Assay for Carcinogenicity

Test Agent[a]	Carcinogenicity Strain[b]	Transgenic Tissue[c]	Transgenic Result	Transgenic Reference
Mutagenic carcinogens				
1,3-Butadiene[2,2]	B6C3F1	lung	+	Recio et al., 1992
7,12-Dimethylbenzanthracene[4;5,13]	C57Bl/6, DBA/2	skin	+	Thompson et al., 1992; Ashby et al., 1993b
S-7,12-Dimethylbenzanthracene[6,6]	albino	skin	+	Ashby et al., 1993b
Diethylnitrosamine[3,3]	C57Bl/6	liver	+	Suzuki et al., 1994
Dimethylnitrosamine[3,3]	C3H, Swiss	liver	+	Tinwell et al., 1994a
Ethylnitrosourea[3,3]	B6C3F1	bone marrow	+	Douglas et al., 1993; Myhr, 1991; Suzuki et al., 1993
MNNG[1,1]	ICR	skin	+	Myhr, 1991
Mitomycin C[7,7]	C57Bl/6	bone marrow	+	Suzuki et al., 1993
Procarbazine[10,1]	CDF1, Swiss	bone marrow	+	Myhr, 1991

Nonmutagenic carcinogens				
Acrylamide[9;1,8]	A/J	bone marrow	+	Myhr, 1991; Hoorn et al., 1993
Methylclofenapate[11,12]	B6C3F1, C57Bl	liver	-	Lefevre et al., 1994
Nonmutagenic noncarcinogens				
Acetone	not reported	skin	-	Thompson et al., 1992

[a] Mutagenicity is defined by the result in the *Salmonella*/microsome test and carcinogenicity is defined by the result in mouse bioassays. The first number following the chemical name indicates the reference for the *Salmonella* results. The second number or set of numbers following the chemical name indicates the reference for the carcinogenicity results. The references are coded as follows: 1- IARC, 1987b; 2- IARC, 1987a; 3- IARC, 1978; 4- NTP, 1991; 5- Nesnow et al. (1986); 6- Ashby et al., 1993b; 7- IARC, 1976; 8- Registry of Toxic Effects of Chemical Substances (1993); 9- IARC, 1986; 10- Parodi et al., 1981; 11- Lefevre et al., 1994; 12- Stanley et al., 1994; 13- DiGiovanni et al., 1984.

[b] A relevant but not comprehensive list of strains in which the chemical was reported to be carcinogenic (references in footnote a).

[c] The tissue listed for each chemical is a tumor target. All transgenic studies were conducted in adult male mice.

Table 6. Summary of Transgenic Mouse Mutation Assay Results According to Rodent Carcinogenicity and *Salmonella*/Microsome Test Results

	Carcinogen[a]		Noncarcinogen	
	SAL +[b]	SAL -	SAL +	SAL -
Transgenic				
Big Blue® *(lacI)*				
+	10[c]	2	0	0
-	2	4	1	2
MutaMouse™ *(lacZ)*				
+	9	1	0	0
-	0	1	0	1

[a] Carcinogenic in the mouse
[b] SAL, *Salmonella*/microsome test
[c] Number of chemicals, from Table 4 (Big Blue®) or Table 5 (MutaMouse™).

transgenic result is consistent with the profiles of these chemicals from other gene mutation assays. Another liver carcinogen that was negative in the transgenic mutation assay was phenobarbital, whose very weak mutagenicity in the *Salmonella*/microsome assay has not been explained to date (Albertini and Gocke, 1992; Ashby et al., 1988); classic DNA-damaging properties have not been detected for phenobarbital.

One point of concern about the responses in the *lacI* transgenic assay in terms of carcinogenicity predictivity is with 1-(2-chloroethyl)-3-(4-methylcyclohexyl)-1-nitrosourea (MeCCNU), a mutagenic carcinogen which induced no increase in MF. The negative response in the report on MeCCNU (Ashby et al., 1993a) could be due to the short expression time (7-10 days) relative to recovery of target cell regrowth. Another plausible explanation for the negative transgenic result would be if MeCCNU is a crosslinking agent, like structurally related compounds (Bodell and Pongracz, 1993). Cross linking agents may not be detected in the mutation assay if the crosslinks are blocks to DNA replication because the damaged target gene may not be replicated as efficiently either *in vivo* or *in vitro* and mutant phage would not be produced and recovered. These factors need to be taken into account to understand the performance of the assay.

In the *lacZ* system, the single noncarcinogen was negative and ten of the eleven carcinogens were positive, including one nonmutagenic carcinogen (acrylamide). Thus, the *lacZ* transgenic assay is slightly more predictive of carcinogenicity than the Salmonella/microsome test for this set of chemicals. This result may be somewhat unexpected in that the genetic background of MutaMouse™ (Balb/c x DBA/2) is unlike the strains in which most of the chemicals were tested for carcinogenicity. In most cases, the carcinogenicity of the chemicals in the Balb/c x DBA/2 genetic background is not known. The positive correlation reported here is possibly reflective of the potency of the carcinogens tested (independent of mouse strain) or the susceptibility of MutaMouse™ to mutagenic agents.

Table 7 shows the positive and negative predictivity of the transgenic mouse assays. In the *lacI* assay, the specificity (# noncarcinogens negative/# noncarcinogens tested) and the positive predictivity (# carcinogens positive/# positive results) are 100% for this set of chemicals. The sensitivity (# carcinogens positive/# carcinogens tested) and the negative predictivity (# noncarcinogens negative/# negative results), however, are 67% and 33%, respectively. It is possible that the sensitivity and negative predictivity could be improved by using the standardized protocols and optimized study designs. The overall concordance [(carcinogens positive + noncarcinogens negative) ÷ (carcinogens + noncarcinogens tested)] for this set of chemicals is 71%. Thus, a positive result in this assay is meaningful in terms of predicting carcinogenicity in rodents but, at this stage in the evaluation, a negative result may not be meaningful without additional data. This conclusion is similar to that drawn by others from an analysis of carcinogenic and *lacI* mutagenic potencies (Shephard et al., 1994). It is necessary to define what other information may be required to demonstrate that a negative is meaningful in terms of predicting rodent carcinogenicity.

The *lacZ* system shows 100% specificity and positive predictivity for carcinogenicity with 91% sensitivity and 50% negative predictivity for the set of 12 chemicals listed. Thus, based on this preliminary analysis, a positive result in the *lacZ* system, like the *lacI* system, is predictive of carcinogenicity but a negative result is not wholely predictive. This favorable assessment has been observed previously early in the evaluation of other genotoxicity tests (McCann et al., 1975), depending on the size and composition of the data base, but especially when the data base is comprised primarily of strong carcinogens, as in the *lacI* and *lacZ* databases used in these examples. Clearly, a full evaluation of the predictivity of both transgenic assays for carcinogenicity will require the analysis of a larger number of chemicals, including diverse carcinogens and noncarcinogens.

One of the primary advantages of the transgenic mutation assays is that one can assess tissue-specific mutagenesis. For example, to predict heritable effects, mutagenesis in germ cells can be assessed directly. It is possible, however, that studies in germ cells would require study designs different from somatic cell studies to assess mutagenesis in the appropriate germ cell populations. In the interest of efficiency for routine testing, it is useful to know whether mutagenesis in somatic cells can predict heritable effects. A brief assessment of the predictivity of somatic cell mutation in the transgenic assays for heritable effects is possible at this time. Results from the mouse specific locus test (MSL) are compared with the transgenic mutation results in Table 8. Only the 13 chemicals for which data are available from both a transgenic assay in somatic cells and

Table 7. Characteristics of the Transgenic Mouse Mutation Assays for Predicting Rodent Carcinogenicity

Characteristic	Response	
Big Blue® (lacI)		
Sensitivity[a]	67%	(12/18)
Specificity[b]	100%	(3/3)
+ Predictivity[c]	100%	(12/12)
- Predictivity[d]	33%	(3/9)
Overall Concordance[e]	71%	(15/21)
Overall Concordance for the *Salmonella*/microsome test for this set of chemicals	67%	(14/21)
MutaMouse™ (lacZ)		
Sensitivity[a]	91%	(10/11)
Specificity[b]	100%	(1/1)
+ Predictivity[c]	100%	(10/10)
- Predictivity[d]	50%	(1/2)
Overall Concordance[e]	92%	(11/12)
Overall Concordance for the *Salmonella*/microsome test for this set of chemicals	83%	(10/12)

[a] Percentage of carcinogens with a positive result in the transgenic mutation assay.
[b] Percentage of noncarcinogens with a negative result in the transgenic mutation assay.
[c] Percentage of positive results in the transgenic mutation assay that are carcinogens.
[d] Percentage of negative results in the transgenic mutation assay that are noncarcinogens.
[e] Percentage of chemicals tested for which the transgenic mutation results agree with the carcinogenicity results.

the MSL are listed. Most of the chemicals tested in both assays were positive in both assays. The exceptions are benzo[a]pyrene and urethane, which are positive in the transgenic assay but negative in the MSL, and methyl methanesulfonate, which is negative in the transgenic assay but positive in the MSL. These may be cases of tissue-specificity in the transgenic assay as mutations in germ cells were not evaluated in these

Table 8. Chemicals Tested in the *lacZ* or *lacI* Transgenic Mouse Mutation Assays in Somatic Cells that have also been Tested in the Mouse Specific Locus Test

Chemical	MSL[a]	TG[b]	Strain[c]	Tissue	TG Reference
Acrylamide	-/+	+	*lacZ*	bone marrow	Myhr, 1991
Chlorambucil	-/+	+	*lacZ*	bone marrow	Myhr, 1991
Diethylnitrosamine	-/(-)	+	*lacZ*	liver	Suzuki et al., 1994
Ethyl methanesulfonate	-/+	+	*lacZ*	bone marrow, liver	Suzuki et al., 1994
Mitomycin C	+/(+)	+	*lacZ*	bone marrow	Suzuki et al., 1993
Procarbazine	+/+	+	*lacZ*	bone marrow	Myhr, 1991
Benzo[a]pyrene	-/(-)	+	*lacI*	spleen	Kohler et al., 1991
Cyclophosphamide	-/+	+	*lacI*	spleen	Kohler et al., 1991
Ethyl nitrosourea	+/+	+	*lacI*	spleen[d]	Kohler et al., 1991
Ethylene oxide	-/+	+	*lacI*	lung, spleen[d]	Sisk et al., 1994b
Methyl methanesulfonate	(+)/+	-	*lacI*	liver	Mirsalis et al., 199
Methyl nitrosourea	+/+	+	*lacI*	spleen[d]	Provost et al., 199
Urethane	-/-	+	*lacI*	lung	Shephard et al., 19

[a] MSL: mouse specific locus test results. Data are from Bentley et al., 1994. Responses in spermatogonial/post-spermatogonial stages are reported, respectively. + or -, data are conclusively positive or negative; (+) or (-), mutants or no mutants were observed, respectively, but results are inconclusive (see Bentley et al., 1994).

[b] TG: transgenic mouse mutation assay results.

[c] Strain of transgenic mouse in which test was conducted: *lacZ*: MutaMouse™ (*lacZ*) transgenic mice; *lacI*: Big Blue® (*lacI*) transgenic mice. Adult male mice were used for all transgenic experiments except for urethane, where adult female mice were used.

[d] Tested in transgenic germ cells, with positive result: ethyl nitrosourea (Provost and Short, 1994), methyl nitrosourea (Provost et al., 1993); with negative result: ethylene oxide (Sisk et al., 1994b).

three studies.A large collaborative investigation of germ cell mutagenesis in the transgenic assays is underway (Ashby, 1995). It is anticipated that these studies will address in detail the ability of the transgenic assays in germ cells to predict heritable effects.

Summary of Accomplishments on Validation

Altogether, much progress has been made in the evaluation of the transgenic mouse mutation assays. The assays are qualitatively reproducible. Induced mutations in the target gene reflect the types of mutations induced in an endogenous gene as tested for a limited number of compounds. Multiple genotoxicity endpoints can be detected in one set of transgenic mice and responses are similar to those in the nontransgenic mice with similar genetic backgrounds, showing the transgenic mice are not grossly biologically perturbed by the presence of the transgene. Finally, based on the limited and possibly biased set of data available, the assays show good positive predictivity for carcinogenicity. The negative predictivity of the assays requires further investigation.

STUDY DESIGN

Study Design Issues

Two important tools to develop study designs for the mutation assays in transgenic mice are the appropriate statistical methods and knowing the experimental parameters that affect the detection of mutations. Methods and considerations for the statistical analyses are discussed elsewhere (Gorelick and Thompson, 1994; Piegorsch et al., 1994; Carr and Gorelick, 1994; Carr and Gorelick, 1995; Piegorsch et al., 1995) and therefore will not be discussed in detail here, except to underscore the importance of involving the statisticians early in the development of experimental designs and considering their recommendations. In addition, the publication of individual animal MF data (numbers of mutants and total pfu for each animal) will ensure as much data as possible are accessible for use in the development of appropriate statistical methods. It is this work that will determine ultimately the cost and the sensitivity of the transgenic mutation assays.

Some experimental parameters that may affect the induction and detection of mutations include exposure route, the number of exposures, dosage, target tissue, and expression time. Progress has been made in assessing the impact of these parameters on MF. In particular, MF depends on the number of exposures. For example, higher MFs were detected after subchronic compared with acute exposures to BP and to ENU (Kohler et al., 1991a; Myhr, 1991). Secondly, dose-response relationships have been reported for a number of chemicals (Gunz et al., 1993; Shephard et al., 1993; Mirsalis et al., 1993b; Sisk et al., 1994a). It has also been reported that spontaneous and induced MFs are tissue-specific (O'Kelly et al., 1994; Provost et al., 1994). Finally, the induction of MF is dependent on expression time (Provost et al., 1993; Mirsalis et al., 1993b, Hoorn et al., 1993) and this dependence may be tissue-specific.

The mutation assays in transgenic mice may not be routine in the sense that one study design (e.g., exposure route, number of exposures, expression time, target tissue, etc.) will probably not be suitable for the detection of all mutagens. It is likely that one will have to integrate information from other toxicity, metabolism or pharmacology studies and from the anticipated human exposures to insure that any particular study design is appropriate from a biological standpoint. Clearly, this petition for additional safety information makes the use of these assays more complicated than a routine *in vitro* mutation assay. The power of the transgenic mutation assays for use in routine chemical safety assessments, however, *is* the fact that mutation *can* be determined in the whole animal in any tissue of interest after various exposure scenarios.

On-going efforts

A concerted effort is needed to validate further the transgenic mutation assays for carcinogen detection with different chemicals, including carcinogens and noncarcinogens. This effort may be best achieved by using multiple exposures to the chemical dosages used in mouse carcinogen bioassays (Shephard et al., 1994). A series of studies to determine MFs in tumor target as well as nontarget tissues would be informative in that if carcinogen treatments increase the MF in nontarget tissues, then one or a few surrogate tissues may be used for screening new agents. This outcome would be necessary for the successful application of these assays in routine screening since it is not possible to know *a priori* the tumor target tissue without conducting the bioassay. On the other hand, if carcinogen treatment increases the MF only in tumor target tissues, these assays will probably be most useful as tools to study carcinogenic mechanisms. As these data are collected, it will be important also to maintain a data base of the studies and results. One possibility is that this may be tied into a data base of mutational spectra, which is under development (deBoer, 1995). The transgenic mutation assays will be most useful when both a positive result *and* a negative result are both meaningful. To develop a data set that supports this is the challenge ahead of us.

CONCLUSIONS

The transgenic mouse strains used for mutation assays do not appear to be unusual in their susceptibility to chemically-induced mutation. In these mouse models, it is possible to detect increases in MF induced by a variety of agents, and the mutational spectra recovered are consistent with the types of DNA damage formed by these chemicals. Furthermore, the mutational spectra for the chemicals analyzed so far are comparable between the transgenes and endogenous genes, including those genes that are biologically relevant for carcinogenesis. These and other transgenic models are likely to be useful for predicting *in vivo* mutagenicity and for mechanistic studies of mutation *in vivo.* In particular, genetic crosses between transgenic mouse strains used for mutation analysis and strains susceptible to carcinogenesis [e.g., p53 knockout mice (Donehower et al., 1992)] may offer unique opportunities to study the effects of susceptibility genes on mutation and carcinogenesis.

ACKNOWLEDGEMENTS

I am grateful to M. Aardema, E. Thompson and J. Ashby for continued discussions on the topics discussed herein.

REFERENCES

Albertini S, Gocke E (1992): Phenobarbital: Does the positive result in TA1535 indicate genotoxic properties? Environ Mol Mutagen 19:161-166.

Ashby J (1995): Transgenic germ cell mutation assays: a small collaborative study. Environ Mol Mutagen 25:1-3.

Ashby J, Short JM, Jones NJ, Lefevre PA, Provost GS, Rogers BJ, Martin EA, Parry JM, Burnette K, Glickman BW, Tinwell H (1994): Mutagenicity of o-anisidine to the bladder of *lacI-* transgenic B6C3F1 mice: absence of ^{14}C or ^{32}P bladder DNA adduction. Carcinogenesis 15:2291-2296.

Ashby J, Tinwell H, Burnette K, Lefevre PA (1993a): Results for the Big Blue transgenic assay using two genotoxins and a peroxisome proliferator. Environ Mol Mutagen 21 (Suppl 22):4.

Ashby J, Brusick D, Myhr BC, Jones, NJ, Parry JM, Nesnow S, Paton D, Tinwell H, Rosenkranz HS, Curti S, Gilman D, Callander RD (1993b): Correlation of carcinogenic potency with mouse-skin ^{32}P-postlabeling and MutaMouse lacZ-mutation data for DMBA and its K-region sulphur isostere: comparison with activities observed in standard genotoxicity assays. Mutat Res 292:25-40.

Ashby J, Callander RD, Paton D, Zeiger E, Ratpan F (1988): Weak and unexpected mutagenicity to *Salmonella* of the rat hepatocarcinogen methapyrilene. Environ Mol Mutagen 12:243-252.

Bentley K, Sarrif AM, Cimino MC, Auletta AE (1994): Assessing the risk of heritable gene mutation in mammals: *Drosophila* sex-linked recessive lethal test and tests measuring DNA damage and repair in mammalian germ cells. Environ Mol Mutagen 23:3-11.

Bodell WJ, Pongracz K (1993): Chemical synthesis and detection of the cross-link 1-[N^3-(2'-deoxycytidyl)]-2-[N^1-(2'-deoxyguanosinyl)]ethane in DNA reacted with 1-(2-chloroethyl)-1-nitrosourea. Chem Res Toxicol 6:434-438.

Brown CD, MacNeela HP, Wong B, Fennell TR (1994): DNA and hemoglobin adduct dosimetry in normal and *lacI* transgenic mice exposed to ethylene oxide. Proc Am Assoc Cancer Res 35:566.

Carr GJ, Gorelick NJ (1995): Statistical design and analysis of mutation studies in transgenic mice. Environ Mol Mutagen 25:246-255.

Carr GJ, Gorelick NJ (1994): Statistical tests of significance in transgenic mutation assays: Considerations on the experimental unit. Environ Mol Mutagen 24: 276-282.

de Boer JG (1995): A software package for the management of sequencing projects using *lacI* transgenic animals. Environ Mol Mutagen 25:256-262.

DiGiovanni J, Prichett WP, Decina PC, Diamond L (1984): DBA/2 mice are as sensitive as SENCAR mice to skin tumor promotion by 12-O-tetradecanoylphorbol-13-acetate. Carcinogenesis 5:1493-1498.

Donehower LA, Harvey M, Slagle BL, McArthur MJ, Mongomery CA Jr., Butel JS, Bradley A (1992): Mice deficient for p53 are developmentally normal but susceptible to spontaneous tumors. Nature 356:215-221.

Douglas GR, Gingerich JD, Gossen JA (1993): Time-course and sequence spectra of ethylnitrosourea-indcued *lacZ*- mutations in transgenic mouse somatic and germ cells. Environ Mol Mutagen 21 (Suppl 22):18.

Dycaico MJ, Provost GS, Kretz PL, Ransom SL, Moores JC, Short JM (1994): The use of shuttle vectors for mutation analysis in transgenic mice and rats. Mutat Res 307: 461-478.

EPA (1988): in Registry of Toxic Effects of Chemical Substances (1993) published by U.S. National Institute for Occupational Safety and Health, U.S. Department of Health and Human Services, Public Health Service, CDC, U.S. Printing Office, Publication numbers 87 through 114.

Gibson D, O'Kelly JA, Aardema MJ, Gorelick NJ (1995): Comparison of assessment of micronuceli and mutations in *lacI* transgenic mice. Environ Mol Mutagen 25 (Supple.25):18.

Gold LS, Manley NB, Slone TH Garfinkel GB, Rohrbach L, Ames BN (1993): The fifth plot of the carinogenic potency database: results of animal bioassays published in the general literature through 1988 and by the National Toxicology Program through 1989. Environ Health Perspect 100:65-135.

Gorelick, NJ (1995a): Introduction: Update on Transgenic Mouse Mutation Assays. Workshop Proceedings from the 1994 Environmental Mutagen Society Meeting. Environ Mol Mutagen 25:216-217.

Gorelick, NJ (1995b): Overview of mutation assays intransgenic mice for routine testing. Environ Mol Mutagen 25:218-230.

Gorelick, NJ, O'Kelly JA, Gu M, Glickman BW (1995): Mutational spectra in the *lacI* gene from 7,12-dimethylbenzanthracene (DMBA)-treated and untreated transgenic mice. Mol Carcinogen: *in press*.

Gorelick NJ, Thompson ED (1994): Overview of the workshops on statistical analysis of mutation data from transgenic mice. Environ Mol Mutagen 23:12-16.

Gossen JA, DeLeeuw WJF, Verwest A, Lohman PHM, Vijg J (1991): High somatic mutation frequencies in lacZ transgene integrated on the mouse X-chromosome. Mutat Res 250:423-429.

Gossen JA, DeLeeuw WJF, Tan CHT, Zwarthoff EC, Berends F, Lohman PHM, Knook DL, Vijg J (1989): Efficient rescue of integrated shuttle vectors from transgenic mice: A model for studying mutations *in vivo*. Proc Natl Acad Sci USA 86:7971-7975.

Gunz D, Shephard SE, Lutz WK (1993): Can nongenotoxic carinogens be detected with the *lacI* transgenic mouse mutation assay? Environ Mol Mutagen 21:209-211.

Hoorn AJW, Custer LL, Myhr BC, Brusick D, Gossen J, Vijg J (1993): Detection of chemical mutagens using MutaMouse: a transgenic mouse model. Mutagenesis 8:7-10.

International Agency for Research on Cancer (1987b): "IARC Monographs on the evaluation of carcinogenic risks to humans, Supplement 7." Lyon, France: International Agency for Research on Cancer.

International Agency for Research on Cancer (1987a): "IARC Monographs on the evaluation of carcinogenic risks to humans: Genetic and related effects, Supplement 6." Lyon, France: International Agency for Research on Cancer.

International Agency for Research on Cancer (1986): "IARC Monographs on the evaluation of the carcinogenic risk of chemicals to humans: Some chemicals used in plastics and elastomers, Vol 39." Lyon, France: International Agency for Research on Cancer, pp 41-66.

International Agency for Research on Cancer (1983): "IARC Monographs on the evaluation of the carcinogenic risk of chemicals to humans: Polynuclear Aromatic Compounds, Part 1: Chemical, Environmental and Experimental data. Vol 32." Lyon, France: International Agency for Research on Cancer, pp 211-224.

International Agency for Research on Cancer (1982): "IARC Monographs on the evaluation of the carcinogenic risk of chemicals to humans: Some aromatic amines, anthraquinones and nitroso compounds and inorganic fluorides used in drinking water and dental preparations. Vol 27." Lyon, France: International Agency for Research on Cancer, pp 63-80.

International Agency for Research on Cancer (1978): "IARC Monographs on the evaluation of the carcinogenic risk of chemicals to humans. Some *N*-Nitroso compounds. Vol 17." Lyon, France: International Agency for Research on Cancer.

International Agency for Research on Cancer (1976): "IARC Monographs on the evaluation of carcinogenic risk of chemicals to man. Some naturally occurring substances. Vol 10." Lyon, France: International Agency for Research on Cancer.

International Agency for Research on Cancer (1974): "IARC Monographs on the evaluation of carcinogenic risk of chemicals to man: Some anti-thyroid and related substances, nitrofurans and industrial chemicals. Vol 7." Lyon, France: International Agency for Research on Cancer, pp 253-260.

Kohler SW, Provost GS, Fieck A, Kretz PL, Bullock WO, Putman DL, Sorge JA, Short JM (1991a): Analysis of spontaneous and induced mutations in transgenic mice using a lambda ZAP/*lacI* shuttle vector. Environ Mol Mutagen 18:316-321.

Kohler SW, Provost GS, Fieck A, Kretz PL, Bullock WO, Sorge JA, Putman DL, Short JM (1991b): Spectra of spontaneous and mutagen-induced mutations in the *lacI* gene in transgenic mice. Proc Natl Acad Sci USA 88:7958-7962.

Layton AD, Cross FT, Lutze LH, Steigler GL, Stillwell LS, Jostes RF (1994): Sequence analysis of *lacI* mutations obtained from lung cells of radon-exposed Big Blue™ transgenic mice. Environ Mol Mutagen 23 (Suppl 23): 37.

Lefevre PA, Tinwell H, Galloway SM, Hill R, Mackay JM, Elcombe CR, Foster J, Randall V, Callander RD and Ashby J (1994): Evaluation of the genetic toxicity of the peroxisome proliferator and carcinogen methyl clofenapate, including assays using MutaMouse and Big Blue transgenic mice. Human and Exptl Toxicol 13:764-775.

Lichtenauer-Kaligis EGR, van der Velde-van Dijke I, den Dulk H, van de Putte P, Giphart-Gassler M, Tasseron-de Jong JG (1993a): Genomic position influences spontaneous mutagenesis of an integrated retroviral vector containing the *hprt* cDNA as target for mutagenesis. Human Mol Genetics 2:173-182.

Lichtenauer-Kaligis EGR, Thijssen J, den Dulk H, van de Putte P, Tasseron-de Jong JG, Giphart-Gassler M (1993b): Genome wide spontaneous mutation in human cells determined by the spectrum of mutations in *hprt* cDNA genes. Mutagenesis 8:207-220.

McCann J, Choi E, Yamasaki E, Ames BN (1975): Detection of carcinogens as mutagens in the Salmonella/microsome test: Assay of 300 chemicals. Proc Natl Acad Sci USA 72:5135-5139.

Mirsalis JC, Monforte JA, Winegar RA (1994): Transgenic animal models for measuring mutations *in vivo*. Crit Rev Toxicol 24:255-280.

Mirsalis JC, Hamer MD, O'Loughlin KG, Winegar RA, Short JM (1993a): Effects of nongenotoxic carcinogens on hepatic mutations in *lacI* transgenic mice. Environ Mol Mutagen 21 (Suppl 22):48.

Mirsalis JC, Provost GS, Matthews CD, Hamner RT, Schindler JE, O'Loughlin KG, MacGregor JT, Short JM (1993b): Induction of hepatic mutations in *lacI* transgenic mice. Mutagenesis 8:265-271.

Monroe TJ, Mitchell MA (1993): In vivo mutagenesis induced by CC1065 and adozelesin DNA alkylation in a transgenic mouse model. Cancer Res 53:5690-5696.

Morrison V, Ashby J (1994): A preliminary evaluation of the performance of the Muta™Mouse (*lacZ*) and Big Blue™ (*lacI*) transgenic mouse mutation assays. Mutagenesis 9:367-375.

Myhr BC (1991): Validation studies with Muta™Mouse: A transgenic mouse model for detecting mutations *in vivo*. Environ Mol Mutagen 18:308-315.

National Toxicology Program (1991): "Sixth annual report on carcinogens." U.S. Department of Health and Human Services, Public Health Service.

Nesnow S, Argus M, Bergman H, Chu K, Firth C, Helmes T, McGaughy R, Ray V, Slaga TH, Tennant R, Weisburger E (1986): Chemical carcinogens. A review and analysis of the literature of selected chemicals and the establishment of the Gene-Tox Carcinogen data base. A report of the U.S. Environmental Protection Agency Gene-Tox Program. Mutat Res 185:1-195.

O'Kelly JA, Young RR, Putman DL, Gibson DP, Aardema MJ, Gorelick NJ (1994): Tissue specificity of mutation in ethylnitrosourea (ENU)-treated Big Blue mice. Environ Mol Mutagen 23 (Suppl 23):50.

Parodi S., DeFlora S, Cavanna M, Pino A, Robbiano L, Bennicelli C, Brambilla G (1981): DNA-damaging activity *in vivo* and bacterial mutagenicity of sixteen hydrazine derivatives as related quantitatively to their carcinogenicity. Cancer Res 41:1469-1482.

Piegorsch WW, Margolin BH, Shelby MD, Johnson A, French JE, Tennant RW, Tindall KR (1995): Study design and sample sizes for a *lacI* transgenic mouse mutation assay. Environ Mol Mutagen 25:231-245.

Piegorsch WW, Lockhart AM, Margolin BH, Tindall KR, Gorelick NJ, Short JM, Carr GJ, Thompson ED, Shelby MD (1994): Sources of variability in data from a lacI transgenic mouse mutation assay. Environ Mol Mutagen 23:17-31.

Provost GS, Rogers BJ, Dycaico MJ, Mirsalis JC, Short JM (1994): Evaluation of mutagenic and nonmutagenic compounds using lacI transgenic rodents. Environ Mol Mutagen 23 (Suppl 23):55.

Provost GS, Short JM (1994): Characterization of mutations induced by ethylnitrosourea in seminiferous tubule germ cells of transgenic B6C3F$_1$ mice. Proc Natl Acad Sci USA 91:6564-6568.

Provost GS, Kretz PL, Hamner RT, Matthews CD, Rogers BJ, Lundberg KS, Dycaico MJ, Short JM (1993): Transgenic systems for *in vivo* mutation analysis. Mutat Res 288:133-150.

Provost GS, Kohler SW, Putman DL, Short JM (1992): ENU induced germ cell mutations in lambda/*lacI* C57BL/6 and B6C3F1 transgenic mice. Environ Mol Mutagen 19 (Suppl 20):51.

Questions and Answers (1993): Updated worldwide regulatory guidelines for genotoxicity testing. *Environ Mol Mutagen* (1993) 21:46-57.

Recio L, Osterman-Golkar S, Csanady GA, Turner MJ, Myhr B, Moss O, Bond JA (1992): Determination of mutagenicity in tissues of transgenic mice following exposure to 1,3-butadiene and N-ethyl-N-nitrosourea. Tox Appl Pharm 117:58-64.

Registry of Toxic Effects of Chemical Substances (1993): published by U.S. National Institute for Occupational Safety and Health, U.S. Department of Health and Human Services, Public Health Service, CDC, U.S. Printing Office, Publication numbers 87 through 114.

Rogers BJ, Provost GS, Young R, Putman DL, Short JM (1995): Intralaboratory optimization and standardization of mutant screening conditions used for a lambda/*lacI* transgenic mouse mutagenesis assay. Mutat Res 327:57-66.

Rogers BJ, Provost GS, Young R, Buchanan M, Putman DL, Short JM (1993): Optimization and standardization of mutant screening conditions used for the Big Blue transgenic mouse mutagenesis system. Environ Mol Mutagen 21 (Suppl 22):58.

Schmezer P, Eckert C, Liegibel UM (1994): Tissue-specific induction of mutations by streptozotocin in vivo. Mutat Res 307:495-499.

Shephard SE, Lutz Wk, Schlatter C (1994): The *lacI* transgenic mouse mutagenicity assay: quantitative evaluation in comparison to tests for carcinogenicity and cytogenetic damage in vivo. Mutat Res 306:119-128.

Shephard SE, Sengstag C, Lutz WK, Schlatter C (1993): Mutations in liver DNA of *lacI* transgenic mice (Big Blue) following subchronic exposure to 2-acetylaminofluorene. Mutat Res 302:91-96.

Sisk SC, Pluta LJ, Bond JA, Recio L (1994a): Molecular analysis of *lacI* mutants from bone marrow of B6C3F1 transgenic mice following inhalation exposure to 1,3-butadiene. Carcinogenesis 15:471-477.

Sisk SC, Preston RJ, Recio L (1994b): Determination of circulating micronuclei and mutant frequency in lung, spleen, and germ cells of male B6C3F1 *lacI* transgenic mice after inhalation exposure to ethylene oxide. Environ Mol Mutagen 23 (Suppl 23):62.

Stanley LE, Backburn DR, Devereaux S, Foley J, Lord PG, Maronpot RR, Orton TC and Anderson MW (1994): *Ras* mutations in methylclofenapate-induced B6C3F1 and C57BL/10J mouse liver tumors. Carcinogenesis 15:1125-1131.

Suzuki T, Hayashi M, Ochiai M, Nagao M, Sofuni T (1995): In vivo mutagenicity of 2-amino-3,4-diemthylimidazo[4,5-*f*]quinoline in *lacI* transgenic mice (Big Blue®). Environ Mol Mutagen 25(Suppl 25):51.

Suzuki T, Hayashi M, Sofuni T (1994): Initial experiences and future directions for transgenic mouse mutation assays. Mutat Res 307:489-494.

Suzuki T, Hayashi M, Sofuni T, Myhr BC (1993): The concomitant detection of gene mutation and micronucleus induction by mitomycin C in vivo using *lacZ* transgenic mice. Mutat Res 285:219-224.

Takehiko N, Michiko M (editors) (1991): "Mutagenicity tests using microorganisms: Collection of data." Bukyo-ku, Japan: Life-Science Information Center Corporation.

Tao KS, Urlando C, Heddle JA (1993a): Comparison of somatic mutation in a transgenic versus host locus. Proc Natl Acad Sci USA 90:10681-10685.

Tao KS, Urlando C, Heddle JA (1993b): Mutagenicity of methyl methanesulfonate (MMS) in vivo at the *Dlb-1* native locus and a *lacI* transgene. Environ Mol Mutagen 22:293-296.

Tennant RW, Margolin BH, Shelby MD, Zeiger E, Haseman JK, Spalding J, Caspary W, Resnick M, Stasiewicz S, Anderson B, Minor R (1987): Prediction of chemical carcinogenicity in rodents from in vitro genetic toxicity assays. Science 236:933-941.

Thompson ED, Gorelick NJ, Binder RL, Myhr BC, Putman DL (1992): Interlaboratory comparisons of dimethylbenzanthracene-induced mutations in skin of Muta^{TM}Mouse and the Big Blue^{TM} mouse. Environ Mol Mutagen, 19 (Suppl 20):64.

Tinwell H, Lefevre PA, Ashby J (1994a): Response of the MutaMouse lacZ/galE- transgenic mutation assay to DMN: comparisons with the corresponding Big Blue (lacI) responses. Mutat Res 307:169-173.

Tinwell H, Lefevre PA, Ashby J (1994b): Mutation studies with dimethyl nitrosamine in young and old *lacI* transgenic mice. Mutat Res 307:501-508.

U.S. Food and Drug Administration, Draft Toxicological Principles for Safety Assessment of Direct Food Additives and Color Additives Used in Food ("Redbook II"), 58 FR 16536, March 29, 1993.

Ushijima T, Okonogi H, Hosoya Y, Ochiai M, Wakabayashi K, Suzuki T, Sofuni T, Sugimura T, Nagao M (1995): Effect of tissue-specific mutational spectra on tissue-specific carcinogenicity: an extensive study of DNA adduct levels, cell proliferation rate, mutation frequencies, mutational spectra and carcinogenicity using Big Blue mice fed MeIQ. Environ Mol Mutagen 25(Suppl 25):54.

Walker VW, Gorelick NJ, O'Kelly JA, Craft TR, deBoer J, Glickman BW, Skopek TR (1994): Frequency and spectrum of ethylnitrosourea induced mutation at the *hprt* and *lacI* loci in splenic T-cells of exposed Big Blue mice. Environ Mol Mutagen 23 (Suppl 23):71.

Winegar RA, Lutze LH, Hamer JD, O'Loughlin KG, Mirsalis JC (1994): Radiation-induced point mutations, deletions and micronuclei in *lacI* transgenic mice. Mutat Res 307:479-487.

Young RR, Rogers BJ, Provost GS, Short JM and Putman DL (1993): Interlab comparison of liver spontaneous mutant frequency from lambda/*lacI* transgenic mice. Environ Mol Mutagen 21 (Suppl 22):79.

Zeiger E, Haseman J, Shelby MD, Margolin BH, Tennant R (1990): Evaluation of four in vitro genetic toxicity tests for predicting rodent carcinogenicity: confirmation of earlier results with 41 additional chemicals. Environ Mol Mutagen 16 (Suppl 18):1-14.

Genetics and Cancer Susceptibility:
Implications for Risk Assessment, pages 109–140

CYTOCHROME P-450 AND ACETYLTRANSFERASE EXPRESSION AS BIOMARKERS OF CARCINOGEN-DNA ADDUCT LEVELS AND HUMAN CANCER SUSCEPTIBILITY

Alaa F. Badawi, Scott J. Stern, Nicholas P. Lang, and Fred F. Kadlubar

National Center for Toxicological Research (HFT-100), Jefferson, AR 72079, USA (A.F.B., F.F.K.) and Arkansas Cancer Research Center, Little Rock, AR 72205 USA (S.J.S., N.P.L.)

SUMMARY

Carcinogen–DNA adducts are generally regarded as relevant biomarkers of carcinogen exposure and their levels in target tissues have often been predictive of tumor incidence in experimental animals. Thus, human risk assessment procedures have utilized dose–response models that assume proportional relationships between carcinogen exposure and cancer susceptibility, even though wide inter–individual variations in human metabolic activating enzymes have now been clearly established. To evaluate these approaches, we have examined the relationship between carcinogen exposure, DNA adduct levels, metabolic activation phenotypes, and cancers of the larynx, urinary bladder, and colon.

Cigarette smoking is a strong risk factor for cancers of the larynx and urinary bladder. In the larynx, the DNA adducts appear to be derived predominantly from polycyclic aromatic hydrocarbons (PAHs) and are evident only in tissue from smokers. However, adduct levels appear to be determined primarily by expression of cytochrome

P450 (CYP) 2C9/10, which varies $>$10–fold in different individuals. This CYP catalyzes the metabolic activation of benzo (α) pyrene (BP) to a 9–hydroxy–BP–DNA adduct that accounts for up to 25% of the putative PAH adducts formed *in vivo*. For the urinary bladder, putative aromatic amine (AA)–DNA adducts are predominant and are significantly elevated in current smokers. Rapid CYP1A2 and slow acetyltransferase (NAT2) phenotypes have been previously implicated in the activation (*N*–oxidation) and detoxification (*N*–acetylation) of AAs for human bladder carcinogenesis. Data now indicate that NAT1, which is expressed in human urothelium and catalyzes the *O*-acetylation of *N*-hydroxy arylamines, is significantly correlated with DNA adduct levels and is bimodally distributed in this tissue. Colo–rectal cancer risk, which has been associated with exposure to heterocyclic amines (HAs) in cooked foods, is strongly elevated in individuals with the combined rapid phenotypes for CYP1A2 and NAT2. These enzymes are uniquely responsible for HA *N*–oxidation and subsequent *O*-acetylation, forming DNA adducts that are found in human colon.

These studies indicate that cancer risk assessment procedures should be redesigned to include biomarkers of susceptibility, especially those involved in carcinogen bioactivation.

INTRODUCTION

The techniques developed for measuring DNA adduct levels and other biomarkers in human populations have been applied primarily to heavily exposed 'at–risk' subjects. However, where exposures are unknown, the identification of a predictive correlation between specific biomarkers and disease incidence could also provide a practical and effective epidemiological tool that could lead to the identification of etiological factors as well as an understanding of the basic mechanisms of the disease (Ehernberg and Tronqvist, 1992).

Identification of the agents involved in the process of cancer formation in humans is critical for a reliable assessment of human cancer risk . It is well known that human populations come into a contact with various chemicals that are also classified as potent carcinogenic agents (Doll and Peto, 1981). Aromatic and heterocyclic amines, polycyclic aromatic hydrocarbons (PAH), and *N*–nitroso compounds are among those chemical agents that are widespread in the environment, largely as consequence of human activity, and are thought to contribute to the incidence of certain occupationally and environmentally related cancers. Sources of human exposure to carcinogenic aromatic amines and amides include the workplace, tobacco smoke, cooked foods, and environmental pollution (for review, see Kadlubar, 1987). For example, 4,4'–methyl-ene–*bis*(2–chloroaniline) (MOCA) is an aromatic amine that is widely used in plastic polymer industry, and human exposure to this compound is well documented (Ward *et al.*, 1987). Moreover, it constitutes the largest potential exposure to a known carcinogen in the workplace environment (Cocker *et al.*, 1990). MOCA is known to induce various types of cancer in experimental animals and has been associated with urinary bladder cancer in humans (Kaderlik *et al.*, 1993). Likewise, aromatic amines present in cigarette smoke appear to account for the majority of DNA adducts detected in the urothelium of smokers and are considered to be the primary etiological agents in human urinary bladder cancer (Talaska *et al.*, 1993; Bartsch *et al.*, 1993). Evidence on the health consequences of tobacco smoking has accumulated rapidly, with retrospective and prospective studies demonstrating that the risk of developing different types of cancer (*e.g.*, lung, larynx, oral cavity, esophagus, pancreas, kidney, and bladder) is increased among smokers as compared to non–smokers (IARC, 1986). Direct evidence for the causal association of cigarette smoking with bladder cancer, for example, comes from analyses that have shown an increase of 4–aminobiphenyl (4–ABP)–DNA adducts in the bladder of cigarette smokers relative to non–smokers (Talaska *et al.*, 1991a).

The carcinogenic PAH's are formed mainly as a result of pyrrolytic processes, particularly incomplete combustion of organic materials, as well as of natural processes such as carbonization. These potent carcinogens are also found in substantial quantities in some foods, depending on the methods of cooking, preservation and storage (IARC, 1986), and in the main and side streams of cigarette smoke (Hemminki, 1990). Heterocyclic amines are formed in cooked meat and fish and can be released into the environment as combustion products (Hemminki, 1990; see below).

It is a generally accepted hypothesis that the carcinogenic potency of many of these chemicals is dependent upon their metabolic biotransformation to electrophilic active intermediates that can lead to the modification of cellular DNA, forming covalent adducts (Miller and Miller, 1981). DNA adduct formation is generally regarded as a critical, initiating event in the multistep process of chemical carcinogenesis (Hemminki, 1990). The enzyme systems responsible for such bioactivation/detoxification are, therefore, important factors in the interaction between humans and xenobiotics (Miles and Wolf, 1991); and changes in expression of these enzyme systems frequently alter the metabolism of chemical carcinogens (Guengerich, 1991) and consequently their DNA–binding potential. The extent of formation, accumulation, and persistence of DNA adducts, which generally correlate with the carcinogenic potencies of various chemicals, often depend on the individual's proficiency in metabolizing these agents to their active forms (Gelboin, 1980; Saffhill *et al.*, 1985; Beland and Kadlubar, 1990).

Assuming the absence of exogenous/endogenous factors that can alter the capacities of the enzymes responsible for carcinogen metabolism, differences in expression of these enzymes may be due primarily to their polymorphic distribution in human populations. Indeed, many of the enzymes and cofactors involved in intermediary metabolism were identified and the diagnosis of several human disease states were found to be based on dysfunction of metabolic pathways. Furthermore, the heritable (genotypic) nature of many of these diseases could often be attributed to specific mutations or translocations in the genome such that a necessary enzyme either was not expressed, was aberrant, or was expressed in a manner uncoordinated with normal tissue requirements. In contrast, other diseases were quickly identified to be a consequence of continued host interaction with environmental factors (phenotypic) such that changes in nutrient intake, life style, occupation, *etc.*, presented an effective means for resolving many health problems. Consequently, individuals may be either 'slow', 'intermediate', or 'rapid' metabolizers for a given substance. The same should also apply for metabolic polymorphisms involved in carcinogen activation or detoxification (Farber, 1980); and there is now sufficient epidemiologic evidence for the association between the metabolic polymorphisms and certain types of human cancer (Caporaso *et al.*, 1991; see below). Thus, individual variations in the capacity to form DNA adducts, due to genetic or environmentally-induced polymorphisms, are likely to be major determinants of individual susceptibility to chemical carcinogenesis (Kadlubar, 1994a).

Using this approach, the quantitation of human DNA-carcinogen adducts should assist in providing estimates of cancer risk. This could be done by relating the levels of particular DNA adducts in the target tissue to the known tumor incidence in this tissue, followed by an estimation of the probability of developing cancers later in the same individual (Poirier, 1994). However, there are several processes that first must be validated in humans: 1) that DNA adduct concentrations can serve as a biomarker of dose to a target tissue in the environmental dose range (Poirier *et al.*, 1991; Gaylor *et al.*, 1992); 2) that the adduct levels measured are at steady-state and represent accurate biomonitoring of exposure, upon which risk estimation can be based; and 3) that the risk associated with relative adduct levels can be used as a quantitative biomarker and be incorporated into risk determinations obtained from classical epidemiology (Lawley, 1994). In this regard, current attempts to use DNA adducts as biomarkers for human risk assessment have suggested that various factors other than DNA damage, *e.g*, cell proliferation and DNA repair (Badawi *et al.*, 1991; 1994), are equally important in the process of carcinogenesis (Lawley, 1994). Nevertheless,, other reports (*e.g*, Poirier *et al.*, 1991; Kadlubar, 1991; Badawi *et al.*, 1992a; Poirier and Beland, 1992; Kadlubar, 1994b) have suggested that DNA adduct quantification could serve as a tool for predicting tumorigenic outcomes. Even though DNA adduct measurements can only estimate recent exposures, they may well be predictive of lifetime exposures. Moreover, the effects of single *vs.* multiple doses on tumor initiation are probably additive at low (*i.e.*, environmental) exposures. As the relationship between dose and risk becomes better understood, then cancer risk estimates based on biomonitoring of DNA adduct levels could be combined with relative risks obtained from susceptibility studies, *e.g.*, metabolic polymorphisms involved in carcinogen bioactivation (*vide supra*).

This review was undertaken in an attempt to examine the advances made recently in our understanding of the possible relationships between carcinogen exposure, DNA adduct levels, metabolic phenotypes, and cancers of the larynx, urinary bladder and colon. Such information could lead to a more systematic and accurate approach for quantitation of human cancer risk from complex exposures and could also assist in constructing a dose–response model for estimating risks from exposure to a specific carcinogen.

METABOLIC POLYMORPHISMS IN HUMAN CARCINOGENESIS

Heritable differences in foreign compound metabolism have been recognized now for about 40 years (Kalow, 1962), with rare phenotypes or genotypes usually occurring in 1–40% of the population. A number of polymorphisms exist in xenobiotic–metabo lizing enzymes; for example, human polymorphisms occur with the cholinesterases, arylesterases, aldehyde hydrogenases, alcohol dehydrogenases, flavin-containing monooxygenases, *S*-oxidases, cytochromes P450, acetyltransferases, UDP–glucuronosyl-transferases, and sulfotransferases (Kalow, 1991). Such polymor-phisms are often associated with various pathological disorders, and they may also be manifested upon exposure to certain environmental factors (Gonzalez ang Gelboin, 1993). Several drug/carcinogen metabolizing systems are also known to play a role in the etiology of human cancers. These include: the polymorphic *N*-acetyltransferase (NAT2) in bladder and colorectal cancers (Kadlubar *et al.*, 1992), aryl hydrocarbon hydroxylase (AHH) in lung cancer (Kellermann *et al.*, 1973), debrisoquine hydroxylase in lung cancer (Caporaso *et al.*, 1989), and glutathione–*S*–transferase Mu1–1 (GSTM1) in human lung (Kihara *et al.*, 1994), urinary bladder (Daly *et al.*, 1993; Brockmöller *et al.*, 1994; Lin *et al.*, 1994a), colon (Singhal *et al.*, 1992), and breast (Zhong *et al.*, 1993) cancers. Moreover, studies of the genotypes for human cytochromes P450 (CYPs) have now been performed in racially diverse populations and ethnic differences in genotype/phenotype appear to predict individual susceptibility to a variety of human cancers (Butler *et al.*, 1992; Stern *et al.*,1993; Cosma *et al.*, 1993; Lang *et al.*,1994; Degawa *et al.*,1994; Kelsey *et al.*,1994; Sivaraman *et al.*, 1994; London *et al.*, 1994; Tefre *et al.*, 1994; Uematsu *et al.*,1994). Among the most studied CYPs in this respect is the polymorphism for CYP1A2, which has been found recently to be associated with increased risk to human colorectal (Lang *et al.*, 1994) and urinary bladder cancer (Butler *et al.*, 1992). In addition, polymorphisms in CYP1A1 (Cosma *et al.*, 1993) have been found to contribute to high risk for human lung (Kelsey *et al.*, 1994), laryngeal (Degawa *et al.*, 1994; Stern *et al.*, 1993), and colon (Sivaraman *et al.*, 1994) cancers; while higher cancer risks have been noted for specific CYP2D6 genotypes in lung cancer (London *et al.*, 1994; Tefre *et al.*, 1994) and for CYP2E1 in gastrointestinal (Gonzalez and Gelboin, 1993) and lung (Uematsu *et al.*, 1994) cancer. The molecular bases for most of these polymorphisms have been shown to be due to mutations in the structural genes that results in unstable enzymes or enzymes with altered catalytic activities. However, polymorphic expression might be also due to regulatory factors controlling gene expression. Sequencing CYP genes using polymerase chain reaction (PCR) techniques can now determine any structural gene changes that might be associated with either slow or rapid carcinogen–metabolizing enzyme phenotype. Ultimately, this procedure can be expected to be used for diagnostic assays that can determine cancer risk.

Genetically–based differences in drug metabolism is associated with many human diseases (*e.g.*, Vesell, 1985; Badawi and Mostafa, 1993). An example is the association between the polymorphisms in NATs and CYP1A2 and susceptibility to various types of human cancers (see Kadlubar *et al.*,1992; Kadlubar, 1994a; Kaderlik and Kadlubar, 1995). These two drug/carcinogen–metabolizing enzyme systems are involved in the metabolic biotransformation of aromatic amines (Kadlubar, 1994b). As with many other carcinogenic agents, aromatic amines were found to be metabolically activated to reactive electrophiles that can form carcinogen–DNA adducts (Kadlubar, 1994a). Studies concerning the metabolism of these agents in experimental animal and in human tissues strengthened the role of aromatic amines in urinary bladder and colorectal carcinogenesis (Turesky *et al.*, 1991; Kadlubar *et al.*, 1991; Bartsch *et al.*, 1993). Further support of these hypotheses have been also obtained by the detection and quantification of aromatic amine–DNA and protein adducts in bladder and colon tissues (Kaderlik and Kadlubar, 1995; see below).

Aromatic amines are activated by *N*-hydroxylation, primarily in the liver. *N*-Acetylation is a competing detoxification reaction catalyzed by NATs. These enzymes are coded in humans by two distinct genes, designated NAT1 and NAT2 (Kadlubar, 1991). High activities of the latter one has been correlated with increased risk of colorectal cancer and decreased susceptibility to bladder cancer (Kadlubar, 1991). NAT2 exhibits a polymorphism that is due to point mutations in the coding regions of an intronless gene and allows the detection of phenotypically slow and rapid metabolizers. Slow acetylators are homozygous for the slow acetylator gene while rapid acetylators are either heterozygous or homozygous for the rapid acetylator gene. Acetylation phenotype can be measured by administration of several different compounds, including sulfamethazine and caffeine (Bulm *et al.*, 1991). The molar ratios of acetylated and nonacetylated metabolites in urine or blood are then determined (Weber and Hein, 1985). This approximation has allowed the identification of slow and rapid acetylation phenotypes. However, the predominance of the mutations (M1 and M2) in two alleles of NAT2 gene has now facilitated the development of a simple DNA amplification assay to genotype most (80–90%) individuals (Bulm *et al.*, 1991). Slow acetylator individuals, who possess NAT2 alleles with point mutations (Kadlubar, 1994a; Lin *et al.*, 1994b), produce proteins that are either poorly expressed, unstable or have partially reduced catalytic activities. The prevalence of these slow NAT2 genotypes was also found to vary significantly from one human population to another (for review see Kadlubar, 1994a).

Slow acetylators are at higher risk for bladder cancer, particularly those who are occupationally exposed to aromatic amines (Cartwright *et al.*, 1982; Mommsen and Aagaard, 1986; Caporaso *et al.*, 1991). Furthermore, higher levels of 4-ABP hemoglobin adducts were found in slow acetylators as compared to the rapid acetylators who smoked the same quantity and type of cigarettes (Bartsch *et al.*, 1993). Since the highest levels of adducts were found in individuals with rapid *N*-oxidation (CYP1A2) and slow *N*-acetylation (NAT2) phenotype (Bartsch *et al.*, 1983), determination of phenotypes and genotypes may provide a better prediction and assessment of human cancer risk. It may be relevant here to mention that NAT1, which codes for the acetyltransferase activity originally thought to be monomorphic, has also recently been shown to be a polymorphic gene, when tested in human peripheral blood (Weber and Vatsis, 1993; Vatsis and Weber, 1993) and in urinary bladder tissue (Badawi *et al.*, 1995a). Rapid acetylators, on the other hand, are at increased risk of colon cancer (Ilett *et al.*, 1987; 1994; Wohlleb *et al.*, 1990; Kirlin *et al.*, 1991).

Simultaneous determination of NAT2 and CYP1A2 phenotypes has been accomplished by using different caffeine metabolites as specific probes for hepatic CYP1A2 and NAT2 (Butler *et al.*, 1989; 1992). Except in a Japanese population, analysis of CYP1A2 distribution emerged as a trimodality (slow, intermediate and rapid metabolizers) in humans (see Kadlubar, 1994a). This polymorphism could be due to point mutations in the gene(s) controlling CYP1A2; however, differences in DNA sequences between slow, intermediate and rapid CYP1A2 metabolizers have not yet been detected. A wide variation in metabolic proficiency for CYP1A2 across racial/ethnic groups was indicated and it was similar to those observed for NAT2 in the same studied populations. Metabolic phenotyping of CYP1A2 has been evaluated by using caffeine metabolism, phenacetin *O*-deethylation and theophylline 1-demethylation (see Kadlubar *et al.*,1992; Kadulbar, 1994a). CYP1A2 is a caffeine 3-demethylase and also converts 1,7-dimethylxanthine to 1-methylxanthine, while NAT2 converts 1,7-dimethylxanthine to 5-acetylamino-6-formylamino-3-methyl-uracil (AFMU), and xanthine oxidase produces 1-methylurea from 1-methylxanthine. Thus, a number of enzymes can potentially and simultaneously be monitored by caffeine metabolism, *e.g.* CYP1A2 and NAT2. Applying these procedures, the urinary ratio of [1,7-dimethylxanthine (17X) + 1,7-dimethyluric acid (17U)] / [caffeine (137X)], taken at 4-5 hours after caffeine ingestion, was used to determine CYP1A2 phenotypes (Butler *et al.*, 1992) in subjects from Arkansas (n= 101), Italy (n=95) and China (n=78). In nonsmokers, CYP1A2 activity was not normally distributed and appeared trimodal (12–13% slow, 51–67% intermediate and 20–37% rapid) in the different populations. Cigarette smoking induced CYP1A2 by increasing the caffeine metabolite ratio in the smokers of blonde tobacco, in contrary to the black tobacco smokers (Butler *et al.*, 1992). These differences were interpreted to be due to the genetic polymorphism in the CYP1A2 gene or in a regulatory gene, from individual differences in exposure to inducing agents, as well as from other epigenetic factors. Therefore, the procedures involving caffeine metabolic phenotyping are suitable for use in epidemiological studies and may provide a means for assessing the human cancer risk due to exposure to aromatic amines (Caporaso *et al.*, 1989).

Metabolic polymorphism, both in NAT and in CYP1A2, is expected to affect the levels of DNA adduct in the target tissue (Flamming *et al.*, 1992a; b). In a recent study (Vineis *et al.*, 1994), levels of DNA adducts in bladder cells and 4–ABP-hemoglobin adducts were determined in 79 individuals, together with the acetylation phenotypes and genotypes. Among the slow acetylators, levels of 4–ABP–hemoglobin adducts were significantly higher compared to those present in rapid acetylators. This study indicated that clearance of low–dose carcinogen is decreased in the genetically based slow acetylator phenotype. Such genetic modulation of low–dose environmental risks is relevant to human cancer risk assessment procedures. In general, regardless of either of the smoking status or the tissue origin, biomonitoring studies have shown that slow acetylators have significantly higher concentrations of bladder DNA– and hemoglobin–adducts as compared to that in rapid acetylators (see Yu *et al.*, 1994; Kaderlik and Kadlubar, 1995).

At the present time, the relationship between carcinogen exposure, DNA adducts levels, metabolic activation phenotypes, and cancer (of the larynx, urinary bladder and colon) have been examined and can be used to assess the role of carcinogen exposure and individual susceptibility in cancer risk estimation.

LARYNGEAL CANCER

Numerous epidemiologic, pathologic, and clinical studies have firmly established that cigarette smoking is causally related to laryngeal cancer (US Department of Health and Human Services, 1982). Approximately 82% of the laryngeal cancer incidence and 87% of the mortality is directly attributable to cigarette smoking (Newcomb and Carbone, 1992). In 1995, an estimated 11,600 new cases of laryngeal cancer and 4,090 deaths will occur; this represents about a 70% increase over the past 35 years (Wingo *et al.*, 1995). Cigarette smoking is the principal risk factor for laryngeal cancer (Wynder and Stelman, 1979), and a strong dose response for this tumor is observed with a greater number of cigarettes smoked producing a greater risk of cancer (US Department of Health and

Human Services, 1982; Wynder and Stelman, 1979).

Alcohol is an independent and important determinant factor in laryngeal cancer risk. The combined effect of smoking and alcohol consumption increases the risk of laryngeal cancer by 75% over the risk associated with smoking or alcohol drinking alone (Newcomb and Carbone, 1992). Since food rarely reaches the laryngeal mucosa, direct tissue exposure to dietary carcinogens is unlikely. The mucosa of the larynx is, then, readily and frequently exposed to tobacco smoke particles and vapor containing chemical carcinogens, with alcohol probably serving as a cocarcinogenic stimulus (Degawa *et al.*, 1994). Cigarette smoke is a complex mixture of carcinogenic agents, including PAHs, *N*-nitroso compounds, and aromatic amines. However, several studies have implicated the role of PAHs in the etiology of human laryngeal cancer. A strong correlation between the induction of aryl hydrocarbon hydroxylase (AHH) in human lymphocytes and the susceptibility to cancer of the larynx has been reported in at least four studies (Trell *et al.*, 1976; Korsgaarsd *et al.*, 1984; Andereasson *et al.*, 1987; Degawa *et al.*, 1994). Moreover, oral and nasal mucosa, which are adjacent to the laryngeal mucosa, have been shown to metabolize PAHs (Murphy and Hecht, 1985; Hecht *et al.*, 1993) and to contain variable levels of CYPs (Chen *et al.*, 1993; Degawa *et al.*, 1994). Smoking-related DNA adducts were also detected in oral (Dunn and Stich, 1992) and laryngeal mucosa (Degawa *et al.*, 1994).

Recently, the smoking-related DNA adduct levels in the larynx tissues, from smokers and non/ex-smokers having laryngeal cancer, were studied in relation to the levels of carcinogen- metabolizing enzymes (Degawa *et al.*, 1994). DNA adducts were evident only in smokers and the chromatographic profiles of the adducts suggested that they were derived from PAHs but not from aromatic amines or *N*-nitroso compounds. In contrast to the lack of CYP1A2-dependent 4-ABP *N*-oxidation (Stern *et al.*, 1993) by the laryngeal microsomal fraction, relatively high AHH activities (28-30 pmol/30 min/mg protein) were observed (Degawa *et al.*, 1994). Several CYPs have now been shown to possess AHH activity (*i.e.* BP 3- and 9-hydroxylation), including 1A1, 1A2, 3A4, and the 2C family. Accordingly, total DNA adduct levels in the larynx correlated best with levels of CYP2C9/10*, followed by CYP3A4 and CYP1A1 (r = 0.90, 0.76, 0.72, respectively, $p<0.05$; see Figure 1). Thus, DNA adduct levels appeared to be determined primarily by expression of CYP2C9/10, which varied >10-fold in different individuals. It should also be mentioned here that the laryngeal CYP1A1 levels represented the highest yet found in human extrahepatic tissues. CYP2C9/10, which is

---

* CYP2C9 and CYP2C10 are allelic variants whose gene products differ by only two amino acids; tentatively identified from its migration pattern using authentic CYP2C markers (Badawi *et al.*, unpublished data).

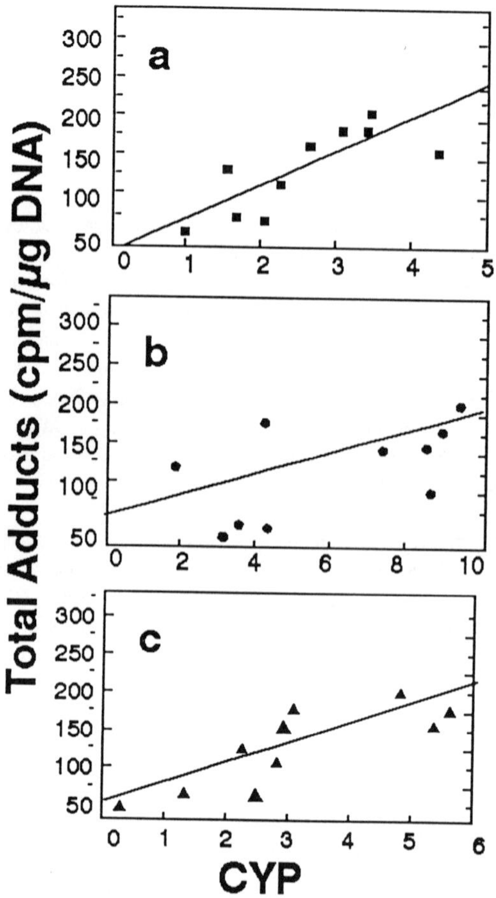

Figure 1. Correlation between total adduct levels (cpm/μg DNA) and (a) CYP1A1, (b) CYP3A4, and (c) CYP2C9 in human larynx. Correlation coefficients (r), using best-fit analysis, were 0.72 ($p<0.05$), 0.76 ($p<0.05$), and 0.90 ($p<0.01$), respectively.

a major component of the CYP2C subfamily, is known to catalyze the tolbutamide hydroxylation (Guengerich *et al.*, 1991) and to metabolically activate BP to its 9-hydroxy derivative. 9-Hydroxy-BP was also shown as the major metabolite formed by the human larynx microsomal incubations (Degawa *et al.*, 1994). Accordingly, 9-hydroxy-BP-DNA adducts accounted for up to 25% of the putative PAH adducts formed *in vivo* in the human larynx. Moreover, laryngeal microsomes showed high activities of NAT1 but not NAT2 (Stern *et al.*, 1993; Degawa *et al.*, 1994). These measurable activities of NAT1 were not correlated with total DNA adducts, which is consistent with the absence of aromatic amine DNA adducts in this tissue (*vide supra*).

The analysis of H-*ras* mutations in human larynx showed mutations in approximately 60% of specimens; both tumor and non-tumor specimens exhibited mutations in codons 12, 13, and 61. Specifically, a single common point mutation, a transversion in codon 61 (Gln→Glu) occurred in about 30% of the studied cases, all of whom were smokers, but not necessarily in tumor tissues (Stern *et al.*, 1993). Thus, these biomarker studies provide strong evidence for the role of tobacco smoke-derived PAHs in laryngeal cancer. Moreover, the data suggest that in smokers the primary determinant of DNA damage and perhaps cancer susceptibility is determined by expression of the enzymes catalyzing their bioactivation.

COLORECTAL CANCER

Colorectal cancer is the second leading cause of cancer death in United States. In 1995, an estimated 138,200 new cases of colon/rectum cancer and 55,300 deaths will occur. Although genetic and dietary factors have been strongly associated with colorectal cancer, there is increasing evidence that exposure to food-borne heterocyclic amines, which undergo metabolic activation to form mutagenic DNA adducts (Sugimura and Sato, 1983; Sugimura, 1986), may contribute substantially to the induction of this disease (Friesen *et al.*, 1994). The formation of this group of carcinogenic agents takes place mainly during cooking and/or pyrolysis of food or food products that are rich in animal protein. Several studies have suggested a causal association between meat consumption and colon cancer (*e.g.*, Potter and McMichael, 1986; Willett *et al.*, 1990). 2-Amino-1-methyl-6-phenylimidazo[4,5-*b*] pyridine (PhIP), which is a heterocyclic amine that induces colon tumors in rats, accounts for more than 85% of the mutagenic activity associated with fried beef (Felton and Knize, 1991) and is formed consistently in grilled fish, tobacco smoke, beer and wine.

In addition to the variation in exposure to chemical carcinogens, individual susceptibility to colon cancer have been suggested to be attributed to the variability in the metabolic proficiency of heterocyclic amines, *i.e.*, the polymorphism in NAT2 and

CYP1A2 (Lang *et al.*,1994; Ilett *et al.*, 1987; Lang *et al.*, 1986). The initial bioactivation step of heterocyclic amines involves hepatic *N*–oxidation, catalyzed by CYP1A2, to form the corresponding *N*–hydroxy derivative. Subsequent *O*–acetylation, by NAT2, of the latter intermediate, in the liver or in the colon, forms the *N*–acetoxy derivative that reacts covalently with DNA (Kadlubar *et al.*, 1991; Kaderlik and Kadlubar, 1995). The findings that polymorphic NAT is expressed in a phenotypically dependent manner in colorectal mucosa (Ilett *et al.*, 1994) indicates that this tissue has the capacity to participate in the latter bioactivation step. However, the *N*–acetoxy derivative (*e.g.*, *N*–acetoxy–PhIP) was found to be stable enough to be transported from the liver *via* the blood to the colon, forming DNA adducts that may lead to the initiation of colon cancer (Kaderlik *et al.*, 1994). Therefore, individuals exposed to heterocyclic amines and having the rapid *N*–oxidation phenotype with the rapid *O*–acetylation phenotype should have the highest levels of DNA adducts in their colon epithelium with a consequent high risk of developing colon cancer (Lang *et al.*, 1994).

Accordingly, in a recent study (Lang *et al.*, 1994), the CYP1A2 and NAT2 phenotypes were determined in 205 controls and 75 colon cancer/colon polyp patients. Applying the caffeine phenotyping procedures for CYP1A2 and NAT2 (Butler *et al.*, 1992), the urinary ratio of (17X+17U)/137X was used to determine CYP1A2 phenotypes, while the raio of AFMU/1–methylxanthine (1X) was used to determine the NAT2 phenotypes. The prevalence of rapid CYP1A2 and rapid NAT2 phenotypes were each slightly greater in cancer patients *versus* healthy controls (Lang *et al.*, 1994). However, the combined rapid–rapid phenotypes of CYP1A2/NAT2 was found in 35% of the cases, which was significantly higher than the frequency of 16% that was observed in controls (p=0.002). The CYP1A2 phenotype was clearly influenced by smoking status, demonstrating a mean CYP1A2 level that was nearly double that seen in nonsmokers, with an apparent ethnic variation (Lang *et al.*, 1994). The acetylation rate (NAT2), which is much higher in rapid *versus* slow acetylators (Ilett *et al.*, 1994), was also significantly higher in cases (1.4-1.6 for AFMU/1X) as compared to the healthy controls (1.1-0.99, p = 0.04). Therefore, metabolic phenotype, particularly rapid–rapid CYP1A2/NAT2, combined with exposure to food–borne carcinogenic heterocyclic amines are important risk factors in human colorectal cancer.

A pilot survey (Friesen *et al.*, 1994) of human tissue DNA samples, including pancreas, colon, and urinary bladder, was carried out by two independent methods, alkaline hydrolysis–gas chromatography/mass spectrometry and ^{32}P–postlabelling. Both methods provided evidence for the presence of heterocyclic amines (PhIP)–DNA adducts in colon samples, but not in the samples from human pancreas or urinary bladder. The issue of relating the phenotypes of NAT2 and CYP1A2 to the extent of DNA adduct formation in human colon and their role in subsequent development of cancer is clearly an area for further investigation.

URINARY BLADDER CANCER

Urinary bladder cancer is the sixth most prevalent cancer in the United States and accounts for about 8% of all cases of human cancer. In 1995, an estimated 50,500 new cases of bladder cancer and 11,200 deaths will occur (Wingo *et al.*, 1995). Nearly 50% of all bladder cancer deaths were attributable to tobacco smoking in men, with a lower percent in women (Newcomb and Carbone, 1992; Silverman *et al.*, 1992). However, in tropical and subtropical countries, where *Schistosoma haematobium* is highly endemic, the proportional incidence of bladder cancer is higher than the figures reported from many Western countries (for reviews see Badawi *et al.*, 1992a; 1995b; Badawi and Mostafa, 1992; 1993). In these areas, bladder neoplasm is the first type of cancer reported in males and second only to the breast cancer in females with an overall rate of incidence of about 30.8% among all other types of cancer (see Badawi *et al.*, 1995b).

Epidemiological studies of cancer of the urinary bladder began in the year 1895 when Rehn published his first observation on the excessive occurrence of bladder cancers among aniline–dye workers, and was confirmed later by Case *et al,* (Case *et al.*, 1954). Since then, a large volume of evidence has accumulated documenting the relationship of bladder cancer to certain industrial exposures and the known carcinogenic effects of occupationally encountered chemicals. For example, the analysis of published case–control studies concluded that about 19% of male and 6% of female bladder cancers were attributable to occupational exposures to identified industrial carcinogens (Vineis and Simonato, 1986; Jones *et al.*, 1992), *e.g.*, 4,4'–methylene *bis*(2–chloroaniline), 2–naphthylamine, or *o*–toluidine (IARC, 1980; Ward *et al.*, 1991), substances that have been implicated in an increased bladder cancer incidence of 30-fold, or more (Rubino *et al.*, 1982).

There is also epidemiological evidence that cigarette smoking is causally associated with bladder cancer (Vineis, 1992). As demonstrated in more than 30 case–control studies and in 10 cohort studies, cigarette smoking is now accepted as a major cause of urinary bladder cancer (for review see Silverman *et al.*, 1992). In 1991, smoking was responsible for the development of more than 4,200 new cases of urinary bladder cancer in United States. Evidence on the consequences of cigarette smoking has accumulated rapidly, with retrospective and prospective studies demonstrating that the risk of developing different types of cancer (*e.g.*, lung, larynx, oral cavity, esophagus, pancreas, kidney and bladder) is increased among smokers as opposed to non–smokers (Vineis, 1992; Burnham; 1989). Habitual exposure to cigarette smoke may contribute to more than half of bladder cancers in men in certain regions of the world (Newcomb and Carbone, 1992; Silverman *et al.*, 1992). Human exposure to 4–ABP, which was earlier identified as an occupational carcinogen, also occurs *via* tobacco smoke and may represent an important contributing risk for urinary bladder carcinogenesis (Kaderlik and Kadlubar, 1995). The presence of 4–ABP– hemoglobin adducts and 4–ABP–DNA adducts in human bladder have been established and are characteristic, to some extent, of the exposure to tobacco smoke (see Table 1 and references therein). Direct evidence for the causal association of cigarette smoking with bladder cancer comes from analyses that have shown an increase of 4–ABP (Kadlubar *et al.*, 1988; Kadlubar, 1991; Talaska *et al.*, 1991a; 1991b; 1993), PhIP (Peluso *et al.*, 1991), and 8–oxoguanine (Loft *et al.*, 1992)–modified DNA among cigarette smokers relative to nonsmokers (Table 1).

Exposure to several other agents is known to carry a defined risk of bladder cancer. These agents include benzidine, the immunosuppressive and antineoplastic agent cyclophosphamide, the chemotherapeutic agent chlornaphazine that was previously used for leukaemias and Hodgkin's disease, and analgesic mixtures containing phenacetin (IARC, 1987). On the other hand, much less well defined risks for bladder cancer have been associated with exposure to the volatiles of coal tar (IARC, 1987), excessive coffee drinking (IARC, 1991), beverages made with chlorinated water (Cantor *et al.*, 1987), industrial exposure to formaldehyde vapour (Fayerweather *et al.*, 1983), and inconclusively for isoniazid (IARC, 1987). Although the epidemiological evidence for the carcinogenicity of saccharin to the bladder provides little evidence of excess cancers, it is carcinogenic in laboratory animals and will promote the effects of initiating agents such as nitrosamines in the rat bladders (IARC, 1987). This carcinogenecity seems to occur through the mechanism of increased bladder cell turnover secondary to increased urinary pH and sodium ion concentrations.

There are several sources of information that indicate aromatic amines as causative agents in bladder carcinogenesis in smokers. Examination of DNA adducts in the biopsies of 42 subjects with bladder cancer (Talaska *et al.*, 1991a) showed that *N*–(deoxyguanosin–8–yl)- 4–aminobiphenyl (*N*–dG8– ABP) is one of the major adducts in smokers and was found to be strongly related to smoking status. Several individual DNA adducts were also significantly elevated in the urothelium of smokers as compared to non–smokers. In another study (Vineis *et al.*, 1990), ABP–hemoglobin adducts correlated well with the number of cigarettes smoked, with urinary cotinine and nicotine, and with the type of tobacco. Among smokers, of 12 DNA adducts that could be quantified separately, two were clearly correlated with both the number of cigarettes smoked and the levels of ABP–hemoglobin adducts; one of these two exhibited a chromatographic pattern similar to that of *N*–dG8–ABP (Talaska *et al.*, 1991b) and was linearly correlated with levels of ABP–hemoglobin adducts. Therefore, it not unreasonable to suggest that 4–ABP, and perhaps other arylamines, may play an important role in huamn bladder carcinogenesis initiated by smoking. Indeed, *N*–dG8–PhIP (Peluso *et al.*, 1991), 8–oxo–guanosine (Loft *et al.*, 1992), and various other unspecified aromatic amine–DNA adducts (*e.g.* Talaska *et al.*, 1993; Badawi *et al.*,

1995) were found to be elevated in the urothelial mucosa of smokers as opposed to non-smokers (see Table 1). These data further implicate the association between cigarette smoking and DNA damage and suggest a molecular basis for the initiation of human bladder carcinogenesis by smoking (*vide infra*) in which aromatic amines are involved. In addition, *N*-(deoxyadenosin-8-yl)- MOCA (*N*-dA8-MOCA) (Kaderlik *et al.*, 1993), O^6-methyldeoxyguanosine (O^6-MedG) (Badawi *et al.*, 1991; 1992b; 1994), and ochratoxin-A related DNA adducts (OAT-DNA) (Pfohl-Leszkowicz *et al.*, 1993) were associated with increased risk of human bladder cancer presumably induced by occupational, parasitic, and dietary exposures, respectively. These adducts were found in higher levels in cancer cases *versus* controls (Table 1), further strengthing the association of these environmental factors with human bladder cancer.

The DNA binding and the carcinogenicity of aromatic amines is a consequence of their metabolic activation by complex, competing pathways (see above). The formation of electrophilic intermediates in the liver through *N*-hydrox-ylation is catalyzed in humans predominantly by CYP1A2. The *N*-hydroxy metabolite of arylamines, such as *N*-hydroxy-ABP, then enters the circulation, reacts covalently with the hemoglobin or is filtered into the bladder lumen where it it can undergo an acid-catalyzed reaction with urothelial DNA (Kadlubar, 1991; Bartsch *et al.*, 1993). This reaction produces a C-8 substituted deoxyguanosine adduct as well as other minor adducts and has been considered to be the critical event in the initiation of human bladder carcinogenesis (Miller and Miller, 1981). The *N*-acetylation reaction, catalyzed by hepatic NATs is, however, a competing pathway leading to the detoxification of the amine.

Since CYP1A2 and NATs mediate the activation and detoxification of ABP and exhibit polymorphisms, studies have been carried out to determine whether or not individual variation in aromatic amine-DNA adduct formation is due to a particular metabolic phenotypes. Studies concerning aromatic amine-induced bladder carcinogenesis in humans occupationally exposed to the carcinogenic agents has demonstrated that humans at highest risk of bladder cancer are probably those with the rapid CYP1A2 and slow NAT2 phenotypes (Kadlubar *et al.*, 1992). *N*-Acetylation and *N*-oxidation phenotypes, assigned on the basis of urinary caffeine metabolism procedures (Butler *et al.*, 1992; see above), have been examined in relation to aromatic amine exposure and hemoglobin adduct levels. These studies (Kadlubar, 1991; Bartsch *et al.*, 1993) indicated that smoking subjects with the slow NAT2/rapid CYP1A2 phenotypes exhibit 50% higher 4-ABP-hemoglobin adduct levels as compared to rapid NAT2/slow CYP1A2 individuals; the other phenotypic combination gave intermediate values.

Recently, the enzyme which has long been thought to code for the monomorphic *N*-acetyltransferase activity (NAT1), was shown to be regulated by a polymorphic gene when tested in human peripheral blood (Weber and vatsis, 1993; Vatsis and Weber,

TABLE 1: Detection of DNA Adducts in Human Urinary Bladder[1]

SOURCE OF EXPOSURE	DNA ADDUCT	ADDUCT LEVEL (μmole/mole N)[2]	No. OF CASES	DETECTION METHODS	REF.[4]
BACKGROUND	*N*-dG8-ABP	0.110	9	^{32}P	1, 2
		0.135	21	^{32}P	3, 4
		0.360	8	GC-NICI-MS	5
	O^6-MedG	0.046	12	RIA	6-8
		n.d.	33	RIA	9
	N-dG8-PhIP	+[3]	1	^{32}P	10
		n.d.	6	^{32}P/GC-MS	11
	8-OH-dG	0.591*	83	HPLC-GC-MS	12
	Unspecified aromatic adducts	0.378	9	^{32}P	1, 2
		0.513	21	^{32}P	3, 4
		0.270	5	^{32}P	13
		0.621	27	^{32}P	14

TABLE 1: Detection of DNA Adducts in Human Urinary Bladder (Cont.)

SOURCE OF EXPOSURE	DNA ADDUCT	ADDUCT LEVEL (μmole/mole N)[2]	No. OF CASES	DETECTION METHODS	REF.[4]
SMOKING	*N*-dG8-ABP	0.385	13	^{32}P	1, 2
		0.216	18	^{32}P	3, 4
		1.539	4	^{32}P	15
	N-dG8-PhIP	++[4]	2	^{32}P	10
	8-OH-dG	0.844*	85	HPLC-GC-MS	12
	Unspecified aromatic adducts	1.242	13	^{32}P	1, 2
		0.648	18	^{32}P	3, 4
		2.670	16	^{32}P	16, 17
		0.918	8	^{32}P	13
OCCUPATIONAL	*N*-dA8-MOCA	139.32	1	^{32}P	18
PARASITIC INFECTION	O^6-MedG	0.134	46	RIA	6-8
DIET	OAT-DNA	0.484	5	^{32}P	19

[1]Abbreviations used: *N*-dG8-ABP, *N*-(deoxyguanoosine-8-yl)-4-aminobiphenyl; *O*[6]-MedG, O[6]-methyldeoxyguanosine; *N*-dG8-PhIP, N-(deoxyguanosin-8-yl)-2-amino-1-methyl-6-phenylimidazo[4,5-b]pyridine; 8-OH-dG; 8-hydroxy-guanosine; *N*-dA8-MOCA; *N*-(deoxyadenosin-8-yl)-4-amino-3-chlorobenzyl alcohol; OAT-DNA, ochratoxin-A related DNA adducts; ^{32}P, ^{32}P-postlabelling; GC-NICI-MS; gas chromatography with negative ion chemical ionization mass spectrometry; RIA, radioimmunoassay; HPLC-GC-MS, high pressure liquid chromatography with gas chromatography mass spectrometry; n.d., not detected.

[2]Data were calculated from the original paper in μmol adduct per mole normal nucleotide using the assumption that 100 μg DNA contains ~70 nmol of each normal nucleotide except in (*) were the previous assumption was applied together with the apporoximation that a somatic mammalian cell will contain about 5,500x10^6 nucleotide pairs in ~6pg DNA.

[3]DNA adducts were detected in levels corresponded to the smoking status but not discussed in the original text.

[4]References cited: (1) Talaska *et al.*, 1991a; (2) Kadlubar, 1991; (3) Talaska *et al.*, 1991b; (4) Talaska *et al.*, 1993; (5) Lin and Lay *et al.*, 1994; (6) Badawi *et al.*, 1991; (7) Badawi *et al.*, 1992b; (8) Badawi *et al.*, 1994; (9) Souliotis *et al.*, 1992; (10) Peluso *et al.*, 1991; (11) Friesen *et al.*, 1994; (12) Loft *et al.*, 1992; (13) Cuzick *et al.*, 1990; (14) Badawi *et al.*, 1995b; (15) Kadlubar *et al.*, 1988; (16) Randerath *et al.*, 1989; (17) Randerath and Randerath, 1993; (18) Kaderlik *et al.*, 1993; and (19) Pfohl-Lezkowicz, 1993.

1993). NAT1 is expressed in human urothelial mucosa (Frederickson *et al.*, 1994) and also catalyzes the *O*–acetylation of *N*–hydroxy arylamines, but not *N*–hydroxy heterocyclic amines. Data on phenotyping and genotyping of NAT1, using PCR techniques (*vide supra*), now indicate that this enzyme is bimodally distributed in human urinary bladder in a manner that is significantly correlated with the DNA adducts in this tissue. Individuals with the rapid NAT1 'at risk' genotype were found to have 2–fold higher levels of DNA adducts ($p=0.05$) as compared to those with slow 'protective' NAT1 genotype (Badawi *et al*, Bell *et al*, manuscripts in preparation).

It is clear that the metabolic phenotyping and/or genotyping of any enzyme, that is involved in the process of carcinogen activation (or detoxification) and is polymorphically distributed, could influence the DNA adduct formation in urothelial cells and could ultimately lead to alterations in bladder cancer risk. Therefore, cancer risk assessment procedures should be redesigned to include biomarkers of susceptibility, especially those involved in carcinogen biotransformation.

BIOMARKERS IN EPIDEMIOLOGY: QUANTITATIVE APPROACHES

Quantitative cancer risk estimation requires the establishment of a mathematical relationship between tumor incidence and exposure to a carcinogen. However, carcinogen exposure in a human population is usually difficult to quantify. Often, humans can only be classified as 'not exposed' or 'exposed' to a carcinogen, without a measure of the amount of exposure other than perhaps years of exposure. Accordingly, cancer risk estimates are generally based on animal bioassays where known quantities of chemicals are administered. Obviously, such studies do not duplicate the human environment containing thousands of chemicals; thus, the relevance of animal studies for humans must always be critically evaluated.

Biomarkers (*e.g.*, specific DNA adducts) provide a way to measure human exposure to chemical carcinogens. Moreover, DNA adducts can provide a measure of the dose to the carcinogen target site (DNA) required for biologically-based dose-response models. Then, it may be possible to establish a relationship between tumor incidence and exposure as measured by adduct levels. Many factors influence carcinogen exposure, such as sex, race, age, tobacco smoking, alcohol consumption, occupation, and diet. Thus, a fairly homogeneous population for these risk factors is necessary to establish a quantitative relationship by statistical regression techniques between tumor risk and exposure to a specific carcinogen or class of carcinogens. However, even in a relatively homogeneous population, it has become apparent that there are large inter-individual variations and that this problem is exacerbated further in heterogeneous populations derived from multi-racial and multi-ethnic origins. Nevertheless, it may be possible to stratify individuals into relatively homogeneous subgroups and/or to account for their effects by multiple regression techniques. The latter procedure may not be successful where exposure is also associated with these susceptibility factors for cancer risk.

On the other hand, DNA adducts from a specific organ may be inaccessible and a good surrogate adduct may not be available. These circumstances can be partially abrogated by the combinations of exposure information (epidemiology) and metabolic activation or detoxification potential (phenotyping). A case-control study using these methods to test the hypothesis that heterocyclic amine exposure and efficient heterocyclic amine activation combine to increase the risk of colon neoplasia demonstrates the value of this approach (Lang *et al.*, 1994). The univariate analysis of the data is supplemented with the use of logistic regression analysis to identify those variables most important in defining risk in this study. This provides the investigator with a model which can then be tested prospectively on a new group of individuals. This model can then be used to assess the value of any intervention in a cohort study by the effect of the intervention on reducing observed events (tumors) below the expected level.

The logistic regression model (Hosmer and Lemeshow, 1989) is also useful because it can be used to provide the probability (*P*) of an event. This is illustrated by the equation:

$$P(\text{Colon neoplasia}) = e^{f(x)}/(1+ e^{f(x)}),$$

where, $$f(x)=b0+b1*Age+b2*MeatWellDone+b3*BothRapid,$$

where (b) is the value of the Y intercept; taken from our study on colon cancer or polyps (Lang *et al.*, 1994). The values calculated for the coefficients are inserted into the equation to give a set of curves that show the probability of an event, in this case colon neoplasia, for different combinations of the risk factors - age, phenotype, and meat cooking preference (Figure 2). This statistical treatment allows the impact of dietary practices (which can be changed) relative to phenotypic factors or age (which cannot be

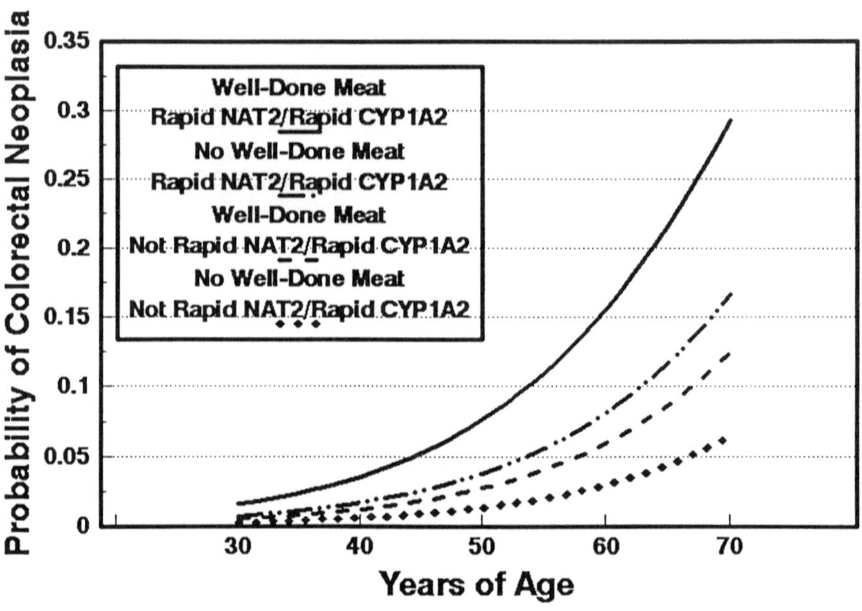

Figure 2. Probability of developing colorectal cancer as a function of age, exposure, and combined rapid CYP1A2–NAT2 phenotypes.

changed) to be clearly evident. Moreover, this study on colon neoplasia suggests that dietary changes will not bring the risk to zero. In fact, other practices such as increased cruciferous vegetable consumption may be capable of a further reduction in the probability of colon neoplasia. Such hypotheses are indeed testable using the logistic regression model as discussed above. Therefore, if a relationship can be established between biomarkers of exposure and susceptibility to a carcinogen or class of carcinogens as measured by adduct levels, it should be possible to predict the probability of cancer for individual subgroups. The effectiveness of an intervention could then be assessed in terms of tumor risk for an individual or the subpopulation as a whole. Furthermore, subpopulations of high or low risk could possibly be identified on the basis of adduct level.

REFERENCES

Andereasson L, Bjorlin G, Hocherman M, Korsgaard R, Trell E (1987): Laryngeal cancer, aryl hydrocarbon hydroxylase inducibility and smoking: A follow up study. ORL 49:187–192.

Badawi AF, Cooper DP, Mostafa MH, Aboul-Azm T, Margison GP, O'Connor PJ (1991): O^6–Alkylguanine–DNA–alkyltransferase activity in relation to the promutagenic damage in bladder DNA from humans predisposed to bladder cancer associated with schistosomiasis. Eur J Cancer 27:46.

Badawi AF, Mostafa MH, O'Connor PJ (1992a): Involvement of alkylating agents in schistosome–associated bladder cancer: the possible basic mechanisms of induction. Cancer Lett 63:171–188.

Badawi AF, Mostafa MH, Aboul-Azm T, Haboubi NY, O'Connor PJ, Cooper DP (1992b): Promutagenic methylation damage in bladder DNA from patients with bladder cancer associated with schistosomiasis and from normal individuals. Carcinogenesis 13: 877– 881.

Badawi AF, Mostafa MH (1992): Schistosomiasis: some health and socieconomic aspects in the Egyptian environment. Ramazzini Newslett 3:33–44.

Badawi AF, Mostafa MH (1993): Possible mechanisms of alteration in the capacities of carcinogen metabolizing enzymes during schistosomiasis and their role in bladder cancer induction. J Int Med Res 21:281–305.

Badawi AF, Cooper DP, Mostafa MH, Aboul-Azm T, Barnard B, Margison GP,

O'Connor PJ (1994): O^6–alkylguanine–DNA–alkyltransferase activity in schistosomiasis- associated human bladder cancer. Eur J Cancer 30:1314–1319.

Badawi AF, KR Kaderlik, CH Teitel, FF Kadlubar (1995b): Role of aromatic amine acetylation phenotype in carcinogen–DNA adduct formation in the human urinary bladder. Proc Am Assoc Cancer Res 36:913.

Badawi AF, Mostafa MH, Probert A, O'Connor PJ (1995b): Role of schistosomiasis in huamn bladder cancer: evidence of association, etiological factors and basic mechanisms of carcinogenesis. Eur J Cancer Prevention 4: 45-59.

Bartsch H, Malaveille C, Friesen M, Kadlubar FF, Vineis P (1993): Black (air–cured) and blond (flue–cured) tobacco cancer risk: IV. Molecular dosimetry studies implicates aromatic amines as bladder carcinogens. Eur J Cancer 8:1199–1207.

Beland FA, Kadlubar FF (1990): Metabolic activation and DNA adducts of aromatic amines and nitroaromatic hydrocarbons. In Cooper CS, Grover PL (eds.): "Chemical carcinogenesis and muta-genesis, vol I." Berlin: Springer–Verlag, pp 267–325.

Blum M, Demierre A, Grant DM, Hein M, Meyer UA (1991): Molecular mechanisms of slow acetylation of drugs and carcinogens in humans. Proc Natl Acad Sci USA 88:5237–5241.

Brockmöller J, Kerb R, Darkoulis N, Staffeldt B, Roots I (1994): Glutathione *S*–transferase M1 and its variants A and B as host factors of bladder cancer susceptibility. Cancer Res 54:4103–4111.

Burnham N (1989): Bladder cancer: detection, prevention and therapeutics. Am Pharmacol 29:33–8.

Butler MA, Iwasaki M, Guengerich FP, Kadlubar FF (1989): Human cytochrome P–450_{PA} (P–4501A2), the phenacetin *O*–deethylase, is primarily responsible for the hepatic 3– demethylation of caffeine and *N*–oxidation of carcinogenic arylamines. Proc Natl Acad Sci USA 86:7696–7700.

Butler MA, Lang NP, Young JF, Caporaso NE, Vineis P, hayes RB, Teitel CH, Massengill JP, Lawsen MF, Kadlubar FF (1992): Determination of CYP1A2 and NAT2 phenotypes in human populations by analysis of caffeine urinary metabolites. Pharmacogenetics 2:116–127.

Cantor KP, Hoover R, Hartge P, Masen TJ (1987): Bladder cancer, drinking water sources and tap water consumption: A case-control study. J Natl Cancer Inst 79:1269-79.

Caporaso N, Hayes RB, Dosemeci M, Hoover R, Ayesh R, Hetzel M, Idle J (1989): Lung cancer risk, occupational exzposure, and the debrisoquine metabolic phenotype. Cancer Res 49:3675-3679.

Caporaso N, Landi MT, Vineis P (1991): Relevance of metabolic polymorphisms to human carcinogenesis: evaluation of epidemiologic evidence. Pharmacogenetics 1:4-19.

Cartwright RA, Glashan RW, Rogers JJ, Barham-Hall D, Ahmed RA, Higgins E, Kahan MA (1982): The role of *N*-acetyltransferase in bladder carcinogenesis: a pharmacogenetic epidemiological approach to bladder cancer. Lancet 2:842-845.

Case RAM, Hosker ME, McDonald DB, Pearson JT (1954): Tumours of the urinary bladder in workmen engaged in the manufacture and use of certain dyestuff intermediates in the British Chemical Industry, Part I. Br J Indust Med 11:75-104.

Chen Y, Sparks DL, Ding X, Getchell TV (1993): Immunohistochemical localization of a cytochrome P-450 isozyme in human nasal mucosa: age-related trends. Ann Otol Rhinol Laryngol 102:368-374.

Cocker J, Boobis AR, Wilson HK, Gompertz D (1990): Evidence that *N*-glucuronide of 4,4'-methylenebis(2-chloroaniline) (MbOCA) is a major urinary metabolite in man: implications for biological monitoring. Br J Ind Med 47:154-161.

Cosma G, Crofts F, Taioli E, Toniolo P, Garte S (1993): Relationship between genotype and function of human CYP1A1 gene. J Toxicol Envirn Health 40:309-316.

Cuzick J, Routledge MN, Jenkins D, Garner RC (1990): DNA adducts in different tissues of smokers and non-smokers. Int J Cancer 45:673-678.

Daly AK, Thomas DJ, Cooper J, Pearson WR, Neal DE, Idle JR (1993): Homozygous deletion of gene for glutathione *S*-transferase M1 in bladder cancer. Br Med J 307:481.

Degawa M, Stern SJ, Martin MV, Guengerich FP, Fu PP, Ilett KF, Kaderlik RK, Kadlubar FF (1994): Metabolic activation and carcinogen-DNA adduct detection in human larynx. Cancer Res 45:4915-4919.

Doll R, Peto R (1981): The causes of cancer. J Natl Cancer Inst 66:1191-1308.

Dunn BP, Stich HF (1992): ^{32}P–Postlabelling analysis of aromatic DNA adducts in human oral mucosal cells. Carcinogenesis 7:1115–1120.

Ehrenberg L and Tornqvist M (1992): Use of biomarkers in epidemiology: quantitative aspects. Toxicol Lett 64/65:485–492.

Farber E (1980): Toxicological significance of liver hypertrophy produced by inducers of drug–metabolizing enzymes. In "Environmental chemicals, enzyme function and human disease, Ciba Foundation Symposium No. 76" Amsterdam: Excerpta Medica, pp 261– 270.

Fayerweather WE, Pell S, Bender JR (1983): Case–control study of cancer deaths in Du Point Workers with potential exposure to formaldehyde In Clary, JJ, Gibson JE, Waritz RS (eds): "Cancer epidemiology and mechanisms" New York: Marcel Dekker, pp. 47–113.

Felton JS, Knize MG (1991): Occurrence, identification and bacterial mutagenicity of heterocyclic amines in cooked food. Mutat Res 259:205–217.

Flammang TJ, Couch LH, Levy GN, Weber WW, Wise CK (1992a): DNA adduct levels in carcinogenic rapid and slow acetylator mouse strain following chronic administration of 4–aminobiphenyl. Carcinogenesis 13:1887–1891.

Flammang TJ, Yerokun T, Bryant MS, Couch LH, Kirlin WG, Lee KJ, Ogolla F, Ferguson RJ, Talaska G, Hein DW (1992b): Hemoglobin adducts and hepatic– and urinary bladder–DNA adduct levels in rapid and slow acetylator Syrian inbred hamsters administered 2–aminofluorene. J Pharmacol Exp Therap 260:865–871.

Frederickson SM, Messing EM, Reznikoff CA, Swaminathan S (1994): Relationship between in vivo acetylator phenotypes ans cytosolic *N*–acetyltranmsferase and *O*–acetyltransferase activities in human urothelial cells. Cancer Epidemiol Biomarkers Prev 3:25–32.

Friesen MD, Kaderlik K, Lin D, Garren L, Bartsch H, Lang NP, Kadlubar FF (1994): Analysis of DNA adducts of 2–amino–1–methyl–6–phenylimidazo[4,5–*b*] pyridine in rat and human tissues by alkaline hydrolysis and gas chromatography/ electron capture mass spectrometry: validation by comparison with ^{32}P–postlabelling. Chem Res Toxicol 7:733– 739.

Gaylor DW, Kadlubar FF, Beland FA (1992): Application of biomarkers to risk assessment. Environ Health Presp. 98:139–141.

Gelboin HV (1980): Benzo(a)pyrene metabolism, activation and carcinogenesis: role and regulation of mixed-function oxidases and related enzymes. Physiol Rev 60: 1107-1166.

Gonzalez FJ, Gelboin HV (1993): Role of human cytochrome P-450s in risk assessment and susceptibility to environmetally based diseas. J Toxicol Environ Health 40:289-308.

Guengerich FP, Brian WR, Sari MA, Ross JT (1991): Expression of mammailan cytochrome P-450 enzymes using yeast-basd vectors. Methods Enzymol 206:130-145.

Guengerich FP (1991): Reactions and significance of cytochrome P450 enzymes. J Biol Chem 226:10019-10022.

Hecht SS, Carmella SG, Murphy SE, Foiles PG, Chung FL (1993): Carcinogen biomarkers related to smoking and upper aerodigestive tract cancer. J Cell Biochem 17F:27-35.

Hemminki K (1990): Exposure to chemical carcinogens. In Cooper CS, Grover PL (eds.): "Chemical carcinogenesis and mutagenesis, vol I" Berlin: Springer-Verlag, pp 33-62.

Hosmer DW and Lemeshow S (1989): Applied Logistic Regression. New York: John Wiley & Sons.

IARC, International Agency for Research on Cancer Working Group (1980): An evaluation of chemicals and industrial processes associated with cancer in humans based on human and animal data; IARC Monographs Vols. 1-20. Cancer Res 40:1-12.

IARC, International Agency for Research on Cancer (1986): IARC monographs on the evaluation of carcinogenic risk chemicals to humans, vol. 38. Tobacco smoking. Lyon: International Agency for Research on Cancer.

IARC, International Agency for Research on Cancer Working Group (1987): Monographs on the evaluation of carcinogenic risks in humans. Overall evaluations of carcinogenicity: an updating of volumes 1-42, Lyon: International Agency for Research on Cancer.

IARC, International Agency for Research on Cancer Working Group (1991): Monographs on the evaluation of carcinogenic risks in humans. Coffee, tea, mate, methylxanthine and methylglyoxal. Volume 51, Lyon: International Agency for Research on Cancer.

Ilett KF, David BM, Dethon P, Castleden WM, Kwa R (1987): Acetylation phenotype in colorectal carcinoma. Cancer Res 47:1466–1469.

Ilett KF, Ingram DM, Carpenter DS, Teitel CH, Lang NP, Kadlubar FF, Minchin RF (1994): Expression of monomorphic and polymorphic *N*-acetyl transferases in human colon. Biochem Pharmacol 47:914–917.

Jones RF, Debiec-Rychter M, Wang CY (1992): Chemical carcinogenesis of the urinary bladder: a status report. J Cancer Res Clin Oncol 118:411–419.

Kaderlik KR, Talaska G, DeBord DG, Osorio AM, Kadlubar FF (1993): 4,4'-Methylene- bis(2-chloroaniline)-DNA adduct analysis in human exfoliated urothelial cells by ^{32}P- postlabelling. Cancer Epidemiol Biomarkers Prev 2:63–69.

Kaderlik KR, Minchin RF, Mulder GJ, Ilett KF, Kadlubar FF (1995): Metabolic activation pathway for the formation of DNA adducts of the carcinogen 2-amino-1-methyl-6-phenylimidazo[4,5-*b*]pyridine (PhIP) in rat extrahepatic tissues. Carcinogenesis: in press.

Kaderlik KR, Kadlubar FF (1995): Metabolic polymorphisms and carcinogen DNA-adduct formation in human populations. Pharmacogenetics: in press.

Kadlubar FF (1987): Metabolism and DNA binding of carcinogenic aromatic amines. ISI Atlas of Science: Pharmacology 1:129–132.

Kadlubar FF, Talaska G, Lang NP, Benson RW, Roberts DW (1988): Assessment of exposure and susceptibility to aromatic amine carcinogens. In Bartsch H, Hemminki K, O'Neill IK (eds): "Methods for detecting DNA damaging agents in humans: Applications in cancer epidemiology and prevention" Lyon: IARC Sci Publ No 89:199–174.

Kadlubar FF (1991): Carcinogenic aromatic amine metabolism and DNA adduct detection in human. In Ernster L (ed): "Xenobiotics and cancer" London: Taylor & Francis Ltd., pp 329–338.

Kadlubar FF, Dooley KL, Teitel CH, Roberts DW, Benson RW, Butler MA, Bailey JR, Young JF, Skipper PW, Tannenbaum SR (1991): Frequency of urination and its effects on metabolism, pharmacokinetics, blood hemoglobin aduuct formation, and liver and urinary bladder DNA adduct levels in beagle dogs administered the carcinogen 4-aminobiphenyl. Cancer Res 51:4371–4377.

Kadlubar FF, Butler MA, Kaderlik KR, Chou H-C, Lang NP (1992): Polymorphisms of aromatic amine metabolism in humans: relevance for human carcinogenesis. Environ Health Presp 98:69–74.

Kadlubar FF (1994a): Biochemical individuality and its implications for drug and carcinogen metabolism: recent insights from acetyltansferase and cytochrome P4501A2 phenotyping and genotyping in humans. Drug Metabolis Rev 26:37–46.

Kadlubar FF (1994b): DNA adducts of carcinogenic aromatic amines. In Hemminki K, Dipple A, Shuker DEG, Kadlubar FF, Segerback D, Bartsch H (eds.): "DNA adducts, identificationand biological significance" Lyon: IARC Sci Publ No. 125, pp 199–216.

Kalow, W (1962): Pharmacogenetics:Heredity and the response to drugs. Philadelphia: W.B. Saunders.

Kalow, W (1991): Interethenic variation of drug metabolism. Trends Pharmacol Sci 12:102–107.

Kellermann G, Shaw CR, Luyten-Kellermann M (1973): Aryl-hydrocarbon hydroxylase inducibility and bronchogenic carcinoma. New Eng J Med 289:934–937.

Kelsey KT, Wiencke JK, Spitz MR (1994): A race-specific genetic polymorphism in the CYP1A1 gene is not associated with lung cancer in African Americans. Carcinognesis 15:1121–1124.

Kihara M, Kihara M, Noda K (1994): Lung cancer risk of GSTM1 null genotype is dependent on the extent of tobacco smoke exposure. Carcinogenesis 15:415–418.

Kirlin WG, Ogolla F, Andrews AF, Trinidad A, Ferguson RJ, Yerkun T, Mpezo M, Hein DW (1991): Acetylator genotype-dependent expression of arylamine *N*-acetyltransferse in human colon cytosol from non-cancer and colorectal cancer patients. Cancer Res 51:549–555.

Korsgaard R, Trell E, Kitzing P, Hood B, Norden G, Simonsson B, Stiksa G (1984): Aryl hydrocarbon hydroxylase inducibility and smoking habits in patients with laryngeal carcinomas. Acta Otolaryngol 98:368–373.

Lang NP, Chu DZJ, Hunter CF, Kendall, DC, Flamming TJ, Kadlubar FF (1986): Role of aromatic amine acetyltransferase in human colorectal cancer. Arch Surg 121:1259–1261.

Lang NL, Butler MA, Massengill J, Lawson M, Stotts RC, Hauer-Jensen M, Kadlubar FF (1994): Rapid metabolic phenotypes for acetyltransferase and cytochrome P4501A2 and putative exposure to food-borne heterocyclic amines increase the risk for colorectal cancer or polyps. Cancer Epidemiol Biomarkers Preven 3:675–682.

Lawley PD (1994): From fluorescence spectra to mutational spectra, a historical overview of DNA-reactive compounds. In Hemminki K, Dipple A, Shuker DEG, Kadlubar FF, Segerbäck D, Bartsch H (eds.): "DNA adducts, identification and biological significance" Lyon: IARC Sci Publ No. 125, pp 3–22.

Lin HJ, Han C-Y, Bernstein DA, Hsiao W, Lin BK, Hardy S (1994a): Ethnic distribution of the glutathione transferase Mu 1-1 (*GSTM1*) null genotype in 1473 individuals and application to bladder cancer susceptibility. Carcinogenesis 15:1077–1081.

Lin HJ, Han C-Y, Lin BK, Hardy S (1994b): Ethnic distribution of slow acetylator mutations in the polymorphic *N*-acetyltransferase (NAT2) gene. Pharmacogenetics 4:125–134.

Lin D, Lay JO, Jr, Bryant MS, Malaveille C, Friesen M, Bartsch H, Lang NP, Kadlubar FF (1994): Analysis of 4-aminobiphenyl-DNA adducts in human urinary bladder and lung by alkaline hydrolysis and negative ion gas chromatography-mass spectrometry. Environ Health Prespectives 102:11–16.

Loft S, Vistisen K, Ewertz M, Tjonneland A, Overvard K, Poulsen HE (1992): Oxidative DNA-damage estimated by 8-hydroxyguanosine excretion in man: Influence of smoking, gender and body mass index. Carcinogenesis 13:2241–1147.

London SJ, Daly AK, Thomas DC, Caporaso NE, Idle JR (1994): Methodological issues in the interpretation of studies of the CYP2D6 genotype in relation to lung cancer risk. Pharmacogenetics 4:107–108.

Miles JS, Wolf CR (1991): Developments and prespectives on the role of cytochrome P450s in chemical carcinogenesis. Carcinogenesis 12:2195–2199.

Miller EC, Miller JA (1981): Searches for ultimate chemical carcinogens and their reactions with cellular macromolecules. Cancer 47:2327–2345.

Mommsen S, Aagaard J (1986): Susceptibility in urinary bladder cabcer: acetyltransferase phenotypes and related risk factors. Cancer Lett 32:199–205

Murphy SE, Hecht SS (1985): Dual-lable high-performance liquid chromatographic assay for femtomole levels of benzo[a]pyrene metabolites. Anal Biochem 146:442–447.

Newcomb PA, Carbone PP (1992): The health consequences of smoking: cancer. Med Clin N Am 76:305–331.

Peluso M, Castegnaro M, Malaveille C, Friesen M, Garren L, Hautefeuille H, Vineis P, Kadlubar FF, Bartsch H (1991): ^{32}P–Postlabelling analysis of urinary mutagens from smokers of black tobacco implicates 2-amino-1-methyl-6- phenylimidazo[4,5-b] pyridine (PhIP) as a major DNA-damaging agent. Carcinogenesis 12:713–717.

Pfohl-Leszkowicz A, Grosse Y, Castegnaro M, Nicolov IG, Chernozemsky IN, Bartsch H, Betbeder Am, Creppy EE, Dirheimer G (1993): Ochratoxin A-related DNA adducts in urinary tract tumours of Bulgarian subjects. In Phillips DH, Castegnaro M, Bartsch H (eds): "Postlabelling methods for detection of DNA adducts" Lyon: IARC Sci Publ No 124, pp 141–148.

Poirier MC (1994): Human exposure monitoring, dosimetry, and cancer risk assessment: The use of antisera specific for carcinogen–DNA adducts and carcinogen–modified DNA. Drug Metabolism Rev 26:87–109.

Poirier MC, Fullerton NFM, Kinouchi T, Smith BA, Beland FA (1991): Comparison between DNA adduct formation and tumourigenesis in livers and bladders of mice chronically fed 2-acetylaminofluorene. Carcinogenesis 12:895–900.

Poirier MC, Beland FA (1992): DNA adduct measurments and tumour incidence during chronic carcinogen exposure in animal models: implications for DNA adduct-based human cancer risk assessment. Chem Res Toxicol 5:749–755.

Potter JD, McMichael AJ (1986): Diet and cancer of the colon and rectum: a case-control study. J Natl Cancer Inst 76:557–569.

Randerath E, Miller RH, Mittal D, Avitts TA, Dunsford HA, Randerath K (1989): Covalent DNA damage in tissues of cigarette smokers as determined by ^{32}P-postlabelling assay. J Natl Cancer Inst 81:341–347.

Randerath E, Randerath K (1993): Monitoring tobacco smoke-induced DNA damage by ^{32}P-postlabelling. In: Postlabelling methods for detection of DNA adducts. Phillips DH, Castegnaro M, Bartsch H (eds). IARC Sci Publ No 124, pp 305–314, IARC, Lyon.

Rubino GF, Scansetti G, Pioltto G (1982): The carcinogenic effects of aromatic amines:

an epidemiological study on the role of *o*–toluidine and 4,4'– methylene bis(2–methylaniline) in inducing bladder cancer in man. Environ Res 27:241–5.

Saffhill R, Margison GP, O'Connor PJ (1985): Mechanisms of carcinogenesis induced by alkylating agents. Biochem Biophys Acta 823:111–145.

Silverman DT, Hartge P, Morrison AS, Devesa SS (1992): Epidemiology of bladder cancer. Hematol Oncol Clin N Am. 6:1–30.

Singhal SS, Saxena M, Awasthi S, Ahmed H, Sharma R, Awasthi YC (1992): Gender related differences in expression and characteristics of glutathione *S*–transferases of human colon. Biochem Biophys Acta 1171:19–26.

Sivaraman L, Leatham MP, Wilkens LR, Lau AF, Marchand LL (1994): CYP1A1 genetic polymorphisms and *in situ* colorectal cancer. Cancer Res 54: 3692–3695.

Souliotis VL, Zongza V, Nikolopoulou V, Dimitriodis GJ (1992): Measurment of O^6–Alkylguanine–typeadducts in DNA and O^6–Alkylguanine–DNA–alkyltransferase repair activity in normal and neoplastic human tissues. Comparative Biochem Physiol 101:269– 275.

Stern SJ, Degawa M, Martin M, Guengerich FP, Kaderlik RK, Ilett KF, Breau R, McGhee M, Montague D, Lyn–Cook B, Kadlubar FF (1993): Metabolic activation, DNA adducts,and H–*ras* mutations in human neoplastic and non–neoplastic laryngeal tissue. J Cell Biochem 17F:129–137.

Sugimura T (1986): Studies on environmental chemical carcinogenesis in Japan. Science 233:312–318.

Sugimura T, Sato S (1983): Mutagens–carcinogens in foods. Cancer Res 43: 2415–2421.

Talaska G, Al–Juburi AZSS, Kadlubar FF (1991a): Smoking related carcinogen–DNA adducts in biopsy samples of human urinary bladder: identification of *N*–(deoxyguanosin– 8–yl)–4–aminobi phenyl as a major adduct. Proc Natl Acad Sci USA 88:5350–5354.

Talaska G, Schamer M, Skipper P, Tannenbaum S, Caporaso N, Unruh L, Kadlubar FF, Bartsch H, Malaveille C, Vineis P (1991b): Detection of carcinogen–DNA adducts in exfoliated urothelialcells of cigarette smokers: association with smoking, hemoglobin adducts and urinary mutagenicity. Cancer Epidemiol Biomarkers Prev 1:61–66.

Talaska G, Schamer M, Skipper P, Tannenbaum S, Caporaso N, Kadlubar F, Bartsch H, Vineis P (1993): Carcinogen-DNA adducts in exfoliated urothelial cells: techniques for noninvasive human monitoring. Environ Health Presp 99:289–291.

Tefre T, Daly AK, Armstrong M, Leathart JBS, Idle JB, Brogger A, Borresen A-L (1994): Genotyping of CYP2D6 gene in Norwegian lung cancer patients and control. Pharmacogenetics 4:47–57.

Trell E, Krosgaard R, Hood B, Kitzing P, Nordern G, Simonsson BG (1976): Aryl hydrocarbon hydroxylase inducibility and laryngeal carcinomas. Lancet 2:140.

Turesky RJ, Lang NP, Butler MA, Teitel CH, Kadlubar FF (1991): Metabolic activation of carcinogenic heterocyclic aromatic amines by human liver and colon. Carcinogenesis 12:1839–1845.

Uematsu F, Ikawa S, Kikuchi H, Sagami I, Kanamaru R, Abe T, Satoh K, Motomiya M, Watanabe M (1994): Restriction fragment length polymorphism of human CYP2E1 (cytochrome P450IIE1) gene and susceptibility to lung cancer: possible relevance to low smoking exposure. Pharmacogenetics 4:58–63.

US Department of Health and Human Services (1982): The health consequences of smoking: cancer. A Report of the Surgeon General. US Department of Health and Human Services, Public Health Services, Office of the Assistant Secretary for Health, Office of Smoking and Health. DHHS Publication No. (PHS) 82–50179.

Vatsis KP, Weber WW (1993): Structural heterogenicity of Caucasian *N*-acetyl transferase at NAT1 gene locus. Arch Biochem Biophys 301:71–76.

Vesell ES (1985): Genetic host factors: determinants of drug response. New Eng J Med 313:261–262.

Vineis P, Caporaso N, Tannenbaum SR, Skipper PL, Glogowski J, Bartsch H, Coda M, Talaska G, Kadlubar FF (1990): Acetylation phenotype, carcinogen-hemoglobin adducts, and cigarette smoking. Cancer Res 50:3002–3004.

Vineis P, Bartsch H, Caporaso N, Harrington AM, Kadlubar FF, Landi MT, Malaveille C, Shields PG, Skipper P, Talaska G, Tannenbaum SR (1994): Genetically based *N*-acetyltransferase metabolic polymorphism and low-level environmental exposure to carcinogens. Nature (*Lond*) 369:154–156.

Vineis P, Simonato L (1986): Estimates for the proportions of bladder cancer attributable to occupation. Scand J Work Environ Health 12:55–60.

Vineis P (1992): Epidemiological models of carcinogenesis: The example of bladder cancer. Cancer Epidemiol Biomarkers Preven 1:149–53.

Ward E, Smith AB, Halperin W (1987): 4,4'-Methylene-bis(2-chloroaniline): an unregulated carcinogen. Am J Ind Med 12:537–549.

Ward E, Carpenter A, Markowitz S, Roberts D, Halpering W (1991): Excess number of bladder cancer in workers exposed to ortho-toluidine and aniline. J Natl Cancer Inst 83:501–506.

Weber WW, Hein DW (1985): *N*-Acetylation pharmacogenetics. Pharmacol Rev 37:25–79.

Weber WW, Vatsis KP (1993): Individual variability in *p*-aminobenzoic acid *N*-acetylation by human *N*-acetyltransferase (NAT1) of peripheral blood. Pharmacogenetics 3: 209–212.

Willett WC, Stampfer GA, Colditz BA, Rosner BA, Speizer FE (1990): Relation of meat, fat, and fiber intake to the risk of colon cancer in a prospective study among women. New Engl J Med 323:1664–1672.

Wingo, PA, Tong T, Bolden S (1995): Cancer statistics, 1995. CA, Cancer J Clin 45:8–30.

Wohlleb JC, Hunter CF, Blass B, Kadlubar FF, Chu DZ, Lang NP (1990): Aromatic amine acetyltransferase as a marker for colorectal cancer: environmental and demographic associations. Int J Cancer 46:22–30.

Wynder EL, Stellman SD (1979): Impact of long-term filter cigarette usage on lung and larynx cancer risk: A case-control study. J Natl Cancer Inst 62:471–479.

Yu MC, Skipper PL, Taghizadeh K, Tannenbaum SR, Chan KK, Henderson BE, Ross RK (1994): Acetylator phenotype, aminobiphenyl-hemoglobin adduct levels, and bladder cancer risk in white, black and Asian men in Los Angeles, California. J Natl Cancer Inst 86:712–716.

Zhong S, Wyille AH, Barnes D, Wolf CR, Spurr NK (1993): Relationship between the GSTM1 genetic polymorphism and susceptibility to bladder, breast, and colon cancer. carcinogenesis 14:1821–1824.

Genetics and Cancer Susceptibility:
Implications for Risk Assessment, pages 141–157

MOLECULAR EPIDEMIOLOGY

Peter G. Shields, M.D.
Molecular Epidemiology Section
Laboratory of Human Carcinogenesis
National Cancer Institute
Building 37, Room 2C16
Bethesda, MD 20892

INTRODUCTION TO MOLECULAR EPIDEMIOLOGY

The field of molecular epidemiology seeks to identify cancer risk based upon individual exposures and susceptibilities to cancer. The overall goal is to develop, apply and validate biomarkers of cancer risk in order to enhance cancer risk assessments, focus cancer prevention strategies and elucidate mechanisms of carcinogenesis. Our laboratory and others have the immediate objectives of developing assays for determining biologically effective doses of carcinogens and mutagens; develop, apply and validate biomarkers of inherited cancer susceptibility; determine the mutational spectra of key oncogenes and tumor suppressor genes as a marker of exposure and susceptibility; and among the most important, is to assess the relationship between environmental exposure, carcinogen-DNA adducts, inherited susceptibility, mutational spectra and cancer risk. Studies that can identify gene-environment and gene-gene interactions are specifically being developed and implemented.

Two fundamental principles that underlie current studies of molecular epidemiology relate to the complexity of the carcinogenesis process and the fact that individuals vary in response to carcinogenic exposures. For the first, cancer is a multistage process where behind each stage are several genetic events, for which there are a multitude of steps leading to these events. These events might be triggered by exogenous exposures (e.g., chemicals, radiation or viruses), endogenous exposures (e.g., oxy-radicals) or enzymatic errors (e.g., polymerase or recombinase infidelity). Along with each of these triggers, there are yet several other processes that must occur or go awry. For example, for chemical exposures, it is not sufficient for cancer to develop simply from exposure. Before the development of a mutation in a cellular clone with selective survival advantage, a potential carcinogen has to be absorbed, undergo metabolic activation (which frequently requires several enzymatic steps), escape detoxification, be transported to a target organ, adduct a critical protooncogene or tumor suppressor gene, escape DNA repair, escape other mechanisms to control the damage such as cell death, and result in a mutation that affects the function of a critical gene. Thus, the multistage process of carcinogenesis is a very complicated process consisting of multiple steps and pathways.

The consideration of the multistage process of carcinogenesis, along with its multiple inciting events and processes contained within, suggests that our current epidemiological tools are severely limited. Case-control and cohort studies are hindered when trying to identify risk factors against a background of many other factors, steps and events. Important risk factors with large attributable risks (i.e., affecting a large segment or the population)are nevertheless obscured because of other unknown factors, the total of which is greater than the risk factor being studied. Risk factors with large attributable risks might only be associated with small relative risks. Studies will then have limited statistical power, increasing the likelihood of conflicting results among different studies. Small differences in study design or accrual might affect the results of the study, obscuring the importance of the risk factor. Therefore, those risk factors with consistent results among several studies are likely to be strong risk factors observable above a background of other factors.

The second fundamental principle of molecular epidemiology is based upon data demonstrating interindividual variation (Harris, 1989) in response to carcinogen exposure and carcinogenic processes. Currently, investigators tend to study the population as if it were homogeneous in its response to carcinogen exposure and/or the carcinogenic process. Laboratory scientists studying individual genes, for example, will clone genes from only one or two persons. Laboratory animal studies frequently use inbred strains to reduce genetic heterogeneity. Epidemiology studies, utilizing population based statistics, assume that all persons in a study group will respond similarly to a specific exposure. How much these approaches actually approximate the general population's response may be difficult to estimate, especially if a particular study (i.e., the development of a clone or studies of inbred rodents) represents an unknown polymorphic activity or if a response to exposure in an epidemiological study is modified by a genetic polymorphism. In fact, the population is actually quite heterogeneous. Different ages, gender, race, ethnicity, lifestyle (e.g., tobacco use, alcohol, exercise), diet, occupation, and recreational activities all might contribute to significant differences in responses to environmental agents, although the relative effects of these are currently unknown. Equally important are inherited differences in the host's response to specific exposures, such as in one's metabolic capacity to activate or detoxify carcinogens, and/or repair DNA damage.

The study of the population as a homogeneous group might limit the ability to identify new risk factors, gene-environment interactions or gene-gene interactions, because such factors or interactions in a particular susceptible subgroup might be obscured against within a number of subgroups with other factors or interactions. For example, in a study of breast cancer, one group of women might be susceptible to *N*-nitrosamines and develop G→A transitions in the p53 tumor suppressor gene because they have a genetic polymorphism that increases the rate of activation for *N*-nitrosamines. However, another group might be susceptible to polycyclic aromatic hydrocarbons and develop G→T transversions because of a different genetic polymorphism in another gene. If both groups are studied together, then the effects of either group are diluted by the other. In contrast, if the groups were studied independently by classifying them based upon the p53 tumor suppressor gene mutation, or by a particular genetic polymorphism, then the association might be more easily revealed.

An important approach within molecular epidemiology is to build a relationship between an exposure, susceptibility and clinical outcome. Rather than simply seeking associations between an exposure and disease, molecular epidemiology studies a number of intermediate endpoints and biological markers of both exposure and carcinogenesis (Fig. 1). Importantly, these biomarkers are postulated to be biologically linked to both the exposure and disease. By examining several biomarkers, carcinogenic mechanisms and risks might be elucidated. For example, evidence linking exogenous chemical exposures, blood metabolite levels, carcinogen-DNA adduct levels, mutations in critical genes, changes in cellular morphology, development of preneoplastic lesions and clinical cancer to each other provides clear evidence that particular exposure is related to the cancer. Studies that show differences in metabolic capacity (activation and detoxification) and DNA repair relating to the chemical exposure and resultant DNA damage provides further evidence. Separately, when the study of cancer becomes problematic in that latency periods require persons in the general population to be exposed for a long time before a relationship can be established, molecular epidemiological approaches that identify intermediate biomarkers of DNA damage or other cellular changes might suggest earlier intervention prior to the formation of clinical cancer. Although, at the current time, excepting some lesions that precede cancer, little is known about the actual risks of intermediate biomarkers of carcinogenesis.

Figure 1
Examples of Biomarkers of Exposure and Effect

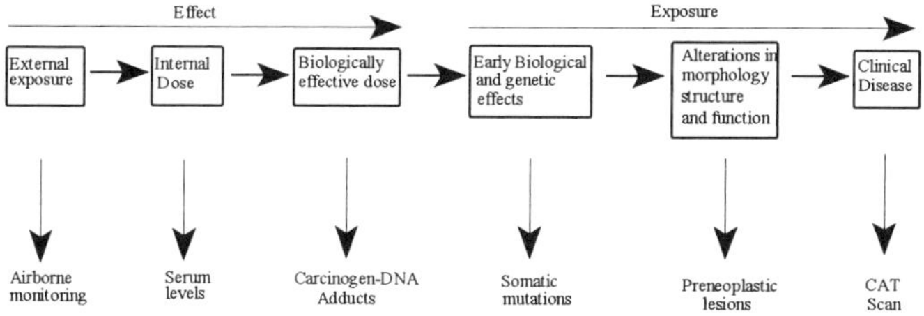

The limitations in identifying cancer risk factors, gene-environment interactions and gene-gene interactions, due to the complexities of multiple carcinogenic processes and population subgroups, require that different and novel types of corroborative molecular epidemiological studies be utilized. For example, when studies provide conflicting evidence for a particular risk factor, other types of studies might lend biological credence to those studies that are positive. Experimental studies, in vitro models and epidemiological studies with alternate hypotheses can be used. Some of these studies from our laboratory and others will be described below.

GENE-ENVIRONMENT AND GENE-GENE INTERACTIONS

Among the most interesting evidence to have come from molecular epidemiological studies are those demonstrating gene-environment and gene-gene interactions. These associations are among the most difficult to demonstrate because of limitations in statistical power, as described above. However, the repeated demonstration of such among different exposures, genes and cancers suggests that these interactions indeed exist. Interestingly, the data in some studies indicate that gene-environment interactions are more pronounced at lower levels of exposures while for others, the interactions occur at higher levels of exposure. Table I summarizes several examples of gene-environment interactions.

One example of an intriguing gene-environment interaction relates to a genetic polymorphism for cytochrome P450 (CYP) 1A1. Several polymorphisms have been identified. The first to be studied (Kawajiri et al., 1990) was for a locus 3' to the last exon of the gene and revealed by an *Msp*1 restriction fragment length polymorphism analysis. However, a change in biological function related to a change in the nucleotide base has not yet been reported. A second polymorphism (Hayashi et al., 1991) is an A→G base substitution responsible for an isoleucine to valine substitution (residue 462) in the catalytic heme binding region. This alteration has been related in vitro to an increased catalytic activity (Kawajiri et al., 1993; Crofts et al., 1994). In Japanese, the presence of the less common (minor) allele at the *Msp*1 site was predictive of the valine substitution (Hayashi et al., 1991; Okada et al., 1995). In this study (Nakachi et al., 1991; Okada et al., 1995), a gene-environment interaction was reported where the risk for lung cancer among persons who were homozygote for the "at risk" allele was greatest in persons who smoked less. In fact, the combination of the "at risk" genotype and light smoking yielded odds ratios similar to having the "lesser risk" genotype and heavier smoking. There also is one report that associates this polymorphism with increased stage of disease (Okada et al., 1995). The implication of this interaction is that in persons who smoke less, inherited susceptibilities can be important, but in heavier smokers, the genetics do not matter. It should be noted, however, that an association of *CYP1A1* polymorphisms and lung cancer risk has only been identified in Japanese, although studies in Western populations are limited due to statistical problems relating to the low prevalence of the "at risk" allele. Several Western studies of the *Msp*1 locus, including Caucasians (Shields et al., 1993; Alexandrie et al., 1994; Tefre et al., 1991; Hirvonen et al., 1992) and African-Americans

(Shields et al., 1993) did not find an increased risk. For the valine substitution, several studies (Hirvonen et al., 1992; Alexandrie et al., 1994) in Northern Europe have thus far not identified an increased risk, although one report from Brazil has found such an association in persons with squamous cell lung cancer (Hamada et al., 1995). The risk for the *CYP1A1* exon 7 genetic polymorphism in Caucasian- or African-Americans have not yet been reported, but the inheritance pattern for the *Msp*1 locus and the valine-substituted locus are different between Caucasian- and African-Americans (unpublished data).

There are several other examples of gene-environment interactions where at lower levels of exposure, the relative risk estimate is greater. One example where an intermediate carcinogenesis biomarker was studied relates to the N-acetyltransferase 2 gene (*NAT2*) and

Table I
Gene-Environment Interactions

1	*CYP1A1* "at risk" allele increases the risk of lung cancer in persons with lower degrees of cigarette use (Nakachi et al., 1991; Okada et al., 1995).
2	N-acetyltransferase 2 slow acetylation genotype increases the level of 4-aminobiphenyl hemoglobin adducts in persons with lower degrees of smoking or are exposed only passively to tobacco smoke (smoking degree reported by measuring urinary cotinine and nicotine levels) (Vineis et al., 1994).
3	*CYP2E1 minor allele* and *CYP2D6* extensive metabolizer genotype increases the level of 7-methyl-deoxyguanosine adducts in human lung tissues in persons with lower exposures to cigarette smoke (smoking degree reported by measuring serum cotinine) (Kato et al., 1995).
4	*CYP2D6* extensive metabolizer phenotype increases the risk of lung cancer in persons exposed to asbestos or polycyclic aromatic hydrocarbons (Caporaso et al., 1989).
5	N-acetyltransferase 2 rapid acetylator and *CYP1A2* rapid acetylator phenotypes increase the risk of colon cancer in persons exposed to dietary heterocyclic amines (Lang et al., 1994).
6	N-acetyltransferase 2 slow acetylation genotype increases the risk of breast cancer in persons with higher levels of cigarette smoking (unpublished data).
7	Glutathione-*S*-transferase M1 null genotype increases the risk of lung cancer among persons with lower degrees of smoking (London et al., 1995).

cigarette smoking. It was originally shown that the level of 4-aminobiphenyl hemoglobin adducts, where 4-aminobiphenyl is a constituent of cigarette smoke, was correlated with levels of cigarette smoking (Vineis et al., 1990). In fact, it was found that the levels correlated with the type of cigarette smoked (black versus blond), but that in all cases, levels were higher in persons who were phenotypically slow acetylators. It was hypothesized that the decreased detoxification by the *NAT2* in the liver led to an increased number of reactive metabolites that were available to adduct hemoglobin. The data have undergone further analysis (Vineis et al., 1994) when levels of cigarette smoking were determined in study subjects by measuring urinary nicotine and cotinine. The analysis suggested that persons with passive tobacco smoke exposure and were slow acetylators were at a proportional greater risk of forming adducts compared to active tobacco smokers.

A polymorphism in the glutathione-*S*-transferase (*GSTM1*) (Mannervik et al., 1992) results in a deletion of the entire gene (Seidegard et al., 1988). Phenotypically, using cultured blood cells and trans-stilbene oxide conjugation, this polymorphism has been related to lung cancer risk in several studies (Seidegard et al., 1990; Nazar-Stewart et al., 1993), although not consistently (Heckbert et al., 1992). The lack of activity also has been associated with increased polycyclic aromatic hydrocarbon-DNA adducts in human lung tissue (Kato et al., 1995), sister chromatid exchange formation (Wiencke et al., 1990; van Poppel et al., 1992) and mutagenicity of human lung microsomes in the Ames' assay (Bartsch et al., 1991). The application of PCR to the study of this gene has revealed an association of the null genotype with lung cancer in several Caucasian groups (Nazar-Stewart et al., 1993; Zhong et al., 1991; Hirvonen et al., 1993), especially squamous cell cancers (Zhong et al., 1991; Hirvonen et al., 1993), although some studies have not found such an association (Brockmöller et al., 1993). There also is a report of an over-representation of the null genotype in European women with squamous cell lung cancer (Alexandrie et al., 1994). In a recent report by London, et al.,(London et al., 1995), the risk for lung cancer was seen only in persons with squamous cell cancer and those with less than 40 pack-years of smoking. However, the literature, reviewed in the same London, et al., paper (London et al., 1995) suggests that there are considerable inconsistencies in this area.

The cytochrome P450 2D6 (*CYP2D6*)gene has been one of the earliest polymorphisms to be associated with lung cancer (Ayesh et al., 1984). This association has been found in other studies (Caporaso et al., 1990), although not consistently (reviewed in Caporaso, et al. (Caporaso et al., 1995)). The activity can be measured phenotypically (Mahgoub et al., 1977; Green-Gallo et al., 1991) or genetically (Heim, Meyer, 1990). While reports suggest that PCR-based assays are adequate to estimate the activity (Heim, Meyer, 1990), there are now over 10 different polymorphisms (Table 2) (Heim, Meyer, 1990; Gonzalez et al., 1988; Saxena et al., 1994; Evert et al., 1994; Johansson et al., 1993; Armstrong et al., 1994; Wang et al., 1993; Kondo et al., 1991; Kagimoto et al., 1990; Hanioka et al., 1990; Gaedigk et al., 1991) identified in this gene, where some decrease activity while others increase activity. Moreover, families have been identified (Johansson et al., 1993) that have inherited amplified copies of the gene that result in significantly increased rates of metabolism. Thus, the firmest associations of *CYP2D6* and lung cancer remains in studies that have measured phenotypes (through the administration of Debrisoquine). A gene-environment interaction for *CYP2D6* and lung cancer has been suggested through several types of analyses. One approach (Caporaso et al., 1995) has been to examine the differences for smoking in studies that report positive and negative associations. It has been suggested (Caporaso et al., 1995) that there is a relationship to smoking where only those studies that use study groups with heavy smokers are the likeliest to reveal the association. Nonetheless, there also is an apparent association of extensive metabolism and increased 7-methyl-deoxyguanosine adducts in human lung tissue (Kato et al., 1995), which appears to be greatest in persons with lowest serum cotinine levels, analogous to studies reported above. Although, the numbers of poor metabolizers in this study were small. Lastly, a gene-environment interaction is suggested in an analysis of lung cancer risk and *CYP2D6* where risks of lung cancer increase significantly in persons who also report occupational exposure to polycyclic aromatic hydrocarbons or asbestos (Caporaso et al., 1989).

The study of gene-gene interactions has been more difficult due to statistical power where low numbers of study subjects with particular combinations of genetic variants decreases. In Japanese, where the rates of *CYP1A1* minor alleles and *GSTM1* null genotypes are greater than in other populations, studies (Hayashi et al., 1992) have been able to assess the combined relationships. The null genotype was additive to the risk of the *CYP1A1* minor allele and increased the cigarette smoking-related lung cancer risk (Kihara, Noda, 1994).

In a study that demonstrates both a gene-gene interaction and gene-environment interaction, Lang and coworkers (Lang et al., 1994) reported that neither *NAT2* or *CYP1A2* independently predicted colon cancer or polyp risk. However the combined rapid-rapid phenotypes was statistically associated with risk, yielding an odds ratio of 2.91 in logistic regression. Moreover, the consumption of well-done meat, in the same logistic regression model yielded a statistically significant odds ratio of 2.08.

CORROBORATIVE STUDIES IN MOLECULAR EPIDEMIOLOGY

While case-control and cohort studies remain the best approaches to determining risk in the general population, other methods and novel studies are needed to corroborate findings from these studies. As described above, case-control and cohort studies lack sensitivity and these methods cannot establish biological or mechanistic relationships. Our laboratory and others have been exploring different approaches, some of which will be described below.

A corroborative laboratory approach that examines intermediate biomarkers of carcinogenesis is essential for providing confirmatory data. We have established a data set of lung tissues from human autopsy donors (n=90) (Kato et al., 1995). These individuals generally died of sudden death, are young and free of cancer. This approach allows us to examine carcinogen-DNA adduct formation where the presence of disease would not alter metabolism

TABLE 2
***CYP2D6* GENETIC POLYMORPHISMS**

Designation	Nucleotide sequence	Amino acid change	*Xba*1 RFLP by Southern Blot	Enzyme Activity	Comments
CYP2D6	WT	--	29	Normal	Wildtype
CYP2D6A	Del A - 2367	Yes	29	Absent	Stop Codon
CYP2D6B	G→T - 1934	Yes	29 or 44	Absent	Splice site defect
CYP2D6C	Del AAG - 2702	Yes	29	?↓↑	Increased lung cancer risk reported
CYP2D6D	Deleted	Yes	11.5	Absent	Entire gene deleted
CYP2D6J	C→T - 188	Yes	42, 44 or 29	?↓	Seen in Chinese; Same as CYP2DCH1
CYP2D6J	G→C - 4268	Yes	42, 44 or 29	?↓	Same as CYP2D6L
CYP2D6L	C→T - 2938	Yes	175, 44, 42 or 29	?↑	Not found in the CYP2D6J so may be linked to amplified gene

TABLE 2 - CONTINUED
***CYP2D6* GENETIC POLYMORPHISMS**

Designation	Nucleotide sequence	Amino acid change	*Xba*1 RFLP by Southern Blot	Enzyme Activity	Comments
CYP2D6L	G→C - 4268	Yes	175, 44, 42 or 29	?↓↑	Same as CYP2D6J, reported along with amplification
CYP2D6L	G→C - 1726	No	175, 44, 42 or 29	--	Not reported in CYP2D6J
CYP2D6CH1	C→T - 188	Yes	29, 42 or 44	↓	Same as CYP2D6J
CYP2D6T	DEL T - 1795	Yes	29	↓	Low frequency in population but occurs in some people with B mutation.

or lifestyle. The tissues from this study set provide an in vivo "snapshot" of the interaction of exposure and the host's capacity to metabolize, detoxify and repair. To date, 7-methyl-2'-deoxyguanosine, 7-ethyl-2'-deoxyguanosine and polycyclic aromatic hydrocarbon-2'-deoxyguanosine adducts have been measured. Associations have been identified relating 7-methyl-2"deoxyguanosine with *CYP2E1* and *CYP2D6* genetic polymorphisms (Kato et al., 1995), supporting a role for these genetic polymorphisms in lung cancer. Also, an association for the polycyclic aromatic hydrocarbon-2'-deoxyguanosine adducts and the *GSTM1* null genotypes was found, providing further evidence for the role of this gene and its genetic polymorphism. Importantly, thee studies have been performed in target tissues. Other studies are now focusing on the relationship of these adducts and genetic polymorphisms to quantity and activity of the proteins involved in metabolism and detoxification.

The findings of *CYP1A1* and increased risk of lung cancer in Japanese at lower levels of tobacco smoke exposure has led us to look for other Oriental populations where similar studies could be conducted. We have decided to focus on Chinese populations from the Peoples Republic of China because of lung cancer patterns there. In that country, the rates of lung cancer among non-smoking women are high (Jin et al., 1993; Fraumeni, Jr., Mason, 1974; MacLennan et al., 1977; International Agency for Research on Cancer, 1992). Epidemiologically, several risk factors have been identified (Wu-Williams et al., 1990; Gao et al., 1987), including exposure to smoke from cooking oils. This smoke has been found to be mutagenic in several different assays (Qu et al., 1992; Shields et al., 1995) and to contain potential human carcinogens such as 1,3-butadiene and aldehydes (Shields et al., 1995). Therefore, we are currently conducting a population-based case-control study of non-smoking women in two Chinese cities (Shanghai and Harbin) that will allow us to examine genetic polymorphisms, exposure to cooking oils and other forms of indoor air pollution and lung cancer risk.

If we hypothesize that specific variants of carcinogen metabolizing genes leads to increased risk of cancer, then the converse variant might lead to a decreased risk of that same cancer. To test this hypothesis, we have performed a pilot study of one hundred men who are older than 65 years of age and have a smoking history of greater than 40 pack-years (average number of packs smoked per day in a life time times the number of years smoked). There are inherent difficulties in studying this hypothesis because the chosen study design actually considers total survival from all diseases, thus limiting the statistical power. Secondly, there is no suitable control population to identify differences in gene frequency. For these reasons, we decided to limit our initial study and seek large differences in gene frequency compared to the rates reported for the general population. The data for several polymorphisms are currently being analyzed.

In a separate attempt to elucidate the importance of genetic polymorphisms, we have established a study set of tumors from individuals from different countries in order to examine an association of specific p53 mutations and genetic polymorphisms. This effort involves over ten different collaborators from four countries and utilizes over four hundred tumors. Previously, it has been reported that persons with the *GSTM1* null genotype had a greater risk

Table 3
Evaluating Cancer Etiology
Sir Austin Bradford-Hill Criteria (Hill, 1965)

Criteria	Explanation
Strength of Association	What is the magnitude of the risk?
Consistency	Are there repeated observations by multiple investigators in different populations?
Specificity	Is the effect specific or are there other known causes
Temporality	Does exposure preceded effect?
Biological gradient	Is there a dose-response relationship?
Biological Plausibility	Is the effect predictable?
Coherence	Is the effect consistent with other scientific data?
Analogy	Do other similar agents act similarly?

G→T transversions (Ryberg et al., 1994). One limitation of this study is that for many individuals, exposure data are not available. Nonetheless, crude associations for transitions and transitions for *GSTM1*, *CYP1A1*, *CYP2D6*, *CYP2E1* and *NAT2* genetic polymorphisms will be determined.

CONCLUSIONS

The field of molecular epidemiology is now firmly established, although, compared to other areas of epidemiology, it remains in its infancy. Many investigators have used a variety of approaches to show that the methods are useful and that gene-environment interactions can be demonstrated. Which applications and genes will be important to the carcinogenic process, and which data will be useful for cancer risk assessments needs to be determined. As with other areas of epidemiology, however, specific guidelines, such as those proposed by Sir Austin Bradford-Hill (Table 3) (Hill, 1965), continue to be useful in identifying cancer risk factors. The elucidation of cancer etiologies will require multiple rigorous corroborative studies examining a variety of endpoints.

ACKNOWLEDGMENTS

The author would like to thank the efforts of the following collaborators and co-investigators who have contributed substantially to the work and ongoing studies cited herein: S. Kato, E.D. Bowman, A.M. Harrington, B. Blomeke, G.E. Trivers, A. Weston, S. Petruzzelli, V.D. Doan, X. Xu, Y.H. Qu, Y.T. Goa, E.,D. Pellizzari, W.J. Blot, J.F. Fraumeni, N.E. Caporaso, M.A. Tucker, B.F. Trump, and C.C. Harris. The author also would like to thank the cooperation of the following hospitals: University of Maryland, Loch Raven Veterans Administration, Union Memorial, St. Agnes, Sinai, Harbor Center, Mercy Medical Center and Northwest Medical Center.

REFERENCE LIST

Alexandrie AK, Sundberg MI, Seidegard J, Tornling G, Rannug A (1994): Genetic susceptibility to lung cancer with special emphasis on CYP1A1 and GSTM1: A study on host factors in relation to age at onset, gender and histological cancer types. Carcinogenesis 15:1785-1790.

Armstrong M, Fairbrother K, Idle JR, Daly AK (1994): The cytochrome P450 CYP2D6 allelic variant CYP2D6J and related polymorphisms in a European population. Pharmacogenetics 4:73-81.

Ayesh R, Idle JR, Ritchie JC, Crothers MJ, Hetzel MR (1984): Metabolic oxidation phenotypes as markers for susceptibility to lung cancer. Nature 312:169-170.

Bartsch H, Petruzzelli S, De Flora S, Hietanen E, Camus AM, Castegnaro M, Geneste O, Camoirano A, Saracci R, Giuntini C (1991): Carcinogen metabolism and DNA adducts in human lung tissues as affected by tobacco smoking or metabolic phenotype: a case-control study on lung cancer patients. Mutat Res 250:103-114.

Brockmöller J, Kerb R, Drakoulis N, Nitz M, Roots I (1993): Genotype and phenotype of glutathione S-transferase class mu isoenzymes mu and psi in lung cancer patients and controls. Cancer Res 53:1004-1011.

Caporaso N, Hayes RB, Dosemeci M, Hoover R, Ayesh R, Hetzel M, Idle JR (1989): Lung cancer risk, occupational exposure, and the debrisoquine metabolic phenotype. Cancer Res 49:3675-3679.

Caporaso N, DeBaun MR, Rothman N (1995): Lung cancer and CYP2D6 (the debrisoquine polymorphism): sources of heterogeneity in the proposed association. Pharmacogen 5:S129-S134.

Caporaso NE, Tucker MA, Hoover R, Hayes RB, Pickle LW, Issaq H, Muschik G, Green-Gallo L, Buivys D, Aisner S, Resau J, Trump BF, Tollerud D, Weston A, Harris CC (1990): Lung cancer and the debrisoquine metabolic phenotype. J Natl Cancer Inst 85:1264-1272.

Crofts F, Taioli E, Trachman J, Cosma GN, Currie D, Toniolo P, Garte SJ (1994): Functional significance of different human CYP1A1 genotypes. Carcinogenesis 15:2961-2963.

Evert B, Griese EU, Eichelbaum M (1994): Cloning and sequencing of a new non-functional CYP2D6 allele: deletion of T1795 in exon 3 generates a premature stop codon. Pharmacogen 4:271-274.

Fraumeni JF, Jr., Mason TJ (1974): Cancer mortality among Chinese Americans, 1950-69. J Natl Cancer Inst 52:659-665.

Gaedigk A, Blum M, Gaedigk R, Eichelbaum M, Meyer UA (1991): Deletion of the entire cytochrome P450 CYP2D6 gene as a cause of impaired drug metabolism in poor metabolizers of the debrisoquine/sparteine polymorphism. Am J Hum Genet 48:943-950.

Gao YT, Blot WJ, Zheng W, Ershow AG, Hsu CW, Levin LI, Zhang R, Fraumeni JF, Jr. (1987): Lung cancer among Chinese women. Int J Cancer 40:604-609.

Gonzalez FJ, Skoda RC, Kimura S, Umeno M, Zanger UM, Nebert DW, Gelboin HV, Hardwick JP, Meyer UA (1988): Characterization of the common genetic defect in humans deficient in debrisoquine metabolism. Nature 331:442-446.

Green-Gallo LA, Buivys DM, Fisher KL, Caporaso N, Slawson RG, Elias G, Didolkar MS, Ivusich WJ, Resau JH (1991): A protocol for the safe administration of debrisoquine in biochemical epidemiologic research protocols for hospitalized patients. Cancer 68:206-210.

Hamada GS, Sugimura H, Suzuki I, Nagura K, Kiyokawa E, Iwase T, Tanaka M, Takahashi T, Watanabe S, Kino I, Tsugane S (1995): The heme-binding region polymorphism of cytochrome P450IA1 (CypIA1), rather than the RsaI polymorphism of IIE1 (CypIIE1), is associated with lung cancer in Rio de Janeiro. CEBP 4:63-67.

Hanioka N, Kimura S, Meyer UA, Gonzalez FJ (1990): The human CYP2D locus associated with a common genetic defect in drug oxidation: a G1934——A base change in intron 3 of a mutant CYP2D6 allele results in an aberrant 3' splice recognition site. Am J Hum Genet 47:994-1001.

Harris CC (1989): Interindividual variation among humans in carcinogen metabolism, DNA adduct formation and DNA repair. Carcinogenesis 10:1563-1566.

Hayashi S, Watanabe J, Nakachi K, Kawajiri K (1991): Genetic linkage of lung cancer-associated MspI polymorphisms with amino acid replacement in the heme binding region of the human cytochrome P450IA1 gene. J Biochem (Tokyo) 110:407-411.

Hayashi SI, Watanabe J, Kawajiri K (1992): High susceptibility to lung cancer in terms of combined genotypes of P450IA1 and Mu-class glutathione S-transferase genes. Jpn J Cancer Res 83:866-870.

Heckbert SR, Weiss NS, Hornung SK, Eaton DL, Motulsky AG (1992): Glutathione S-transferase and epoxide hydrolase activity in human leukocytes in relation to risk of lung cancer and other smoking-related cancers. J Natl Cancer Inst 84:414-422.

Heim M, Meyer UA (1990): Genotyping of poor metabolizers of debrisoquine by allele-specific PCR amplification. Lancet 336:529-532.

Hill AB (1965): The environment and disease: association or causation. Proc Royal Soc Med 58:295-300.

Hirvonen A, Husgafvel-Pursiainen K, Karjalainen A, Anttila S, Vainio H (1992): Point-mutational Msp1 and Ile-Val polymorphisms closely linked in the CYP1A1 gene: lack of association with susceptibility to lung cancer in a Finnish study population. CEBP 1:485-489.

Hirvonen A, Husgafvel-Pursiainen K, Anttila S, Vainio H (1993): The GSTM1 null genotype as a potential risk modifier for squamous cell carcinoma of the lung. Carcinogenesis 14:1479-1481.

International Agency for Research on Cancer (1992): Cancer Incidence in Five Continents, Volume VI. Lyon, France: IARC.

Jin F, Devesa SS, Zheng W, Blot WJ, Fraumeni JF, Jr., Gao YT (1993): Cancer incidence trends in urban Shanghai, 1972-1989. Int J Cancer 53:764-770.

Johansson I, Lundqvist E, Bertilsson L, Dahl ML, Sjoqvist F, Ingelman-Sundberg M (1993): Inherited amplification of an active gene in the cytochrome P450 CYP2D locus as a cause of ultrarapid metabolism of debrisoquine. Proc Natl Acad Sci U S A 90:11825-11829.

Kagimoto M, Heim M, Kagimoto K, Zeugin T, Meyer UA (1990): Multiple mutations of the human cytochrome P450IID6 gene (CYP2D6) in poor metabolizers of debrisoquine. Study of the functional significance of individual mutations by expression of chimeric genes. J Biol Chem 265:17209-17214.

Kato S, Bowman ED, Harrington AM, Blomeke B, Shields PG (1995): Human lung carcinogen-DNA adduct levels mediated by genetic polymorphisms in vivo. JNCI 87:902-907.

Kawajiri K, Nakachi K, Imai K, Yoshii A, Shinoda N, Watanabe J (1990): Identification of genetically high risk individuals to lung cancer by DNA polymorphisms of the cytochrome P450IA1 gene. FEBS 263:131-133.

Kawajiri K, Nakachi K, Imai K, Watanabe J, Hayashi S (1993): The CYP1A1 gene and cancer susceptibility. Crit Rev Oncol Hematol 14:77-87.

Kihara M, Noda K (1994): Lung cancer risk of GSTM1 null genotype is dependent on the extent of tobacco smoke exposure. Carcinogenesis 15:415-418.

Kondo I, Yonaha M, Okano K, Gonzalez FJ, Kanazawa I (1991): Identification of a novel CYP2D6 allele associated with poor metabolism of sparteine in a Japanese population. Pharmacogenetics 1:161-164.

Lang NP, Butler MA, Massengill J, Lawson M, Stotts RC, Hauer-Jensen M, Kadlubar FF (1994): Rapid metabolic phenotypes for acetyltransferase and cytochrome P4501A2 and putative exposure to food-borne heterocyclic amines increase the risk for colorectal cancer or polyps. Cancer Epidemiol Biomarkers Prev 3:675-682.

London SJ, Daly AK, Cooper J, Navidi WC, Carpenter CL, Idle JR (1995): Polymorphism of glutathione S-transferase M1 and lung cancer risk among African-Americans and Caucasians in Los Angeles County, California. JNCI 87:1246-1252.

MacLennan R, Da Costa J, Day NE, Law CH, Ng YK, Shanmugaratnam K (1977): Risk factors for lung cancer in Singapore Chinese, a population with high female incidence rates. Int J Cancer 20:854-860.

Mahgoub A, Idle JR, Dring LG, Lancaster R, Smith RL (1977): Polymorphic hydroxylation of Debrisoquine in man. Lancet 2:584-586.

Mannervik B, Awasthi YC, Board PG, Hayes JD, di Ilio C, Ketterer B, Listowsky I, Morgenstern R, Muramatsu M, Pearson WR, et al (1992): Nomenclature for human glutathione transferases [letter]. Biochem J 282:305-306.

Nakachi K, Imai K, Hayashi S, Watanabe J, Kawajiri K (1991): Genetic susceptibility to squamous cell carcinoma of the lung in relation to cigarette smoking dose. Cancer Res 51:5177-5180.

Nazar-Stewart V, Motulsky AG, Eaton DL, White E, Hornung SK, Leng ZT, Stapleton P, Weiss NS (1993): The glutathione S-transferase mu polymorphism as a marker for susceptibility to lung carcinoma. Cancer Res 53:2313-2318.

Okada T, Kawashima K, Fukushi S, Minakuchi T, Nishimura S (1995): Association between a cytochrome P450 CYPIA1 genotype and incidence of lung cancer. Pharmacogen 4:333-340.

Qu YH, Xu GX, Zhou JZ, Chen TD, Zhu LF, Shields PG, Wang HW, Gao YT (1992): Genotoxicity of heated cooking oil vapors. Mutat Res 298:105-111.

Ryberg D, Kure E, Lystad S, Skaug V, Stangeland L, Mercy I, Borresen AL, Haugen A (1994): p53-mutations in lung tumors. Relationship to putative susceptibility markers for cancer. Cancer Res 54:1551-1555.

Saxena R, Shaw GL, Relling MV, Frame JN, Moir DT, Evans WE, Caporaso N, Weiffenbach B (1994): Identification of a new variant CYP2D6 allele with a single base deletion in exon 3 and its association with the poor metabolizer phenotype. Hum Mol Genet 3:923-926.

Seidegard J, Vorachek WR, Pero RW, Pearson WR (1988): Hereditary differences in the expression of the human glutathione transferase active on trans-stilbene oxide are due to a gene deletion. Proc Natl Acad Sci U S A 85:7293-7297.

Seidegard J, Pero RW, Markowitz MM, Roush G, Miller DG, Beattie EJ (1990): Isoenzyme(s) of glutathione transferase (class Mu) as a marker for the susceptibility to lung cancer: a follow up study. Carcinogenesis 11:33-36.

Shields PG, Caporaso NE, Falk RT, Sugimura H, Trivers GE, Trump BF, Hoover RN, Weston A, Harris CC (1993): Lung cancer, race, and a CYP1A1 genetic polymorphism. Cancer Epidemiol Biomarkers & Prev 2:481-485.

Shields PG, Xu GX, Blot WJ, Fraumeni JF, Jr., Trivers GE, Pellizzari ED, Qu YH, Gao YT, Harris CC (1995): Mutagens from heated Chinese and U.S. cooking oils. J Natl Cancer Inst 87:836-841.

Tefre T, Ryberg D, Haugen A, Nebert DW, Skaug V, Brogger A, Borresen AL (1991): Human CYP1A1 (cytochrome P1450) gene: lack of association between the Msp I restriction fragment length polymorphism and incidence of lung cancer in a Norwegian population. Pharmacogen 1:20-25.

van Poppel G, de Vogel N, van Balderen PJ, Kok FJ (1992): Increased cytogenetic damage in smokers deficient in glutathione S-transferase isozyme mu. Carcinogenesis 13:303-305.

Vineis P, Caporaso N, Tannenbaum SR, Skipper PL, Glogowski J, Bartsch H, Coda M, Talaska G, Kadlubar F (1990): Acetylation phenotype, carcinogen-hemoglobin adducts, and cigarette smoking. Cancer Res 50:3002-3004.

Vineis P, Bartsch H, Caporaso N, Harrington AM, Kadlubar FF, Landi MT, Malaveille C, Shields PG, Skipper P, Talaska G, et al (1994): Genetically based N-acetyltransferase metabolic polymorphism and low-level environmental exposure to carcinogens. Nature 369:154-156.

Wang SL, Huang JD, Lai MD, Liu BH, Lai ML (1993): Molecular basis of genetic variation in debrisoquin hydroxylation in Chinese subjects: polymorphism in RFLP and DNA sequence of CYP2D6. Clin Pharmacol Ther 53:410-418.

Wiencke JK, Kelsey KT, Lamela RA, Toscano WA, Jr. (1990): Human glutathione S-transferase deficiency as a marker of susceptibility to epoxide-induced cytogenetic damage. Cancer Res 50:1585-1590.

Wu-Williams AH, Dai XD, Blot W, Xu ZY, Sun XW, Xiao HP, Stone BJ, Yu SF, Feng YP, Ershow AG, et al (1990): Lung cancer among women in north-east China. Br J Cancer 62:982-987.

Zhong S, Howie AF, Ketterer B, Taylor J, Hayes JD, Beckett GJ, Wathen CG, Wolf CR, Spurr NK (1991): Glutathione S-transferase mu locus: use of genotyping and phenotyping assays to assess association with lung cancer susceptibility. Carcinogenesis 12:1533-1537.

Genetics and Cancer Susceptibility:
Implications for Risk Assessment, pages 159–174

EPIDEMIOLOGY OF SUSCEPTIBILITY TO BREAST CANCER

Barbara S. Hulka, M.D., M.P.H.

Department of Epidemiology, The University of North Carolina, Chapel Hill, NC 27599-7400

Presented at the 8th International Conference on Carcinogenesis and Risk Assessment. Genetics and Susceptibility: Impact on Risk Assessment, Barton Creek Conference Resort in Austin, Texas, November 30 - December 3, 1994.

ABSTRACT

Numerous factors have been noted to be associated with risk of breast cancer. Indicators of endogenous hormonal alterations are among them: early age at menarche and late age at menopause, nulliparity, late age at first full term pregnancy and obesity in postmenopausal women. Other established risk factors are family history of breast cancer, histologic characteristics of benign tissue, mammographic patterns, exogenous hormones and alcohol consumption. Endogenous indicators may be a reflection of enhanced susceptibility, whereas exogenous exposures can have both independent effects on risk and the ability to interact with markers of inherited susceptibility.

In case control studies of breast cancer, family history confers a risk elevation of two to three fold. The higher risk estimate occurs when first degree rather than second degree relatives are affected, or if more than one relative is affected. A relative diagnosed before age 45 increases risk for early-onset breast cancer. These findings have been obtained using either traditional analytic methods for case control data or an alternative strategy, which uses case control status as the predictor variable and models the risk to relatives in a time-dependent fashion. Risk of breast cancer is greater for the mother and sisters of cases than controls. The magnitude of risk increases with 1) decreasing age of diagnosis of the index case 2) additional family members with diagnosed breast cancer and 3) bilateral breast cancer in the index case. Although these two analytic approaches have somewhat different data requirements and may be subject to different biases, the results produced are quite consistent.

Mutated p53 in female family members of patients with Li-Fraumeni syndrome was one of the first identified genetic susceptibility markers for breast cancer. Application of segregation and linkage analyses to pedigrees with multiple affected family members successfully focused the search for BRCA1. Recent cloning and sequencing of BRCA1 will allow for its use in risk assessment, diagnostic evaluation and screening of high risk women. BRCA1 appears to be primarily responsible for early-onset breast cancer in high risk families. Rare alleles of H-ras could account for some of the late-onset cases in unselected populations since at least 85% of breast cancer appears to be sporadic, other genetic markers yet to be identified undoubtedly exist.

RISK PROFILE

Numerous studies have evaluated the effect of various endogenous and exogenous factors on risk of breast cancer. Some authors have attempted to estimate the extent to which these factors can account for the total breast cancer experience of U.S. women. Depending on the specific risk factors used, the population from which the data were obtained, and the mathematical model employed, somewhere between 25 and 55% of total risk may be accounted for with known risk factors (Seidman, 1982; Bruzzi, 1985). Table 1 shows the established breast cancer risk factors, categorized by the magnitude of their effects, i.e., relative risks. The table illustrates the large number of such factors, and the diverse biological and demographic themes which they represent. For a review of breast cancer epidemiology see Kelsey, 1993 and Kelsey and Horn-Ross, 1993.

A modest number of factors exhibit a strong effect on breast cancer risk (relative risk >4.0 or 2.1-4.0). Among these, some suggest a genetic etiology (family history) and others may represent stages in the carcinogenic process (atypical cells in nipple aspirate, atypical hyperplasia in tissue samples and nodular densities in mammograms). The international variation in rates may have some genetic component but not exclusively, since within two to three generations, migrants to the United States assume rates more similar to U.S. rates than to those of their native countries. Radiation to the chest is only relevant with high dose exposures such as those experienced by women who underwent repeated flouroscopies in relation to lung collapse therapy for tuberculosis, or who had radiotherapy in which the field of exposure included the breast. The minimal radiation exposure incurred by mammography is insignificant in risk assessment. Oophorectomy at an early age protects against breast cancer, and as such, provided some of the early support for a hormonal theory of breast cancer carcinogenesis.

Age heads the list of breast cancer risk factors. Rates increase dramatically from young ages (26/100,000 women at ages 30-34) to the middle years (225/100,000 women at ages 50-54) with continuing increases into old age (440/100,000 at ages 70-74) (Hankey, et al., 1993). When age-specific incidence rates are plotted on a log-log scale, a downward inflection in the incidence curve occurs at about age 50 with a deceleration in the rate of increase thereafter. This moderation in the rate of increase is cited as evidence for the importance of sex steroid hormones in carcinogenesis, as age 50 approximates the median age at natural menopause. Menopause results from ovarian failure with depletion of ovarian follicles and cessation of estrogen and progesterone production (Richardson, et al., 1987).

The remainder of table 1 shows factors with modest effects on breast cancer risk (relative risk of 1.1-2.0). The first grouping represents demographic characteristics, some of which may be proxies for life style and reproductive characteristics more directly associated with risk. The effect of socioeconomic status is contrary to that found with many diseases and most cancers; the most deprived segments of society are often the most adversely affected. With breast cancer, women from the highest educational, occupational and income groups experience the highest rates. Some of this excess, but not all, can be explained by the reproductive and life style characteristics noted in the remainder of the table (White, 1987).

Many of the reproductive and menstrual factors are thought to be indicators of hormonal effects on breast cancer risk, and more specifically, on the mitotic activity of epithelial cells in the terminal ducts of the breast lobules (Pike, et al., 1993). It is also postulated that these cells may be most susceptible to carcinogenic insult, and the fixation of molecular alterations through mitogenesis, in the early postmenarchal years prior to a first full-term pregnancy (Russo, et al., 1982). Such observations have been made in the rat model and are consistent with epidemiologic studies, in which early age at first pregnancy has a protective effect against risk of subsequent breast cancer. Obesity may increase risk because of the preferential conversion of androstenedione to estrone in adipose cells, resulting in elevated levels of serum estrone (Cauley, et al., 1989).

FAMILY HISTORY

Many epidemiologic studies have reported on family history of breast cancer as one of many risk factors of interest. More recently, studies have pursued family history as the primary analytic variable and in so doing have obtained more accurate information on familial relationships, utilized data from large data sets and employed analytic methods suited specifically for genetic epidemiologic analysis. The analytic approaches used have varied but may be illustrated by at least three different approaches. First is the standard case control analysis in which "history of breast cancer in relatives of cases and controls" is the exposure variable. Relatives are characterized by type e.g., mother or sister, and genetic distance from the index case, usually first or second degree relatives. The analytic method is commonly logistic regression analysis with the odds ratio as an estimate of the relative risk. An estimate of the attributable risk can also be obtained in that the proportion of controls with affected relatives is known (Slattery and Kerber, 1993; Sattin, et al., 1985; Mettlin, et al., 1990; Schwartz, et al., 1991; Byrne, et al., 1991). A second approach

Table 1. Established risk factors for breast cancer in women

Factor	High-risk group	Low-risk group
	Relative risk > 4.0	
Age	Old	Young
Country of birth	North America, Northern Europe	Asia, Africa
Mother *and* sister with history of breast cancer, especially if diagnosed at an early age	Yes	No
Atypical epithelial cells in nipple aspirate fluid	Yes	No fluid produced
History of cancer in one breast	Yes	No
	Relative risk = 2.1-4.0	
Nodular densities on the mammogram	Densities occupying >75% of breast volume	Parenchyma composed entirely of fat
Mother *or* sister with history of breast cancer	Yes	No
Biopsy-confirmed atypical hyperplasia	Yes	No
Radiation to chest in high doses	Yes	No
Oophorectomy before age 35	No	Yes

Table 1 (continued)

Factor	High-risk group	Low-risk group
	Relative risk = 1.1-2.0	
Socioeconomic status	High	Low
Place of residence	Urban	Rural
Place of residence (within United States)	Northern	Southern
Race/ethnicity		
Breast cancer at 40 years of age	White	Asian
Breast cancer at < 40 years of age	Black	Asian
Religion	Jewish	Seventh-day Adventist, Mormon
Age at first full-term pregnancy	30 years	< 20 years
Age at menarche	11 years	15 years
Age at menopause	55 years	< 45 years
Obesity (postmenopausal)	Obese	Thin
Nulliparity (postmenopausal)	Yes	No
Parity (postmenopausal)	Low	High
Breast feeding (premenopausal)	None	Several years
Long-term use of oral contraceptives		
Breast cancer diagnosed at < 45 years of age	Yes	No
Long-term use of estrogen replacement therapy	Yes	No
Diethylstilbestrol use during pregnancy	Yes	No
Height	Tall	Short
History of primary cancer in endometrium, ovary, colon	Yes	No
Alcohol consumption	Yes	No

Adapted from Kelsey JL (1993a).

using a case control study design considers case or control status as the exposure variable. A Cox proportional hazards model provides a time dependent estimate of risk to relatives of the cases and controls. Thus, either a hazard ratio or a cumulative risk of developing breast cancer up to any given age can be estimated for each type of relative (Claus, et al., 1990; 1994). Lastly, some studies have followed a prospective design (cohort studies) with exposure information, including family history, collected prior to the development of breast cancer, which was subsequently identified through follow-up of subjects (Colditz, et al., 1993; Calle, et al., 1993; Sellers, et al., 1992). In such studies a relative risk is obtained based on person-time of exposure (until the development of breast cancer or closure of the study), or the Cox proportional hazard model provides a time-dependent rate ratio.

The findings from these studies are reasonably consistent. Overall, there appears to be a 2-3 fold increased risk of breast cancer for women who have an affected first degree relative. With only a second degree affected relative, the relative risk estimate is less than 2. Several factors affect these estimates. The earlier the age of diagnosis of the relative the greater the risk to the individual. Illustrating this point are data from Claus et al. who analyzed the Cancer and Steroid Hormone study data, which included 4730 cases and 4688 controls under 55 years of age. The hazard ratio for the mother of a case with breast cancer diagnosed at 50 years of age was 1.7, at 40 years 2.7 and at 30 years 4.3. For none of the rate ratios did the 95% confidence interval overlap one. It should also be noted that for any given family history , the younger the individual at risk the greater the relative risk of breast cancer. Or stated differently, family history of breast cancer exerts a greater effect on risk of early-onset breast cancer than for late-onset disease.

If two first degree relatives are affected, the risk is greater than if only one is affected. Bilateral disease in a relative increases risk more than unilateral disease (Slattery and Kerber, 1993; Mettlin, et al., 1990) although this finding has not appeared in all studies (Claus, et al., 1990; Sattin, et al., 1985). Most studies have shown no significant interaction between established breast cancer risk factors and family history (Colditz, et al. 1993; Calle, et al., 1993; Slattery and Kerber, 1993; Claus, et al. 1990, 1994; Schwartz, et al., 1991; Byrne, et al., 1991; Parazzini, et al., 1992; Mettlin, et al., 1990). The effect of oral contraceptive use on risk of breast cancer was no different among women with or without an affected first degree relative (Murray, et al., 1989). Early age at onset of breast cancer is the strongest indicator of genetic susceptibility and heritable transmission.

Most of these studies have the potential for misclassification of family member breast cancer status, because the information is dependent on subject recall. Particularly for older family members, the cancer diagnoses may have been obscured or not well remembered (Ottman, et al., 1983). Furthermore, in case control studies differential misclassification may occur since cases may be much more aware of family history than controls. The Slattery study is distinctive in this regard in that no information was collected directly from subjects; all data were obtained through record linkage of the Utah geneological data base, Utah cancer registry and department of vital statistics (Slattery and Kerber, 1993). This study also produced higher risk estimates in relation to family history than did most other studies. Current best estimates are that 10-15% of breast cancer may be attributable to family history and that approximately half of that amount (7-8%) may be attributable to one or more dominantly inherited predisposing genes (Ottman, et al., 1986).

Classical epidemiologic studies have to some extent given way to linkage studies using pedigrees, and to the combined epidemiological/laboratory studies made possible through the development of molecular epidemiology. Utilizing these methods it has been possible to localize specific genes, to study their transmission in pedigrees and populations, and to document their presence in large numbers of subjects ascertained through epidemiologic research strategies.

GENETIC MARKERS

Literature exists on a diversity of potential genetic susceptibility markers for breast cancer. Some of these are established, e.g., BRCA1 and p53 in Li-Fraumeni syndrome, occuring in rare high risk families, whereas others, e.g., BRCA2 and BRCA3, are in much earlier stages of characterization. Other genetic alterations may have a greater population impact but their risk to the affected individual is likely to be lower. Examples of the latter are Ataxia-Telangiectasia heterozygotes and carriers of rare alleles of H-ras. Mutations and polymorphisms in the estrogen receptor gene, and in the genes responsible for estrogen metabolism, are also under study. Three of these genetic alterations (BRCA1, p53, and rare alleles of H-ras) are reviewed in the current paper.

BRCA1

BRCA1 is a gene, recently cloned and sequenced, which is responsible for at least 45% of breast cancer in families with multiple cases of early-onset disease (Miki, et al., 1994; Futreal, et al., 1994). Although the gene had previously been localized through linkage analysis to a region of about 4 centiMorgans on chromosome 17q21, identification of it's exact location and sequence has opened up extensive new opportunities for clinical application and scientific inquiry (King, et al., 1993).

BRCA1 is an important inherited susceptibility marker for familial breast cancer, and for families with both breast and ovarian cancer. Carriers of BRCA1 have an 85% chance of developing breast cancer by age 80 and more than 50% of those cases will occur before age 50 (King, et al., 1993). Estimates for the population at large suggest that about 1 in 300 women carry a mutant BRCA1 (Claus, et al., 1991). Overall, BRCA1 accounts for about 4% of breast cancer, or 25% of those cases that occur before age 45 (Biesecker, et al., 1993).

The behavior of BRCA1 is characteristic of a tumor suppressor gene. In pedigree analyses, cancer predisposition segregates as a genetic dominant trait. However, at the level of the somatic cell, a single inherited copy of the mutant allele acts like a recessive gene. Loss or inactivation of the wild type homologue is required for malignant transformation. When loss of heterozygosity (LOH) is observed in tumor tissues, it is the wild type allele that is lost, whereas the mutant allele is retained (Miki, et al., 1994; Kelsell, et al., 1993). However, unlike other tumor suppressor genes, the mutated allele is not found in tumor tissue of sporadic cases.

Linkage analysis was essential to localize BRCA1 to a sufficiently limited area of chromosome 17 so that molecular techniques could be used to finalize the identification. Linkage analysis relies on the existence of multiple large pedigrees, that exhibit a high frequency of early onset breast cancer and segregate BRCA1 susceptibility alleles. Biologically, it is based on linkage disequilibrium between two genetic traits, either two markers or a marker and a disease locus, occuring together on a chromosome more frequently than would be expected by chance (Khoury, et al., 1993). Polymorphic genetic markers in the form of (CA)n repeats (microsatellites) arise at known chromosomal locations as a consequence of DNA replication slippage. These repeat units are numerous throughout the genome and highly polymorphic due to length heterogeneity (Black and Solomon, 1993). Identification of these markers on segregating chromosomes from pedigree members allows for the detection of meiotic recombination events, or crossovers, within the cluster of markers known to be linked to the disease gene. The longer the distance between a marker and a disease gene the greater the opportunity for crossover and observable genetic recombination (Khoury, et al., 1993). Using these techniques, BRCA1 was localized to a 600 kilobase region between markers D17S1321 and D17S1325 on chromosome 17q21.1 (Miki, et al., 1994).

Positional cloning techniques and sequencing (Miki, et al., 1994) allowed for the identification of BRCA1, a large gene with 23 coding exons distributed over some 100 kilobases of genomic DNA (Miki, et al., 1994). Mutations that have been identified are of several different types including frameshift, nonsense and regulatory; neutral polymorphisms have been found as well (Miki, et al., 1994; Futreal, et al., 1994). All mutations identified have been in the germ line of breast cancer cases (mostly from kindreds known to be segregating BRCA1) (Miki, et al., 1994). No somatic mutations have been identified in the tumor tissue of sporadic cases, although such patients have a high frequency of LOH at 17q (30 to 70%). It is possible that BRCA1 may not be important in sporadic breast cancer (Futreal, et al., 1994).

The protein expression product, identified in multiple tissue types including breast and ovary, contains 1863 amino acids and a zinc finger domain in the amino-terminal region. It binds DNA like a transcription factor and may regulate gene expression (Miki, et al., 1994; Futreal, et al., 1994).

Identification of BRCA1 creates problems as well as opportunities. In the absence of one or more first degree relatives who have developed early-onset breast cancer, most women would be advised to refrain from genetic testing. On the other hand, the potential value is enormous for women from high risk families who will now have the opportunity to know their genetic status with great certainty, and thereby, risk for developing breast cancer. For such women, diverse types of counseling will be needed: education and assessment, guidance from multidisciplinary clinical personnel and continuing psychological support for those who screen positive (Biesecker, et al., 1993). For women who screen positive, decisions will have to be made concerning alternative choices. Opting for early detection means intensified surveillance through mammography and clinical examination. Probable prevention may be achieved through prophylactic surgery, bilateral mastectomy and bilateral oophorectomy. Ethical issues will have to be resolved as to who should or could have access to the screening results (confidentiality), and who will bear the costs of genetic screening, surveillance, and surgical intervention.

p53 Germline Mutations

p53 mutations in germline tissue were first identified in affected members of Li-Fraumeni families (Malkin, et al., 1992). Li-Fraumeni syndrome is rare and the mortality for affected family members is high. Families are defined by having a proband with sarcoma and at least two other close relatives with sarcoma or carcinoma (Li, et al., 1988). Breast cancer is one of the many types of sarcomas and carcinomas, which are common in these families. Female family members with germline p53 mutations have an 18-fold excess risk of developing breast cancer before age 45 (Garber, et al., 1991).

Tumor suppressor genes are most frequently identified with familial tumors, e.g., Li-Fraumeni, retinoblastoma, and Wilms tumor. Tumor tissue from persons with a germ line p53 mutation frequently exhibits loss of heterozygosity of the wild type allele. The half-life of mutant p53 is markedly increased relative to the wild type protein. Wild type p53 controls the cell cycle by regulating transcription (Fields and Jang, 1990; Raycroft, et al., 1990) and DNA replication (Iguchi-Ariga, et al., 1988; Kern, et al., 1991).

p53 mutations have been sought in sarcoma patients outside of the rare Li-Fraumeni families. A study of 196 sarcoma patients identified eight with germline p53 mutations, all of which were at different locations and of different types (Toguchida, et al., 1992). At least six of the eight patients were previously known or subsequently found to have a strong personal or familial history of cancer. It was concluded that, at most, 1 to 2% of sporadic sarcomas might have germline p53 mutations, a frequency which would hardly justify the routine screening of such patients.

Of more importance to breast cancer susceptibility is a study of 126 consecutive invasive breast cancer patients under age 40 seen at either of two Cancer Centers in Maryland (Sidransky, et al., 1992). Molecular analyses of exons 5 to 8 from lymphocyte DNA was performed by PCR amplification, cloning and sequencing of pooled clones. The one patient found to have a germline mutation at codon 181 had a sister with the same mutation and a mother and grandmother previously diagnosed with breast cancer. Even in familial breast cancer, p53 is unlikely to be numerically important, except in Li-Fraumeni families.

H-ras

Rare alleles in the minisatellite region of the H-ras oncogene have been shown to be associated with an excess of cancers at various sites. This was first reported by Krontiris in 1985 (Krontiris, et al., 1985) and has been subsequently confirmed in other publications. At least nine studies have specifically addressed polymorphisms of the variable number tandem repeat (VNTR) region in relation to breast cancer (Lidereau, et al., 1986; Honda, et al., 1988; Saglio, et al., 1988; Sheng, et al., 1988; Barkardottir, et al., 1989; Corell and Zoll, 1988; Hall, et al., 1990; Krontiris, et al.,1993; Garrett, et al., 1993). A metaanalysis including most of these studies produced a breast cancer risk estimate (odds ratio) of 1.68 for rare alleles (Krontiris, et al., 1993). This effect may be greater for black women, odds ratio of 4.8, than for white women, odds ratio = 1.9 (Garrett, et al., unpublished data). In the latter analysis, rare alleles were those with a frequency of less than 0.005 in the control series.

The H-ras minisatellite (VNTR) is located on chromosome 11p15.5 about 1 kb downstream from the gene's coding sequences. It is composed of 30 to 100 tandemly repeated units, each of which is 28bp in length (Krontiris, et al., 1993). More than 40 different alleles of approximately 1000 to 3000bp have been observed (Garrett, et al., 1993). Based on the observed frequency of allele lengths in the published control series, alleles are designated as common or rare, with the latter sometimes subdivided into intermediate and rare. The four common alleles, designated a1, a2, a3 and a4, comprise >90% of alleles in whites but <60% of alleles in blacks

(Weston, et al., 1991; Garrett, et al., unpublished data); a2 and a3 are less frequent in blacks. Common alleles appear to serve as the progenitors for the less common ones, since each rare VNTR possesses the markers characteristic of the common allele nearest in size (Kasperczyk , et al., 1990)

The function of the minisatellite is not known with certainty. Rare alleles might be in linkage disequilibrium with other components of the H-ras gene or other nearby pathogenic loci. If so, their function would be only as markers of cancer predisposition (Krontiris, et al., 1993). Alternatively, the minisatellite may function in transcriptional regulation. Members of the NFB family of transcription factors have been observed to bind to the VNTR (Trepicchio and Krontiris, 1992). Furthermore, allelic differences in activity appear; at least some rare alleles possess greater enhancer activity than do the common alleles (Green and Krontiris, 1993). Lastly, rare alleles may be markers for genetic instability manifested as a high VNTR mutation rate, analogous to the microsatellite instability associated with mutations in the DNA mismatch repair gene hMSH2 (Conway, et al., in press).

Through minisatellite variant repeat (MVR) analysis, it has become apparent that VNTRs exhibit sequence variation as well as length variability (Jeffreys, et al., 1991; Armour and Jeffreys, 1992). The expectation is that combined sequence and length allelotyping will improve the specification for VNTRs that are most important for breast cancer risk assessment. Furthermore, MVR analysis should improve identification of progenitor alleles and help to focus on mechanisms of formation of rare alleles.

Krontiris has estimated the breast cancer risk attributable to H-ras rare alleles as 0.09 based on a presumed population frequency of 0.058 (Krontiris, et al., 1993). This implies that 1 out of 11 cancers of the breast, and perhaps at other sites, could result from carrying these alleles. Since the H-ras locus is not linked to breast cancer in high risk families, (Hall, et al., 1990) it is probably not relevant to breast cancer occurrence in selected families with a multigenerational history of early-onset breast cancer. Genes such as BRCA1 or BRCA2 are likely to be segregating in those families (Wooster, et al., 1994; Miki, et al., 1994; Futreal, et al., 1994). This does not, however, preclude a role for H-ras polymorphisms in late-onset breast cancer.

SUMMARY

The established genetic markers of breast cancer susceptibility, BRCA1 and p53 in Li-Fraumeni syndrome, are important because of the scientific and human advancement inherent to their discovery. Knowledge about them makes easier the identification and application of additional susceptibility markers for breast cancer. It should be recognized, however, that these genetic alterations occur in rare families, and although extremely important to members of those families, the markers appear to have little direct relevance to the breast cancer problem in the general poplation of women. Sporadic cases account for about 85% of all breast cancers, and 80% of cases occur in women over the age of 50. The genetic susceptibility component for these cases has yet to be determined. The interaction among established epidemiologic risk factors, exogenous exposures and yet to be identified susceptibility markers should be help to clarify pathogenetic pathways in the majority of breast cancer patients.

Although the levels of scientific inquiry reported in this paper exhibit a broad range from epidemiologic population-based interview studies through family studies and laboratory-based molecular analyses, the divergence among these is lessening. Much epidemiologic etiologic research relies heavily on the collection and analysis of biological samples (blood and tissues), while molecular biologists are developing techniques for analysis of large numbers of human tissues, including those that are parafin embedded formalin fixed. These integrated research endeavours are increasing the preventive and therapeutic applications of research findings in human populations and clinical settings.

REFERENCES

Armour JAL, Jeffreys AJ (1992): Biology and applications of human minisatellite loci. Current Opinion in Genetics and Development 2(6): 850-856.

Biesecker BB, Boehnike M, Calzone K, Market DS, Garber JE, Collins FS, Weber BL (1993): Genetic counseling for families with inherited susceptibility to breast and ovarian cancer. JAMA 269(15):1970-1974.

Black DM, Solomon E (1993): The search for the familial breast/ovarian cancer gene. TIG 9(1):22-26.

Bruzzi P, Green SB, Byar DP, Brinton LA, Schairer C (1985): Estimating the population attributable risk for multiple risk factors using case-control data. Am J Epidemiol 122:904-914.

Byrne C, Brinton LA, Haile RW, Schairer C (1991): Heterogeneity of the effect of family history on breast cancer risk. Epidemiol 2:276-284.

Calle EE, Martin LM, Thun MJ, Miracle HL, Heath CW, Jr (1993): Family history, age, and risk of fatal breast cancer. Am J Epidemiol 138:675-681.

Cauley JA, Gutal JP, Kuller LH, LeDonne D, Powell JG (1989): The epidemiology of serum sex hormones in postmenopausal women. Am J Epidemiol 129(6):1120-1131.

Claus EB, Risch NJ, Thompson WD (1990): Age at onset as an indicator of familial risk of breast cancer. Am J Epidemiol 131:961-972.

Claus EB, Risch N, Thompson WD (1991): Genetic analysis of breast cancer in the cancer and steroid hormone study. Am J Hum Genet 48:232-242.

Claus EB, Risch N, Thompson WD (1994): Autosomal dominant inheritance of early-onset breast cancer. Cancer 73:643-651.

Colditz GA, Willett WC, Hunter DJ, Stampfer MJ, Manson JE, Hennekens CH, Rosner BA, Speizer FE (1993): Family history, age, and risk of breast cancer: Prospective data from the nurses' health study. JAMA 270:388-343.

Conway K, Edmiston S, Hulka BS, Garrett PA, Liu ET (1994): Ha-ras rare alleles in breast cancer susceptibility. In press.

Fields S, Jang SK (1990): Presence of a potent transcription activating sequence in the p53 protein. Science 249:1046-1049.

Futreal PA, Liu Q, Shattuck-Eidens D, Cochran C, Harshman K, Tavtigian S, Bennett M, et al. (1994): *BRCA1* mutations in primary breast and ovarian carcinomas. Science 266:120-122.

Garber JE, Goldstein AM, Kantor AF, Fraumeni JF Jr. (1991): Followup study of twenty-four families with Li-Fraumeni syndrome. Cancer Res 51:6094-6097.

Garrett PA, Hulka BS, Kim YL, Farber RA (1993): HRAS protooncogene polymorphism and breast cancer. Cancer Epidemiol Biomarkers & Prevention 2:131-138.

Garrett PA, Hulka BS, Kim YL, Leight GS, Iglehart JD, Huth JF, Farber RA (1993): Rare *HRAS* alleles and breast cancer: Association and possible racial variation. Submitted to JNCI.

Green M, Krontiris TG (1993): Allelic variation of reporter gene activation by the HRAS1 minisatellite. Genomics 17:429-434.

Hankey BF, Brinton LA, Kessler LG, Abrams J (1993): Breast. In Miller BA, Ries LAG, Hankey BF, Kosary CL, Harras A, Devesa SS, Edwards BK (eds): "SEER

Cancer Statistics Review 1973-1990." Bethesda, MD: National Cancer Institute, pp IV.6.

Iguchi-Ariga SMM, Okazaki T, Itani T, Ariga H (1988): Cloning of the p53 dependent origin of cellular DNA replication. Oncogene 3:509-515.

Jeffreys AJ, MacLeod A, Tamaki K, Neil DL, Monckton DG (1991): Minisatellite repeat coding as a digital approach to DNA typing. Nature 354:204-209.

Kasperczyk A, DiMartino NA, Krontiris TG (1990): Minisatellite allele diversification: The origin of rare alleles at the HRAS1 locus. Am J Hum Genet 47:854-859.

Kelsell DP, Black DM, Bishop DT, Spurr NK (1993): Genetic analysis of the BRCA1 region in a large breast/ovarian family: Refinement of the minimal region containing BRCA1. Hum Mol Genet 2:1823-1828.

Kelsey JL (1993a): Breast cancer epidemiology: Summary and future directions. Epidemiol Rev 15:256-263.

Kelsey JL, Horn-Ross PL (1993b): Breast cancer: Magnitude of the problem and descriptive epidemiology. Epidemiol Rev 15:7-16.

Kern SE, Kinzler KW, Bruskin A, Jarosz D, Friedman P, Prives C, Vogelstein B (1991): Identification of p53 as a sequence-specific DNA-binding protein. Science 252:1708-11.

Khoury MJ, Beaty TH, Cohen BH (1993): Fundamental genetic concepts and approaches. In Khoury MJ, Beaty TH, Cohen BH (eds): "Fundamentals of Genetic Epidemiology." New York: Oxford University Press, pp 44.

King M, Rowell S, Love SM (1993): Inherited breast and ovarian cancer: What are the risks? What are the choices? JAMA 269(15):1975-1980.

Krontiris TG, DiMartino NA, Colb M, Parkinson DR (1985): Unique allelic restriction fragments of the human Ha-*ras* locus in leukocyte and tumour DNAs of cancer patients. Nature 313:369-374.

Krontiris TG, Devlin B, Karp DD, Robert NJ, Risch N (1993): An association between the risk of cancer and mutations in the HRAS1 minisatellite locus. N Engl J Med 329:517-523.

Li FP, Fraumeni JF Jr., Mulvihill JJ, Fraumeni JF, Mulvihill JJ, Blattner WA, Dreyfus MG, Tucker MA, Miller RW (1988): A cancer family syndrome in twenty-four kindreds. Cancer Res 48:5358-5362.

Malkin D, Li FP, Strong LC, Fraumeni JF Jr., Nelson CE, Kim DH, Kassel J, Gryka MA, Bischoff FZ, Tainsky MA, Friend SH (1990): Germ line p53 mutations in a familial syndrome of breast cancer, sarcomas, and other neoplasms. Science 250:1233-1238.

Mettlin C, Croghan I, Natarajan N, Lane W (1990): The association of age and familial risk in a case-control study of breast cancer. Am J Epidemiol 131:973-983.

Miki Y, Swensen J, Shattuck-Eidens D, Futreal PA, Harshman K, Tavtigian S, Liu Q, Cochran C, Bennett LM, Ding W, Bell R, Rosenthal J, Hussey C, Tran T, McClure M, Frye C, Hattier T, Phelps R, Haugen-Strano A, Katcher H, Yakumo K, Gholami Z, Shaffer D, Stone S, Bayer S, Wray C, Bogden R, Dayananth P, Ward J, Tonin P, Narod S, Bristow PK, Norris FH, Helvering L, Morrison P, Rosteck P, Lai M, Barrett JC, Lewis C, Neuhausen S, Cannon-Albright L, Goldgar D, Wiseman R, Kamb A, Skolnick MH (1994): A strong candidate for the breast and ovarian cancer susceptibility gene *BRCA1*. Science 266:66-71.

Murray PP, Stadel BV, Schlesselman JJ (1989): Oral contraceptive use in women with a family history of breast cancer. Obstet Gynecol 73: 977-983.

Ottman R, King M-C, Pike MC, Henderson BE (1983): Practical guide for estimating risk for familial breast cancer. The Lancet (September 3) 2:556-558.

Parazzini F, La Vecchia C, Negri E, Franceschi S, Bocciolone L (1992): Menstrual and reproductive factors and breast cancer in women with family history of the disease. Int J Cancer 51:677-681.

Pike MC, Spicer DV, Dahmoush L, Press MF (1993a): Estrogens, progestogens, normal breast cell proliferation, and breast cancer risk. Epidemiol Rev 15:17-35.

Pike MC, Bernstein L, Spicer DV (1993b): Exogenous hormones and breast cancer. In Niederhuber JE (ed): "Current therapy in oncology. St. Louis: CV Mosby pp 292-303.

Raycroft L, Wu H, Lozano G (1990): Transcriptional activation by wild-type but not transforming mutants of the p53 anti-oncogene. Science 249:1049-1051.

Richardson SJ, Senikas V, Nelson JF (1987): Follicular depletion during the menopausal transition: Evidence for accelerated loss and ultimate exhaustion. J

Clin Endocrinol Metab 65:1231-1237.

Russo J, Tay LK, Russo IH (1982): Differentiation of the mammary gland and susceptibility to carcinogenesis. Breast Cancer Res Treat 2:5-73.

Sattin RW, Rubin GL, Webster LA, Huezo CM, Wingo PA, Ory HW, Layde PM, the Cancer and Steroid Hormone Study (1985): Family history and the risk of breast cancer. JAMA 253:1908-1913.

Schwartz AG, Kaufmann R, Moll PP (1991): Heterogeneity of breast cancer risk in families of young breast cancer patients and controls. Am J Epidemiol 134:1325-1334.

Sellers TA, Kushi LH, Potter JD, Kaye SA, Nelson CL, McGovern PG, Folsom AR (1992): Effect of family history, body-fat distribution, and reproductive factors on the risk of postmenopausal breast cancer. N Engl J Med 326: 1323-1329.

Sidransky D, Tokino T, Helzlsouer K, Zehnbauer B, Rausch G, Shelton B, Prestigiacomo L, Vogelstein B, Davidson N (1992): Inherited p53 gene mutations in breast cancer. Cancer Res 52:2984-2986.

Seidman H, Stellman SD, Mushinski MH (1982): A different perspective on breast cancer risk factors: Some implications of the nonattributable risk. CA-A Cancer J Clin 32:301-313.

Slattery ML, Kerber RA (1993): A comprehensive evaluation of family history and breast cancer risk. JAMA 270: 1563-1568.

Toguchida J, Yamaguchi T, Dayton SH, Beauchamp RL, Herrera GE, Ishizaki K, Yamamuro T, Meyers PA, Little JB, Sasaki MS, Weichelbaum RR, Yandell DW (1992): Prevalence and spectrum of germline mutations of the p53 gene among patients with sarcoma. N Engl J Med 326:1301-1308.

Trepicchio WL, Krontiris TG (1992): Members of the rel/NF-B family of transcriptional regulatory proteins bind the HRAS1 minisatellite DNA sequence. Nucleic Acids Research 20(10):2427-2434.

Weston A, Vineis P, Caporaso NE, Krontiris TG, Lonergan JA, Sugimura H (1991): Racial variation in the distribution of *Ha-ras* alleles. Mol Carcinog 4:265-268.

White E (1987): Projected changes in breast cancer incidence due to the trend toward delayed childbearing. Am J Public Health 77:495-497.

Genetics and Cancer Susceptibility:
Implications for Risk Assessment, pages 175–199

IDENTIFYING GENES AND PROTEINS INVOLVED IN HUMAN DNA REPAIR PROCESSES USING SOMATIC CELL AND MOLECULAR GENETICS

Larry H. Thompson

Biology and Biotechnology Research Program
Lawrence Livermore National Laboratory
Livermore, California 94551

INTRODUCTION

DNA repair processes play a fundamental role in protecting the cellular genome from damage resulting from external radiation or from chemical attack due to normal metabolism or exposure to environmental agents. In addition repair must correct alterations associated with the intrinsic thermodynamic instability of DNA (Lindahl 1993) or mistakes made during replication or recombination. Thus, in terms of genetic integrity, repair processes are vital to preserving gene and chromosome structure, ranging from the individual nucleotides within a gene to the physical continuity of the DNA molecules over megabase regions of a particular chromosome.

Cancer is a disease that can be characterized by genetic instability, the accumulation of mutations, and the abnormal expression of genes that favor cell proliferation and immortalization. In recent years, large numbers of human genes have been identified that play a role in this progressive process, acting in either a dominant (oncogenes) or recessive (tumor suppressor genes) manner. Since DNA repair processes are relatively efficient at low levels of damage, it is those lesions that go unrepaired (or are repaired incorrectly) that lead to mutations affecting proto-oncogenes or tumor suppressor genes, mutations that are critical in initiating and promoting the gradual evolution of malignant cells. In the complex pathways in which cells become increasingly genetically abnormal, chromosomal events play a significant role. Thus, an understanding of how DNA repair and the related processes of DNA replication and recombination maintain chromosome stability is of central importance. It is entirely appropriate to view DNA repair genes as anti-cancer or "tumor-suppressor" genes.

Evidence in support of this view comes from various human DNA repair disorders, in which cancer-proneness is associated with a genetic alteration causing a DNA repair deficiency or an abnormality in the way in which cells respond to, and recover from, DNA damage. In xeroderma pigmentosum (XP), a defect in nucleotide excision repair (NER) results in a very high risk (>1000-fold increase) of skin cancer due to reduced repair of DNA photoproducts associated with exposure to sunlight (Cleaver and Kraemer 1989). In the absence of exposure to bulky base damage, XP cells grow well and do not show overt chromosome instability. However, in several other human disorders, chromosome instability in the form of spontaneous chromosomal breaks and translocations is a unifying characteristic that appears to be the underlying cause of the cancer-proneness of these diseases (German 1990). Each of these disorders also tends to have characteristic hypersensitivity to certain kinds of DNA damage. Ataxia telangiectasia (AT) is noted for its hypersensitivity to ionizing radiation (Thacker 1989), and Fanconi anemia cells are highly sensitive to agents that produce inter-strand DNA crosslinks (dos Santos et al. 1994). Bloom syndrome (BS) cells show various hypersensitivities and have a hallmark trait of extremely high sister chromatid exchanges (Chaganti et al. 1974; German 1993), a form of recombination that is visualized cytologically and may result from DNA duplex breakage and rejoining events occurring during DNA replication (Painter 1980). For more details of the human repair disorders, the reader is referred to a recent review (Friedberg et al. 1995).

During the last decade extraordinary progress has been made in providing insight at the molecular level as to the nature of the genetic and biochemical defects in some of the human repair disorders. Using the cell lines from both the above human disorders and also mutant rodent cell lines generated in the laboratory, it has been possible to identify and characterize many DNA repair genes and begin to understand the biochemical functions of some of the proteins. In this article, we will examine how this approach has been especially successful in elucidating NER and how it should help determine other, still poorly understood, mechanisms that cells possess to cope with either DNA damage or with the intrinsic fragility of their complex genomes.

CLONING OF REPAIR GENES BASED ON CHROMOSOMAL INTEGRATION OF EXOGENOUS DNA

Using the methods of somatic cell genetics, repair deficient cell lines of human or rodent origin were earlier classified into many genetic complementation groups, which pointed to a complex, multigenic basis for several human disorders, especially XP, and the UV-sensitive mutants of Chinese hamster cells. These collections of mutants were characterized as being deficient in NER and were thought to be defective in the early steps of damage recognition and incision in the repair pathway because incision of damaged DNA was generally not observed among the mutants (Zelle and Lohman 1979; Thompson et al. 1982). Historically there was much concern that rodent cells might be a poor model for human cells because of the observation that cyclobutane pyrimidine dimers were inefficiently removed by repair processes in rodent cells, even though the survival after UV exposure was very similar for human and rodent cells. However, with the discovery of preferential repair of active genes (Bohr et al. 1985, 1986), it was possible to reconcile this inter-species difference because of the realization that rodent cells efficiently repair the transcribed strand of active genes (Mellon et al. 1987).

Currently, there are seven complementation groups of XP cells (excluding the XP variant) that are defective in NER (Vermeulen et al. 1991) and 11 groups of rodent mutants that have a phenotype similar to that of XP (Thompson et al. 1981; Stefanini et al. 1991; Riboni et al. 1992; Collins 1993). As will be seen, there is now substantial overlap between the human and rodent groups although unique members curiously persist within each group. With the development of procedures for incorporating foreign DNA into cells, the goal of cloning human DNA repair genes by genetic complementation became possible and advanced rapidly. This approach has been highly successful using the rodent mutants and, more recently, to some extent using human mutant cell lines. Since human cells were found not to efficiently incorporate exogenous DNA into their chromosomes, this feature initially greatly restricted their utility (Hoeijmakers et al. 1987).

The first human gene to be cloned by transfection/complementation was *ERCC1* (excision repair cross complementing, i.e. human into hamster inter-species complementation), by introducing human genomic DNA into a CHO UV-sensitive mutant (Westerveld et al. 1984; van Duin et al. 1986; see Table 1). By tagging the transfecting DNA with a dominant marker gene, the human repair gene could be identified in the genomic DNA of primary and secondary transformants. Cloning of the *ERCC1* gene involved constructing a cosmid library from the DNA of the secondary transformant. By using similar methods, the *ERCC2*, *ERCC3*, *ERCC4*, *ERCC5*, and *ERCC6* genomic sequences were also obtained (see Table 1 for references on cloning and characterization). With the advent of chromosome-specific cosmid libraries (Longmire et al. 1993), it was possible to use a chromosome 16 library as the starting material for transfection and cloning of the *ERCC4* gene since the chromosomal location was known (Liu et al. 1993). However, this approach would clearly not have worked for larger genes, e.g. *ERCC3* and *ERCC6* (Table 1), since cosmids are limited to inserts of ~40 kb.

Among the rodent mutants, surprisingly, no complementation groups have been identified that are equivalent to the XP-A and XP-C groups of xeroderma pigmentosum. Fortunately, however, both the *XPA* and *XPC* genes were cloned by complementing XP cell lines. The mouse XPA gene was cloned in a very large-scale effort by transfection and integration of mouse genomic sequences in XP-A fibroblasts (Tanaka et al. 1989), and then it was used to clone the homologous human sequences (Tanaka et al. 1990).

Mutants that are defective in other pathways of repair have also been used for gene cloning by functional complementation involving chromosomal integration of the transfected DNA. The human *XRCC1* gene was isolated in cosmid clones following transfection of a CHO hamster cell mutant that is hypersensitive to (m)ethyl methanesulfonate, X-rays and chlorodeoxyuridine (Thompson et al. 1990; see Table 3).

In principle, it is possible to use cDNA libraries for transfection and functional complementation of mutants. If functional sequences indeed exist in such libraries, then recovery of the complementing fragments is much easier than the recovery of the much larger genes themselves. We recently used this approach to isolate a cDNA of the *XRCC3* gene, which corrects the CHO mutant irs1SF (Tebbs et al. 1995). The cDNA library employed was prepared in a vector (pEBS7; see *XPC* gene below) that carries the gene for hygromycin B resistance as a selectable marker and has the cytomegalovirus (CMV) promoter for expression of the cDNA insert (Peterson and Legerski 1991). The cDNA was recovered from a secondary transformant by preparing a cosmid library and screening for the linked hygromycin resistance gene.

CLONING OF REPAIR GENES BASED ON EPISOMAL REPLICATION OF COMPLEMENTING cDNA

The first successful cloning of human repair genes by cDNA transfection was done using complementation in human cells. The cloning of the cDNAs for both Fanconi anemia group C (*FAC*) (Strathdee et al. 1992b) and xeroderma pigmentosum group C (*XPC*) (Legerski & Peterson 1992) was accomplished using a transfection strategy based on correction for resistance to UV or mitomycin C. The cDNA sequences were introduced into cells in vectors that replicated episomally from an Epstein Barr Virus (EBV) origin of replication (Peterson and Legerski 1991). Therefore, isolating the complementing plasmids from the transformed cells was relatively straightforward. Interestingly, the functional *XPC* cDNA clone was later shown in a separate cloning study to be lacking the first 160 bp of the open reading frame (Masutani et al. 1994). The *FAC* cDNAs, however, contained the complete open reading frame. This approach holds promise for cloning cDNAs of other repair genes although attempts to use it with AT cells have apparently been unsuccessful (Meyn et al. 1993).

Although EBV vectors are generally considered unable to replicate in rodent cells (Yates et al. 1985), we have obtained evidence that they can replicate at low efficiency. In an effort to obtain transformants by cDNA transfection of the hamster V79 mutant irs1 (see Table 3) with the pEBS7 library described above, we found that the transformants were phenotypically unstable in terms of their mitomycin C resistance and hygromycin B resistance (N. Liu and L. Thompson, unpublished results). Cells grown in the absence of selection rapidly lost the complementing sequences. By preparing a simple extract (Hirt 1967), we could rescue the complementing *XRCC2* cDNA (N. Liu and L. Thompson, unpublished results). These results imply that the EBV plasmid must be replicating at a very low efficiency such that many daughter cells fail to carry a copy of the plasmid.

IDENTIFICATION OF REPAIR GENES BASED ON PROTEIN SEQUENCE

In instances where mutants do not exist for genes of interest, a biochemical approach can lead to identifying the relevant genes. Several examples of this approach have been reported. The DNA ligase I (*LIG1*) gene was cloned by preparing a degenerate probe based on peptide sequence and screening a cDNA library (Barnes et al. 1990). This cDNA was also cloned by screening for cDNAs that complemented a yeast temperature sensitive mutant defective in DNA ligase.

Another strategy to identify repair proteins has been to search for proteins that bind to damaged DNA. One such protein is the UV-DDB (DNA damage binding) protein that binds to UV-irradiated DNA and was observed to be absent in cell lines from some patients of XP group E (Chu and Chang, 1988). The UV-DDB protein from monkey cells was purified, and polypeptide sequence information was used to clone a cDNA encoding the DDB protein (Takao et al. 1993).

Yet another approach is to identify repair proteins by their association with known proteins. While purifying a protein fraction that complemented DNA repair synthesis in cell-free extracts from XP-C cells, Masutani et al. (1994) identified a tightly associated protein, which proved to be encoded by a human homolog (designated *HHR23B*) of the yeast *RAD23* gene. Thus *HHR23B* (and possibly another homolog, *HHR23A*) is presumed to play a role in repair although no mutant phenotype associated with *HHR23B* has been reported.

CHARACTERIZATION OF GENES AND PROTEINS INVOLVED IN NUCLEOTIDE EXCISION REPAIR

The cloning strategies described above led to the characterization of the genes listed in Table 1, which summarizes the genes involved in damage recognition, incision, excision, as well as the ligation step following resynthesis (see Fig. 1 for a somewhat speculative model of the NER process). Xeroderma pigmentosum is the classical DNA repair disorder in which cellular hypersensitivity to UV radiation (e.g. solar exposure) is associated with defective excision repair, hypermutability, and increased susceptibility to skin cancer. The genes for five of the seven complementation groups of XP have been unambiguously identified while groups E and F remain to be fully characterized. The *ERCC4* gene, which may be equivalent to *XPF*, has been cloned (Thompson et al. 1994) and sequenced (L. Thompson, K. Brookman, J. Lamerdin, and A. Carrano, unpublished results), but XP-F cells have not yet been analyzed for mutations in this gene. The *XPE* gene(s) may be equivalent to one or both subunits of the UV-DDB factor (Keeney et al. 1993), whose DNA binding activity was shown to be absent in a minority of XP-E patients (Chu and Chang 1988; Keeney et al. 1992).

Mutations that are implicated as causal for the repair defect and the disease in XP patients have been reported for *XPA* (Satokata et al. 1990, 1992; Nishigori et al. 1993), *XPB* (Weeda et al. 1990; Vermeulen et al. 1994), *XPC* (Li et al. 1993), *XPD* (Frederick et al. 1994; Broughton et al. 1995; Takayama et al. submitted), and *XPG* (Nouspikel and Clarkson 1994). A candidate gene for XPE has been reported (Takao et al. 1993), and the encoded protein has been shown to correct the defect in repair synthesis in members of the XP-E complementation group that have a deficiency in DNA damage binding (DDB) protein (Keeney et al. 1994). Genes given *ERCC* designations represent rodent complementation groups, and most of these correspond to XP and Cockayne syndrome (CS) groups, as indicated in Table 1.

Cockayne syndrome, like XP, involves cellular hypersensitivity to UV radiation due to defective NER, but in this case the defect specifically affects preferential repair of the transcribed strand of active genes (van Hoffen et al. 1993). The *CSB* gene was cloned by complementing a CHO mutant (UV61) having intermediate UV sensitivity, and identification of mutations in the *CSB* alleles of a patient confirmed the involvement of this gene (Troelstra et al. 1992a). A candidate cDNA for the *CSA* gene was recently isolated after correcting CS-A cells by transfection with the pEBS7 episomally replicating library. The observation that rodent cells defective in the homolog of *CSB*(*ERCC6*) have normal repair in a cell-free plasmid repair assay (Reardon et al. 1993) agrees with the interpretation that *ERCC6* is not required for global DNA repair (i.e. repair not coupled to transcription). Three of the complementation groups of XP (XP-B, XP-D, and XP-G) involve overlap with CS in certain patients having some symptoms of both syndromes. These complex phenotypes appear to be due to single-gene mutations in the respective DNA repair genes, as discussed below.

The *ERCC2* (*XPD*) gene is unusual in that it is also involved in another syndrome, known as trichothiodistrophy (TTD), which has the hallmark features of brittle hair/nails and ichthyosis, as well severe growth defects and dysmyelination in the nervous system (Stefanini et al. 1986; Rebora and Crovato 1987). Yet another genetic disorder, Cockayne syndrome, shows similarities with TTD, in terms of growth failure and neurological abnormalities. (See review of TTD and CS by Friedberg et al. 1993). TTD patients can show a wide range of repair deficiencies, like XP, but curiously they do not have elevated skin cancer rates, a feature that is shared with CS patients. A variety of mutations has been identified in the *ERCC2* gene in TTD cell lines (Broughton et al. 1994; C. Weber and K. Takayama, person. comm.), and in some cases the same mutant allele has been identified in both TTD and XP cell lines (Takayama et al. submitted). In some instances XP-D patients also have features of CS, and mutations in the alleles of

Table 1. Nucleotide excision repair genes that have been cloned and characterized

Gene*	Human disease involved	Gene size (kb)	ORF size (aa)	Chromosomal location	References
ERCC1	?	15	297	19q13.2	van Duin et al. 1986, 1987,1989; Mohrenweiser et al. 1989
ERCC4	XP-F?	30	≈ 856	16p13.13	Thompson et al. 1994; Liu et al. 1993; Thompson et al. unpublish.
XPA	XP-A	25	273	9q34.1	Tanaka et al. 1990; Satokata et al. 1993
XPB (*ERCC3*)	XP-B	45	782	2q21	Weeda et al. 1990, 1991; Thompson et al. 1987
XPC	XP-C	?	940	3p25	Legerski & Peterson 1992; Legerski et al. 1994; Masutani et al. 1994
XPD (*ERCC2*)	XP-D	19	760	19q13.2	Weber et al. 1988, 1990; Flejter et al. 1992; Thompson et al. 1989
UV-DDB	XP-E?	?	1140†	11	Chu & Chang 1988; Takao et al. 1993; Keeney et al. 1994
XPG (*ERCC5*)	XP-G	32	1186	13q33	O'Donovan et al. 1993; Sherly et al. 1993; MacInnes et al. 1993 Samec et al. 1994
CSA	CS-A	?	396		Henning et al. 1995
CSB (*ERCC6*)	CS-B	~85	1493	10q11-21	Troelstra et al. 1992a, 1992b, 1993
HHR23B	?	?	409	3p25.1	Masutani et al. 1994
LIG1	BS-like	53	919	19q13.2	Barnes et al. 1990; Noguiez et al. 1992

*By published agreement (Lehmann et al. 1994), the name "*XPB*" is replacing *XPBC* and *ERCC3*, etc.; original names are given in parentheses and may be preferable in certain contexts.

†The DDB cDNA clone reported by Takao et al. (1993) is from monkey cells.

ERCC2 appear to be the basis of these complex phenotypes (Broughton et al. 1995; Takayama et al. submitted).

Except for the CS genes, almost all of the *ERCC* and *XP* genes listed in Table 1 are required for global and transcription coupled repair. The other exception is the *XPC* gene, which is unnecessary for transcription coupled repair (Venema et al. 1990, 1991). The *ERCC1* gene, which was isolated on the basis of complementation of a highly UV sensitive CHO cell mutant, is exceptional in not being associated with any human disease. Thus, it is not so surprising transgenic mice that are homozygous for a disruption mutation in this locus were developmentally impaired and did not survive into adulthood (McWhir et al. 1993). Nor has any human disorder been associated with the *HHR23B* gene. A picture of the involvement of NER in human genetic disorders is becoming increasingly complex with the understanding of the dual roles of several of the genes (i.e. *XPB*, *XPD*) in both repair and transcription. The genetic disorders CS and TTD are now being viewed as transcription disorders, in which the developmental and neurological defects are likely due to alterations in the transcription function of the affected gene, rather than the repair function (Bootsma and Hoeijmakers 1994; Cleaver et al. 1995; Arlett and Lehmann 1995). A puzzling question that remains to be resolved is why CS and TTD patients fail to get skin cancer even though they have repair deficiency and photosensitivity. Answers to this question will likely come with a better understanding of how the mutations in these patients affect transcription and possibly its coupling to DNA repair.

The *LIG1* gene was previously thought to be a candidate for the Bloom syndrome (BS) gene, but it has been ruled out based on the differing chromosomal locations of the *BS* and *LIG1* genes and other criteria (Noguiez et al. 1992; McDaniel and Schultz 1992). However, one immunodeficient patient was identified who possessed point mutations in both alleles of the *LIG1*, which is likely an essential gene (Barnes et al. 1992). The cells from this patient (46BR) show increased UV sensitivity, suggesting that DNA ligase I plays a role in the NER pathway (see Fig. 1) (Teo et al. 1983).

The proteins encoded by the genes shown in Table 1 are summarized in Table 2 in terms of their yeast "homologs" and biochemical functions. It is evident that most of the human proteins are related to proteins in the yeast *Saccharomyces cerevisiae*, but the degree of similarity varies widely. The most highly conserved proteins are the XPB and XPD, which show about ~50% amino acid identity between species. These two proteins are known to be required for cell viability as well as repair because of their involvement in transcription (see below). For example, microinjection of cells with an antibody against the XPB protein resulted in cell death (van Vuuren et al. 1994). The XPC and XPG proteins show limited regions of similarity with the Rad4 and Rad2 proteins , respectively, with overall identity being >25%. In a few instances there is weak cross-species functionality as, for example, shown by the ability of XPD protein to partially correct the essential function of a *rad3* mutant while not correcting defective repair in this mutant (Sung et al. 1993). Also, the Rad10 protein appeared to give a low level of correction of the repair-deficient phenotype of a CHO mutant in complementation group 1 (Lambert et al. 1988).

Considerable progress has been made in identifying the biochemical functions of the individual repair proteins, with the discovery that these proteins often perform their functions as components of multiprotein complexes (see reviews by Aboussekhra and Wood 1994; Sancar 1994). Figure 1 depicts the roles of proteins known to be involved in the steps of damage recognition, incision, excision, polymerization, and ligation in NER. Very recently, reconstitution of both the incision and polymerization stages of this pathway have been performed using only purified proteins (Mu et al. 1995; Aboussekhra et al.

Table 2. Role of individual repair proteins in damage recognition and excision

Protein	kDa	Homologous protein in *S. cerevisiae*	Specific protein function	References
ERCC1	33	Rad10	incision 5' of lesion (predicted)	van Duin et al. 1986; Bardwell et al. 1994
ERCC4	98	Rad1	incision 5' of lesion (predicted)	Thompson et al. unpublished; Bardwell et al. 1994
XPA	31	Rad14	damage recog.; DNA binding	Tanaka et al. 1990; Bankman et al. 1992; Jones & Wood 1993
XPB	89	Rad25 (Ssl2)	3' to 5' helicase; TFIIH subunit	Weeda et al. 1990; Park et al. 1992; Schaeffer et al. 1993; Drapkin et al. 1994; van Vuuren et al. 1994
XPC	106	Rad4	global genome repair	Masutani et al. 1994; Legerski & Peterson 1992; Venema et al. 1990
XPD	87	Rad3	5' to 3' helicase; TFIIH subunit	Weber et al. 1990; Sung et al. 1993; Drapkin et al. 1994; van Vuuren et al. 1994
UV-DDB (XPE?)	124	?	damage recognition	Takao et al. 1993; Patterson & Chu 1989; Keeney et al. 1993; Payne & Chu 1994
XPG	133	Rad2	incision 3' of lesion	Sherly et al. 1993; O'Donovan et al. 1994
CSA	~44	?	transcrpt. coupling	Henning et al. 1995
CSB	168	Rad26	transcrpt. coupling; helicase?	Troelstra et al. 1992
HHR23B	43	Rad23	global genome repair	Masutani et al. 1994

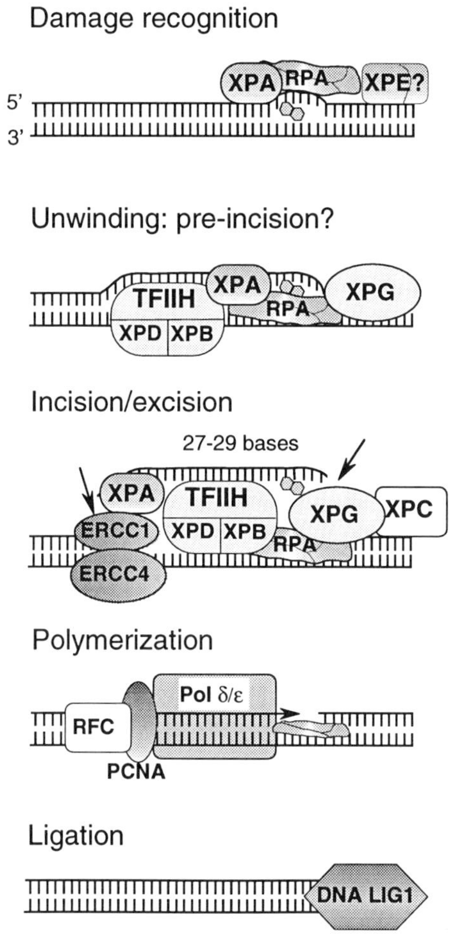

Figure 1. Outline of a model of nucleotide excision repair. Following recognition of damage, DNA unwinding mediated by helicase activity may be necessary for incision on one or both sides of the damaged base(s). Helicase activity may also mediate release of the damaged oligonucleotide. All of the proteins shown here are essential except for XPE (Mu et al. 1995; Aboussekhra et al. 1995). Other proteins (e.g. HHR23) that remain to be identified and characterized may influence the efficiency of the reactions. Some of the known protein interactions are shown, but many details remain to be clarified.

1995). Damage recognition is thought to be mediated by the XPA protein, which exhibits Zn-finger motifs and has an elevated affinity for damaged DNA (Tanaka et al. 1990; Jones and Wood 1993). The XPE-related UV-DDB protein also recognizes a broad spectrum of lesions and may facilitate the recognition process (Payne and Chu 1994). Although this protein is not required to achieve the incision reaction in an in vitro system (Mu et al. 1995), its presence appears to improve the efficiency of the reaction Aboussekhra et al. 1995). Recently the RPA protein (replication protein A, also known as single-strand binding protein), which has single-stranded DNA binding activity and is required for SV40 replication, has also been implicated in damage recognition through a cooperative interaction with XPA (He et al. 1995).

The XPB and XPD proteins have been identified as components of the transcription initiation factor TFIIH, which is required by RNA polymerase II (Gerard et al. 1991; Flores et al. 1992). TFIIH contains approximately eight proteins and is thought to embody XPB and XPD in the form in which they participate in repair as well as in transcription (Drapkin et al. 1994; Schaeffer et al. 1994; Park et al. 1995). Both the XPB and XPD proteins are known to have helicase activity (Schaeffer et al. 1993; Sung et al. 1993), with XPD moving 5' to 3' and XPB moving 3' to 5' on the strand to which it is bound. These helicase activities are implicated in the unwinding that is associated with excision of the damaged oligonucleotide. Helicase activity may also be required to create single-stranded regions that become the substrate for the incision endonucleases. The RPA protein is also required for the incision step (Coverly et al. 1992; Mu et al. 1995; Aboussekhra et al. 1995), perhaps in addition to its role in damage recognition.

The incisions on either side of the damaged base(s) are known be asymmetrically positioned (Huang et al. 1992), with the incision on the 3' side of damage being performed by the XPG nuclease (O'Donovan et al. 1994a, 1994b). An ≈ 30-base oligonucleotide containing the damage is released (Huang et al. 1992; Svoboda et al. 1993), as compared with a 12-mer in *E. coli* (Sancar 1994). The incision on the 5' side of the lesion is predicted to be performed by the ERCC1/ERCC4/XPF complex (van Vuuren et al. 1993; Biggerstaff et al. 1993) complex, based on the finding that the homologous Rad10/Rad1 complex in *Saccharomyces cerevisiae* can incise at a junction between duplex and single-stranded DNA and does so specifically in the strand having a 3' terminus (Bardwell et al. 1994). During global repair, accurate incision also requires the XPC protein (Shivji et al. 1994), which may be necessary for stabilizing the incision produced by the XPG nuclease.

The proteins shown in Fig. 1 may be all that are necessary for a complete incision reaction (Mu et al. 1995). However, Aboussekhra et al. (1995) reported that an additional, unidentified protein (IF7) is needed for incision (as well as the overall repair reaction). Other proteins, such as HHR23B (Masutani et al. 1994) and those represented by the rodent complementation groups 7 through 11 (Hoeijmakers 1993), may enhance the efficiency of the process. A detailed picture of how all these proteins cooperate and interact is just beginning to emerge. Interactions between the XPA protein and ERCC1, RPA, and TFIIH have been reported (Li et al. 1994; Park and Sancar 1994; Park et al. 1995; He et al. 1995), suggesting that the XPA protein plays a key role in recruiting other partners into a multiprotein complex assembled at the site of the lesion. For the coupling of NER to transcription, additional proteins (e.g. CSA and CSB) are required, and a major goal for the future is to develop a cell-free assay in which NER is coupled to transcription.

IDENTIFICATION OF GENES AND PROTEINS INVOLVED IN BASE EXCISION REPAIR AND OTHER MODES OF REPAIR

In analogy with the successful analysis of NER, attempts are being made to dissect repair pathways acting on ionizing radiation damage, DNA crosslinks, and other classes of damage. Table 3 summarizes a number of genes that have been cloned and/or mapped to specific chromosomes and indicates what is known about the biochemical function of the proteins. Mutants, primarily from Chinese hamster lines, which have increased sensitivity to ionizing radiation damage, have been identified (Thacker and Wilkinson 1991; Jeggo et al. 1991; Collins 1993), and human genes that complement these mutations have been given the nomenclature *XRCC* (x-ray repair cross complementing, i.e. interspecies complementation) as suggested by Thompson and Jeggo (1995). The *XRCC1* gene was the first human gene to be identified that corrected a rodent mutant line, CHO EM9, having (slightly) increased x-ray sensitivity (Thompson et al. 1982). The XRCC1 protein is implicated at the ligation step in base excision repair where it appears to form a complex with DNA ligase III, (Caldecott et al. 1994). The cloned *XRCC2* and *XRCC3* cDNAs correct mutants that were isolated as being hypersensitive to ionizing radiation. These mutants have broad-spectrum sensitivity to various types of DNA damage, including extreme hypersensitivity to DNA crosslinking agents. *XRCC3* seems to play a very important role in spontaneous chromosome stability as well as the cellular response to DNA damage (Tebbs et al. 1995), suggesting that the protein might have more than one function. Recent analysis shows that the XRCC3 protein has significant similarity with the Rad51 and Rad57 proteins of *S. cerevisiae* (L. Thompson, J. Lamerdin, and A. Carrano, unpublished results) (however, a much more highly conserved human homolog of Rad51 was previously reported: Shinohara et al. 1993; Yoshimura et al. 1993). A cDNA for *XRCC2* was also recently obtained (N. Liu and L. Thompson, unpublished results) and appears to efficiently correct the V79 mutant irs1.

XRCC4 through *XRCC7* are genes associated with high sensitivity to ionizing radiation and defective double-strand break repair. *XRCC5* and *XRCC6* were recently recognized as the genes encoding the heterodimeric Ku autoantigen (summarized by Troelstra and Jaspers 1994). Ku complexes with, and activates, the SCID protein, which has been identified as the catalytic subunit of the DNA-dependent protein kinase (DNA-PK_{CS}) (Kirchgessner et al. 1995; Blunt et al. 1995).

In ataxia telangiectasia (AT), the human genetic disorder that involves substantial hypersensitivity to ionizing radiation, cell fusion experiments have suggested four complementation groups for AT cell lines (Jaspers et al. 1988) although proof that these groups really represent different genes is lacking. Three putative AT genes have been mapped to a region of the q arm of chromosome 11. However, efforts to clone these genes have not been successful in spite of attempts in several laboratories (Lohrer et al. 1988; Meyn et al. 1993).

Base excision repair is a major pathway that acts on base damage produced by ionizing radiation and simple alkylating agents, as well as spontaneous damage from metabolism (Friedberg et al. 1995). Following removal of altered bases by glycosylases (such as those acting on uracil, 3-methyladenine, thymine glycols, formamidopyrimidine, and G·T mismatches), an apurinic/apyrimidinic (AP) endonuclease, such as APE (HAP1; see Table 3) makes an incision immediately flanking the altered base. Following polymerization (e.g. by Polβ) of one or several nucleotides and removal of the sugar-phos-

Table 3. Genes in other repair pathways that have been cloned or mapped

Gene	Mutant	Chrom. location	Protein function	References
XRCC1 *	EM9	19q13.2-13.3	Ligase III cofactor in BER[#]	Thompson et al. 1990; Caldecott et al. 1994
XRCC2 *	irs1	7q36	not known	Thacker et. al. 1995; Jones et al. 1995
XRCC3 *	irs1SF	14q32.3	chromosome stability	Tebbs et al. 1995
XRCC4	XR-1	5q13-q14	DS[†]-break repair	Stamato et al. 1988; Stamato and Otevrel 1995
XRCC5/Ku86 *	xrs5	2q35	DS-break repair	Hafezparast et al. 1993; Taccioli et al. 1994
XRCC6/Ku70 *	sxi-1	22q13	DS-break repair	Reeves et al. 1989; Griffith et al. 1992 Lee et al. 1995; Boubnov et al. sub.
XRCC7/SCID/ DNA-PK$_{cs}$ *	SCID	8p11.1-11.1	DS-break repair	Kurisama et al. 1994; Kirchgessner et al. 1995
ATA, ATC, ATD	AT-A, -C, -D	11q22-q23	not known	Gatti et al. 1988; Foroud et al. 1991; Lambert et al. 1991; Kodama et al. 1992; Richard et al. 1993
UDG *	-	12	uracil glycosylase	Olsen et al. 1989; Aasland et al. 1990
MPG (MAG) *	(*E. coli*)	16p	Me-purine glycosylase	Samson et al. 1991; Vickers et al. 1993
MGMT *	mex$^-$	10q24.33-qter	Me-Gua-Me-transferase	Tano et al. 1990; Gardner et al. 1991
HAP1 (APE) *	-	14q11.2-12	AP endonuclease	Robson et al. 1991, 1992; Demple et al. 1991
Pol β *	–	8pter-8q22	Polymerization	McBride et al. 1987; Sen Gupta et al. 1986
LIG3 *	-	7	DNA ligase in BER	A. Tomkinson, personal commun.

* Genes and/or cDNAs that have been cloned

[#] BER = base excision repair

[†] DS = double-strand

Table 3 (continuation). Genes in other repair pathways that have been cloned or mapped

Gene	Mutant	Chrom. location	Protein function	References
hRAD51 *	(*S.c.*)[†]	15q15.1	strand transferase?	Shinohara et al. 1993; Yoshimura et al. 1993
hRAD52 *	(*S.c.*)	12p13.3	not known	Pastink et al., person. comm.
hRAD54 *	(*S.c.*)	1p32	not known	Pastink et al., person. comm.
HHR6A *	(*S.c.*)	Xq24-q25	ubiquitin conjugation?	Sung et al. 1990; Koken et al. 1991
HHR6B *	(*S.c.*)	5q23-q31	ubiquitin conjugation?	Sung et al. 1990; Koken et al. 1991
FAC *	FA-C	9q22.3	not known	Strathdee et al. 1992a, 1992b
BS	BS	15q14-qter	not known	McDaniel et al. 1992
hMLH1 *	tumor	3p21	mismatch repair	Papadopoulos et al. 1994; Bronner et al. 1994
hMSH2 *	tumor	2p22-21	mismatch repair	Fishel et al. 1993; Leach et al. 1993
hPMS1 *	tumor	2q31-33	mismatch repair	Nicolaides et al. 1994
hPMS2 *	tumor	7p22	mismatch repair	Nicolaides et al. 1994

* Genes and/or cDNAs that have been cloned

† *Saccharomyces cerevisiae*

phate residue, the repair process is completed by the action of a DNA ligase, either LIGIII (following Polβ) or LIGI (following Polδ/ε) (Lindahl et al. 1995).

Table 3 lists known human genes for uracil glycosylase (*UDG*), methyl purine glycosylase (*MPG*), and methyl-guanine methyltransferase (*MGMT*), which are important for the removal of spontaneous or alkylation-induced damage. These genes encode highly conserved proteins that act in the absence of multiprotein complexes and whose functions are somewhat interchangeable between mammalian cells and bacteria. Although the *APE* gene has been cloned by several laboratories, no mutant lines have been reported. However, expression of antisense *APE* in rat cells resulted in a phenotype of slightly increased sensitivity to methylation damage (Ono et al. 1994). One might predict that such *APE* mutants will be hypersensitive to ionizing radiation. Recently the *LIGIII* cDNA was cloned (A. Tomkinson, J. Chen, I., Husain, and J. Besterman, personal commun.), which should allow for protein overexpression and a much more detailed study of the nature of the interaction of LIG III protein with XRCC1.

In the yeast *S. cerevisiae,* genes in the *RAD52* epistasis group are known to be important in determining sensitivity to ionizing radiation through their role in double strand break repair by homologous recombination (Friedberg et al. 1995). Human and mouse homologs of *RAD51*, *RAD52*, and *RAD54* have been isolated based on sequence conservation, but so far it is unclear whether these homologs are involved in the repair of ionizing radiation damage. The mouse Rad51 protein was found to be present in the synaptonemal complex in mouse meiotic prophase cells, and in cultured human cells discrete nuclear foci were detected by immunofluorescence (Haaf et al. 1995). These foci were more numerous after damage with ionizing radiation and other agents, suggesting an involvement in response to damage.

In *S. cerevisiae* the *RAD6* gene is important for UV mutagenesis and for resistance to both UV and ionizing radiation (Prakash 1989; Cassier-Chauvat and Fabre 1991). The Rad6 protein functions in the conjugation of ubiquitin (Sung et al. 1990), a polypeptide involved in protein degradation and other processes. Based on sequence conservation, two human homologs (*HHR6A* and *HHR6B*) have been identified. It is not yet apparent whether these human genes are involved in DNA repair, but knockout mutations have been made in transgenic mice, which will provide mutant cell lines for analysis (J. Hoeijmakers, personal commun.).

In Bloom syndrome there appears to be a single responsible gene (*BS*), which has been mapped but not cloned. Similarities in the phenotype between the *XRCC1* mutants and Bloom syndrome cells, such as the very high sister chromatid exchanges (Chiganti et al. 1974), suggest that the BS protein may act in the same pathway as XRCC1 protein. In Fanconi anemia (FA) the gene for one of the five complementation groups has been cloned (Strathdee et al. 1992b), but no function has yet been assigned to its protein. Transgenic mice having a knockout mutation in the mouse FAC gene were, surprisingly, developmentally normal and did not show bone marrow failure (Chen et al. 1995).

Finally, in Table 3 are indicated several recently identified genes that are involved in the mismatch repair pathway, all of which have been found to be defective in nonpolyposis colon cancer, perhaps the most common hereditary disease. Defects in this pathway are characterized by great instability of dinucleotide repeats during replication (Parsons et al. 1993) and resistance to simple alkylating agents (Branch et al. 1993; Kat et al. 1993). Thus, mutations in mismatch repair can confer resistance to cell killing by alkylation damage at the expense of a hypermutable phenotype.

CONCLUDING REMARKS

Based on the current rate of progress, we can expect the collection of human repair genes to grow substantially. Additional genes for the poorly understood human repair disorders (AT, BS, and FA) will surely be cloned before long. We can anticipate a much better understanding of how the human homologs of genes in the *RAD6* and *RAD52* epistasis groups are involved in the responses of human cells to DNA damage. For example, do human cells have a pathway for repairing double-strand breaks that involves homologous recombination, or has the Ku/DNA-PK_{CS} system essentially replaced the role of the *RAD52* pathway? Other intriguing issues in mammalian cells include: why some NER-deficient syndromes (XP) are cancer-prone while others (TTD and CS) are not, and why cells have at least three distinct DNA ligases.

The mechanism(s) by which cells repair or circumvent DNA interstrand crosslinks are poorly understood. The extraordinary hypersensitivity (>30-fold) of rodent mutants to the crosslinking agent mitomycin C has been shown for several complementation groups (e.g. the *ERCC1* and *ERCC4* groups of NER as well as the *XRCC2* and *XRCC3* mutants). Many additional complementation groups for mitomycin C sensitivity have been described (Overkamp et al. 1993; Jones 1994). These phenotypes imply highly efficient cellular mechanisms for dealing with these lesions. Analysis of the protein products of the many genes influencing crosslink sensitivity, together with plasmid systems carrying crosslink lesions at defined sites (Bredberg et al. 1995), should provide insight into these processes.

ACKNOWLEDGMENTS

This work was done under the auspices of the U.S. Department of Energy by Lawrence Livermore National Laboratory under contract No. W-7405-ENG-48. I thank Kerry Brookman, Christopher Parris, and Christine Weber for reading the manuscript.

REFERENCES

Aasland R, Olsen LC, Spurr NK, Krokan HE, Helland DE (1990): Chromosomal assignment of human uracil-DNA glycosylase to chromosome 12. Genomics 7:139-141.

Aboussekhra A, Biggerstaff M, Shivji MKK, Vilpo JA, Moncollin V, Podust VN, Protic M, Hubscher U, Egly J-M, Wood RD (1995): Mammalian DNA nucleotide excision repair reconstituted with purified protein components. Cell 80:859-868.

Aboussekhra A, Wood RD (1994): Repair of UV-damaged DNA by mammalian cells and *Saccharomyces cerevisiae*. Curr. Opin. Genet. Dev. 4:212-220.

Arlett CF, Lehmann AR (1995): Xeroderma pigmentosum, Cockayne syndrome, and trichothiodystrophy: sun sensitivity, DNA repair defects and skin cancer. In Eeles R, Ponder B, Horwich A (eds): "Genetic Predisposition to Cancer." London: Chapman and Hall, chapter 12 in press.

Bankmann M, Prakash L, Prakash S (1992): Yeast *RAD14* and human xeroderma pigmentosum group A DNA-repair genes encode homologous proteins. Nature 355:555-558.

Bardwell AJ, Bardwell L, Tomkinson AE, Friedberg EC (1994): Specific cleavage of model recombination and repair intermediates by the yeast Rad1-Rad10 endonuclease. Science 265:2082-2085.

Barnes DE, Johnston LH, Kodama K, Tomkinson AE, Lasko DD, Lindahl T (1990): Human DNA ligase I cDNA: cloning and functional expression in *Saccharomyces cerevisiae*. Proc. Natl. Acad. Sci. U.S.A. 87:6679-6683.

Barnes DE, Tomkinson AE, Lehmann AR, Webster AD, Lindahl T (1992): Mutations in the DNA ligase I gene of an individual with immunodeficiencies and cellular hypersensitivity to DNA-damaging agents. Cell 69:495-503.

Biggerstaff M, Szymkowski DE, Wood RD (1993): Co-correction of the ERCC1, ERCC4 and xeroderma pigmentosum group F DNA repair defects in vitro. EMBO J 12:3685-3692.

Blunt T, Finnie NJ, Taccioli GE, Smith GCM, Demengeot J, Gottlieb TM, Mizuta R, Varghese AJ, Alt FW, Jeggo PA, Jackson SP (1995): Defective DNA-dependent protein kinase activity is linked to V(D)J recombination and DNA repair defects associated with the murine *scid* mutation. Cell 80:813-823.

Bohr VA, Okumoto DS, Hanawalt PC (1986): Survival of UV-irradiated mammalian cells correlates with efficient DNA repair in an essential gene. Proc. Natl. Acad. Sci. U.S.A. 83:3830-3833.

Bohr VA, Smith CA, Okumoto DS, Hanawalt PC (1985): DNA repair in an active gene: removal of pyrimidine dimers from the DHFR gene of CHO cells is much more efficient than in the genome overall. Cell 40:359-369.

Bootsma D, Hoeijmakers JH (1994): The molecular basis of nucleotide excision repair syndromes. Mutat. Res. 307:15-23.

Boubnov NV, Lee SE, Wills ZP, Hall KT, Hendrickson EA, Weaver DT (1995): The Ku p70 gene restores DNA binding, ionizing radiation resistance, and V(D)J recombination proficiency to a mammalian DNA double-strand break repair mutant. submitted.

Branch P, Aquilina G, Bignami M, Karran P (1993): Defective mismatch binding and a mutator phenotype in cells tolerant to DNA damage. Nature 362:652-654.

Bredberg A, Sandor Z, Brant M (1995): Mutational response of Fanconi anaemia cells to shuttle vector site-specific psoralen cross-links. Carcinogen. 16:555-562.

Bronner CE, Baker SM, Morrison PT, Warren G, Smith LG, Lescoe MK, Kane M, Earabino C, Lipford J, Lindblom A, et al. (1994): Mutation in the DNA mismatch repair gene homologue hMLH1 is associated with hereditary non-polyposis colon cancer. Nature 368:258-261.

Broughton BC, Steingrimsdottir H, Weber CA, Lehmann AR (1994): Mutations in the xeroderma pigmentosum group D DNA repair gene in patients with trichothiodistrophy. Nature Genetics 7:189-194.

Broughton BC, Thompson AF, Harcourt SA, Vermeulen W, Hoeijmakers JHJ, Botta E, Stefanini M, King M, Weber C, Cole J, Arlett CF, Lehmann AR (1995): Molecular and cellular analysis of the DNA repair defect in a patient in xeroderma pigmentosum group D with the clinical features of xeroderma pigmentosum and Cockayne syndrome. Am. J. Hum. Genet. 56:167-174.

Caldecott KW, McKeown CK, Tucker JD, Ljungquist S, Thompson LH (1994): An interaction between the mammalian DNA repair protein XRCC1 and DNA ligase III. Mol. Cell. Biol. 14:68-76.

Cassier-Chauvat C, Fabre F (1991): A similar defect in UV-induced mutagenesis conferred by the *rad6* and *rad18* mutations of *Saccharomyces cerevisiae*. Mutat. Res. 254:247-253.

Chaganti RSK, Schonberg S, German J (1974): A manyfold increase in sister chromatid exchanges in Bloom's syndrome lymphocytes. Proc. Natl. Acad. Sci. U.S.A. 71:4508-4512.

Chen M, Cumming R, Krasnoshtein F, Savoia A, Lightfoot J, Santos C, Parker L, Wong J, Joyner A, Buchwald M (1995): Molecular genetics of Fanconi anemia. J. Cell. Biochem. Suppl. 21A:272.

Chu G, Chang E (1988): Xeroderma pigmentosum group E cells lack a nuclear factor that binds to damaged DNA. Science 242:564-567.

Cleaver JE, Kraemer KH (1989): Xeroderma pigmentosum. In. C.R. Scriver, A.L. Beudet, W.S. Sly, and D. Valle (eds.), *The Metabolic Basis of Inherited Disease*, Vol. II, McGraw-Hill, New York, pp. 2949-2971.

Cleaver JE, Speakman JR, Volpe JP (1995): Nucleotide excision repair: Variations associated with cancer development and speciation. Cancer Surveys 25, in press.

Collins AR (1993): Mutant rodent cell lines sensitive to ultraviolet light, ionizing radiation and cross-linking agents: a comprehensive survey of genetic and biochemical characteristics. Mutat. Res. 293:99-118.

Coverley D, Kenny MK, Lane DP, Wood RD (1992): A role for the human single-stranded DNA binding protein HSSB/RPA in an early stage of nucleotide excision repair. Nuc. Acids Res. 20:3873-3880.

Demple B, Herman T, Chen DS (1991): Cloning and expression of APE, the cDNA encoding the major human apurinic endonuclease: definition of a family of DNA repair enzymes. Proc. Natl. Acad. Sci. U. S. A. 88:11450-11454.

dos Santos CC, Gavish H, Buchwald M (1994): Fanconi anemia revisited: old ideas and new advances. Stem Cells 12:142-153.

Drapkin R, Reardon J, Ansari A, Huang JC, Zawel L, Ahn K, Sancar A, Reinberg D (1994): TFIIH, a link between RNA polymerase II transcription and DNA excision repair. Nature 368:769-772.

Fishel R, Lescoe MK, Rao MR, Copeland NG, Jenkins NA, Garber J, Kane M, Kolodner R (1993): The human mutator gene homolog *MSH2* and its association with hereditary nonpolyposis colon cancer. Cell 75:1027-1038.

Flejter WL, McDaniel LD, Johns D, Friedberg EC, Schultz RA (1992): Correction of xeroderma pigmentosum complementation group D mutant cell phenotypes by chromosome and gene transfer: Involvement of the human *ERCC2* DNA repair gene. Proc. Natl. Acad. Sci. U.S.A. 89:261-265.

Flores O, Lu H, Reinberg D (1992): Factors involved in specific transcription by mammalian RNA polymerase II. Identification and characterization of factor IIH. J. Biol. Chem. 267:2786-2793.

Foroud T, Wei S, Ziv Y, Sobel E, Lange E, Chao A, Goradia T, Huo Y, Tolun A, Chessa L, et al. (1991): Localization of an ataxia-telangiectasia locus to a 3-cM interval on chromosome 11q23: linkage analysis of 111 families by an international consortium. Am. J. Hum. Genet. 49:1263-1279.

Frederick GD, Amirkhan RH, Schultz RA, Friedberg EC (1994): Structural and mutational analysis of the xeroderma pigmentosum group D (XPD) gene. Hum. Mol. Genet. 3:1783-1788.

Friedberg EC, Walker GC, Siede W (1995): "DNA Repair and Mutagenesis". Washington, D.C.: American Soc. Microbiol..

Gardner E, Rydberg B, Karran P, Ponder BA (1991): Localization of the human O6-methylguanine-DNA methyltransferase gene to chromosome 10q24.33-qter. Genomics 11:475-476.

Gatti RA, Berkell I, Bodner E, Braedt G, Charmley P, Concannon P, Ersoy F, Foroud T, Jaspers NGJ, Lange K, Lathrop GM, Leppert M, Nakamura Y, O'Connell P, Paterson M, Salser W, Sanal O, Silver J, Sparkes RS, Susi E, Weeks DE, Wei S, White R, Yoder F (1988): Localization of an ataxia-telangiectasia gene to chromosome 11q22-23. Nature 336:577-580.

Gerard M, Fischer L, Moncollin V, Chipoulet JM, Chambon P, Egly JM (1991): Purification and interaction properties of the human RNA polymerase B(II) general transcription factor BTF2. J. Biol. Chem. 266:20940-20945.

German J (1993): Bloom syndrome: a Mendelian prototype of somatic mutational disease. Medicine 72:393-406.

German J (1990): The chromosome-breakage syndromes: rare disorders that provide models for studying somatic mutation. In Spatz, L, Bloom, AD, Paul, NW (eds): "Detection of Cancer Predisposition: Laboratory Approaches." White Plains, NY: March of Dimes Birth Defects Foundation, pp 85-111.

Haaf T, Golub EI, Reddy G, Radding CM, Ward DC (1995): Nuclear foci of mammalian Rad51 recombination protein in somatic cells after DNA damage and its localization in synaptonemal complexes. Proc. Natl. Acad. Sci. U.S.A. 92:2298-2302.

He Z, Henricksen LA, Wold MS, Ingles CJ (1995): RPA involvement in the damage-recognition and incision steps of nucleotide excision repair. Nature 374:566-569.

Henning KA, Bhatia, P, Legerski R, Friedberg EC (1995): Cloning of a candidate gene for Cockayne syndrome group A. J. Cell. Biochem. Suppl. 21A:305.

Hirt B (1967): Selective extraction of polyoma DNA from infected mouse cell cultures. J. Mol. Biol. 26:365-369.

Hoeijmakers JH (1993): Nucleotide excision repair. II: From yeast to mammals. Trends Genet. 9:211-217.

Hoeijmakers JHJ, Odijk H, Westerveld A (1987): Differences between rodent and human cell lines in the amount of integrated DNA after transfection. Exp. Cell Res. 169:111-119.

Huang JC, Svoboda DL, Reardon JT, Sancar A (1992): Human nucleotide excision nuclease removes thymine dimers from DNA by incising the 22nd phosphodiester bond 5' and the 6th phosphodiester bond 3' to the photodimer. Proc. Natl. Acad. Sci. U. S. A. 89:3664-3668.

Jaspers NGJ, Gatti RA, Baan C, Linssen CML, Bootsma D (1988): Genetic complementation analysis of ataxia telangiectasia and the Nijmegen breakage syndrome: a survey of 50 patients. Cytogenet. Cell. Genet. 49:259-263.

Jeggo PA, Tesmer J, Chen DJ (1991): Genetic analysis of ionising radiation sensitive mutants of cultured mammalian cell lines. Mutat. Res. 254:125-133.

Jones CJ, Wood RD (1993): Preferential binding of the xeroderma pigmentosum group A complementing protein to damaged DNA. Biochemistry 32:12096-12116.

Jones NJ (1994): Genetic analysis of mitomycin C-hypersensitive Chinese hamster cell mutants. Mutagen. 9:477-482.

Jones NJ, Zhao Y, Siciliano MJ, Thompson LH (1995): Assignment of the *XRCC2* human DNA repair gene to chromosome 7q36 by complementation analysis. Genomics 26:619-622.

Kat A, Thilly WG, Fang WH, Longley MJ, Li GM, Modrich P (1993): An alkylation-tolerant, mutator human cell line is deficient in strand-specific mismatch repair. Proc. Natl. Acad. Sci. U. S. A. 90:6424-6428.

Keeney S, Chang GJ, Linn S (1993): Characterization of a human DNA damage binding protein implicated in xeroderma pigmentosum E. J. Biol. Chem. 268:21293-21300.

Keeney S, Eker AP, Brody T, Vermeulen W, Bootsma D, Hoeijmakers JH, Linn S (1994): Correction of the DNA repair defect in xeroderma pigmentosum group E by injection of a DNA damage-binding protein. Proc. Natl. Acad. Sci. U. S. A. 91:4053-4056.

Keeney S, Wein H, Linn S (1992): Biochemical heterogeneity in xeroderma pigmentosum complementation group E. Mutat. Res. 273:49-56.

Kirchgessner CU, Patil CK, Evans JW, Cuomo CA, Fried LM, Carter T, Oettinger MA, Brown JM (1995): DNA-dependent kinase (p350) as a candidate gene for the murine SCID defect. Science 267:1178-1183.

Kodama S, Komatsu K, Okumura Y, Oshimura M (1992): Suppression of X-ray-induced chromosome aberrations in ataxia telangiectasia cells by introduction of a normal human chromosome 11. Mutat. Res. 293:31-37.

Koken MH, Reynolds P, Jaspers-Dekker I, Prakash L, Prakash S, Bootsma D, Hoeijmakers JH (1991): Structural and functional conservation of two human homologs of the yeast DNA repair gene *RAD6*. Proc. Natl. Acad. Sci. U. S. A. 88:8865-8869.

Lambert C, Couto LB, Weiss WA, Schultz RA, Thompson LH, Friedberg EC (1988): A yeast DNA repair gene partially complements defective excision repair in mammalian cells. EMBO J. 7:3245-3253.

Lambert C, Schultz RA, Smith M, Wagner-McPherson C, McDaniel LD, Donlon T, Stanbridge EJ, Friedberg EC (1991): Functional complementation of ataxia-telangiectasia group D (AT-D) cells by microcell-mediated chromosome transfer and mapping of the AT-D locus to the region 11q22-23. Proc. Natl. Acad. Sci. U. S. A. 88:5907-5911.

Leach FS, Nicolaides NC, Papadopoulos N, Liu B, Jen J, Parsons R, Peltomaki P, Sistonen P, Aaltonen LA, Nystrom-Lahti M, et al (1993): Mutations of a *mutS* homolog in hereditary nonpolyposis colorectal cancer. Cell 75:1215-1225.

Lee SE, Pulaski CR, He DM, Benjamin DM, Voss M, Um J, Hendrickson EA (1995): Isolation of mammalian cell mutants that are X-ray sensitive, impaired in DNA double-strand break repair and defecfive for V(D)J recombination. Mutat. Res. in press.

Legerski RJ, Liu P, Li L, Peterson CA, Zhao Y, Leach RJ, Naylor SL, Siciliano MJ (1994): Assignment of xeroderma pigmentosum group C (*XPC*) gene to chromosome 3p25. Genomics 21:266-269.

Legerski R, Peterson C (1992): Expression cloning of a human DNA repair gene involved in xeroderma pigmentosum group C. Nature 359:70-73.

Li L, Bales ES, Peterson CA, Legerski RJ (1993): Characterization of molecular defects in xeroderma pigmentosum group C. Nat. Genet. 5:413-417.

Li L, Elledge SJ, Peterson CA, Bales ES, Legerski RJ (1994): Specific association between the human DNA repair proteins XPA and ERCC1. Proc. Natl. Acad. Sci. U. S. A. 91:5012-5016.

Lindahl T (1993): Instability and decay of the primary structure of DNA. Nature 362:709-715.

Lindahl T, Satoh MS, Dianov G (1995): Enzymes acting at strand interruptions in DNA. Phil. Trans. R. Soc. Lond. B 347:57-62.

Liu P, Siciliano J, White B, Legerski R, Callen D, Reeders S, Siciliano MJ, Thompson LH (1993): Regional mapping of human DNA excision repair gene *ERCC4* to chromosome 16p13.13-p13.2. Mutagenesis 8:199-205.

Lohrer H, Blum M., Herrlich P (1988): Ataxia telangiectasia resists gene cloning: an account of parameters determining gene transfer into human recipient cells. Mol. Gen. Genet. 212:474-480.

Longmire JL, Brown NC, Meincke LJ, Campbell ML, Albright KL, Fawcett JJ, Campbell EW, Moyzis RK, Hildebrand CE, Evans GA, et al (1993): Construction and characterization of partial digest DNA libraries made from flow-sorted human chromosome 16. Genet. Anal. Tech Appl. 10:69-76.

MacInnes MA, Dickson JA, Hernandez RR, Learmonth D, Lin GY, Mudgett JS, Park MS, Schauer S, Reynolds RJ, Strniste GF, Yu JY (1993): Human *ERCC5* cDNA-cosmid complementation for excision repair and bipartite amino acid domains conserved with RAD proteins of *Saccharomyces cerevisiae* and *Schizosaccharomyces pombe*. Mol. Cell. Biol. 13:6393-6402.

Masutani C, Sugasawa K, Yanagisawa J, Sonoyama T, Ui M, Enomoto T, Takio K, Tanaka K, van der Spek PJ, Bootsma D, Hoeijmakers JHJ, Hanaoka F (1994): Purification and cloning of a nucleotide excision repair complex involving the xeroderma pigmentosum group C protein and a human homologue of yeast RAD23. EMBO J. 13:1831-1843.

McBride OW, Zmudzka BZ, Wilson SH (1987): Chromosomal location of the human gene for DNA polymerase β. Proc. Natl. Acad. Sci. U.S.A. 84:503-507.

McDaniel LD, Schultz RA (1992): Elevated sister chromatid exchange phenotype of Bloom syndrome cells is complemented by human chromosome 15. Proc. Natl. Acad. Sci. U. S. A. 89:7968-7972.

McWhir J, Selfridge J, Harrison DJ, Squires S, Melton DW (1993): Mice with DNA repair gene (*ERCC-1*) deficiency have elevated levels of p53, liver nuclear abnormalities and die before weaning. Nature Genetics 5:217-224.

Mellon I, Spivak G, Hanawalt PC (1987): Selective removal of transcription-blocking DNA damage from the transcribed strand of the mammalian DHFR gene. Cell 51:241-249.

Meyn MS, Lu-Kuo JM, Herzing LB (1993): Expression cloning of multiple human cDNAs that complement the phenotypic defects of ataxia-telangiectasia group D fibroblasts. Am. J. Hum. Genet. 53:1206-1216.

Mohrenweiser HW, Carrano AV, Fertitta A, Perry B, Thompson LH, Tucker JD, Weber CA (1989): Refined mapping of the three DNA repair genes, *ERCC1*, *ERCC2*, and *XRCC1*, on human chromosome 19. Cytogenet. Cell Genet. 52:11-14.

Mu D, Park C-H, Matsunaga T, Hsu DS, Rearson JT, Sancar A (1995): Reconstitution of human DNA repair excision nuclease in a highly defined system. J. Biol. Chem. 270:2415-2418.

Nicolaides NC, Papadopoulos N, Liu B, Wei YF, Carter KC, Ruben SM, Rosen CA, Haseltine WA, Fleischmann RD, Fraser CM, et al. (1994): Mutations of two PMS homologues in hereditary nonpolyposis colon cancer. Nature 371:75-80.

Nishigori C, Zghal M, Yagi T, Imamura S, Komoun MR, Takebe H (1993): High prevalence of the point mutation in exon 6 of the xeroderma pigmentosum group A-complementing (*XPAC*) gene in xeroderma pigmentosum group A patients in Tunisia. Am. J. Hum. Genet. 53:1001-1006.

Noguiez P, Barnes DE, Mohrenweiser HW, Lindahl T (1992): Structure of the human DNA ligase I gene. Nucleic Acids Res. 20:3845-3850.

Nouspikel T, Clarkson SG (1994): Mutations that disable the DNA repair gene *XPG* in a xeroderma pigmentosum group G patient. Hum. Mol. Genet. 3:963-967.

O'Donovan A, Davies AA, Moggs JG, West SC, Wood RD (1994): XPG endonuclease makes the 3' incision in human DNA nucleotide excision repair. Nature 371:432-435.

O'Donovan A, Scherly D, Clarkson SG, Wood RG (1994): Isolation of active recombinant XPG protein, a human DNA repair endonuclease. J. Biol. Chem. 269:15965-15968.

Ono Y, Furuta T, Ohmoto T, Akiyama K, Seki S (1994): Stable expression in rat glioma cells of sense and antisense nucleic acids to a human multifunctional DNA repair enzyme, APEX nuclease. Mutat. Res. 315:55-63.

Overkamp WJI, Rooimans MA, Neuteboom I, Telleman P, Arwert F, Zdzienicka MZ (1993): Genetic diversity of mitomycin C-hypersensitive Chinese hamster cell mutants: a new complementation group with chromosomal instability. Somat. Cell Mol. Genet. 19:431-437.

Painter RB, Kapp LN (1991): Replication intermediates as substrates for DNA rearrangements. Mutat. Res. 262:21-23.

Papadopoulos N, Nicolaides NC, Wei YF, Ruben SM, Carter KC, Rosen CA, Haseltine WA, Fleischmann RD, Fraser CM, Adams MD, et al. (1994): Mutation of a mutL homolog in hereditary colon cancer. Science 263:1625-1629.

Park C-H, Mu D, Reardon JT, Sancar A (1995): The general transcription-repair factor TFIIH is recruited to the excision repair complex by the XPA protein independent of the TFIIE transcription factor. J. Biol. Chem. 270:4896-4902.

Park CH, Sancar A (1994): Formation of a ternary complex between human XPA, ERCC1, and ERCC4(XPF) excision repair proteins. Proc. Natl. Acad. Sci. U.S.A. 91:5017-5021.

Parsons R, Li GM, Longley MJ, Fang WH, Papadopoulos N, Jen J, de la Chapelle A., Kinzler KW, Vogelstein B, Modrich P (1993): Hypermutability and mismatch repair deficiency in RER+ tumor cells. Cell 75:1227-1236.

Patterson M, Chu G (1989): Evidence that xeroderma pigmentosum cells from complementation group E are deficient in a homolog of yeast photolyase. Mol. Cell. Biol. 9:5105-5112.

Payne A, Chu G (1994): Xeroderma pigmentosum group E binding factor recognizes a broad spectrum of DNA damage. Mutat. Res. 310:89-102.

Peterson C, Legerski R (1991): High-frequency transformation of human repair-deficient cell lines by an Epstein-Barr virus-based cDNA expression vector. Gene 107:279-284.

Prakash L (1989): The structure and function of *RAD6* and *RAD18* DNA repair genes of *Saccharomyces cerevisiae*. Genome 31:597-600.

Reardon JT, Thompson LH, Sancar A (1993): Excision repair in man and the molecular basis of xeroderma pigmentosum syndrome. Cold Spring Harbor Symp. Quant. Biol. 58:605-617.

Rebora A, Crovato F (1987): PIBI(D)S syndrome -- trichothiodystrophy with xeroderma pigmentosum (group D) mutation. J. Am. Acad. Dermatol. 16:940-947.

Riboni R, Botta E, Stefanini M, Numata M, Yasui A (1992): Identification of the eleventh complemenation group of UV-sensitive excision repair-defective rodent mutants. Cancer Res. 52:6690-6691.

Richard CW3d, Cox DR, Kapp L, Murnane J, Cornelis F, Julier C, Lathrop GM, James MR (1993): A radiation hybrid map of human chromosome 11q22-q23 containing the ataxia-telangiectasia disease locus. Genomics 17:1-5.

Robson CN, Hickson ID (1991): Isolation of cDNA clones encoding a human apurinic/apyrimidinic endonuclease that corrects DNA repair and mutagenesis defects in *E.. coli* xth (exonuclease III) mutants. Nucleic Acids Res. 19:5519-5523.

Robson CN, Hochhauser D, Craig R, Rack K, Buckle VJ, Hickson ID (1992): Structure of the human DNA repair gene *HAP1* and its localisation to chromosome 14q 11.2-12. Nucleic Acids Res. 20:4417-4421.

Samec S, Jones TA, Corlet J, Scherly D, Sheer D, Wood RD, Clarkson SG (1994): The human gene for xeroderma pigmentosum complementation group G (*XPG*) maps to 13q33 by fluorescence in situ hybridization. Genomics 21:283-285.

Samson L, Derfler B, Boosalis M, Call K (1991): Cloning and characterization of a 3-methyladenine DNA glycosylase cDNA from human cells whose gene maps to chromosome 16. Proc. Natl. Acad. Sci. U. S. A. 88:9127-9131.

Sancar A (1994): Mechanisms of DNA excision repair. Science 266:1954-1956.

Satokata I, Tanaka K, Miura N, Miyamoto I, Satoh Y, Kondo S, Okada Y (1990): Characterization of a splicing mutation in group A xeroderma pigmentosum. Proc. Natl. Acad. Sci. U. S. A. 87:9908-9912.

Satokata I, Tanaka K, Okada Y (1992): Molecular basis of group A xeroderma pigmentosum: a missense mutation and two deletions located in a zinc finger consensus sequence of the *XPAC* gene. Hum. Genet. 88:603-607.

Schaeffer L, Moncollin V, Roy R, Staub A, Mezzina M, Sarasin A, Weeda G, Hoeijmakers JHJ, Egly JM (1994): The ERCC2/DNA repair protein is associated with the class II BTF2/TFIIH transcription factor. EMBO J. 13:2388-2392.

Schaeffer L, Roy R, Humbert S, Moncollin V, Vermeulen W, Hoeijmakers JH, Chambon P, Egly JM (1993): DNA repair helicase: a component of BTF2 (TFIIH) basic transcription factor. Science 260:58-63.

Scherly D, Nouspikel T, Corlet J, Ucla C, Bairoch A, Clarkson SG (1993): Complementation of the DNA repair defect in xeroderma pigmentosum group G cells by a human cDNA related to yeast *RAD2*. Nature 363:182-185.

Sen Gupta DN, Zmudzka BZ, Kumar P, Cobianchi F, Skowronski J, Wilson SH (1986): Sequence of human DNA polymerase beta mRNA obtained through cDNA cloning. Biochem. Biophys. Res. Commun. 136:341-347.

Shinohara A, Ogawa H, Matsuda Y, Ushio N, Ikeo K, Ogawa T (1993): Cloning of human, mouse and fission yeast recombination genes homologous to *RAD51* and *recA*. Nat. Genet. 4:239-243.

Shivji MK, Eker AP, Wood RD (1994): DNA repair defect in xeroderma pigmentosum group C and complementing factor from HeLa cells. J. Biol. Chem. 269:22749-22757.

Stamato TD, Dipatri A, Giaccia A (1988): Cell cycle-dependent repair of potentially lethal damage in the XR-1 gamma-ray sensitive CHO cell. Radiat. Res. 115:325-333.

Stamato TD, Otevrel T (1995): Regional localization of the human radiation repair gene *XRCC4* to 5q13-q14. Genomics in press.

Stefanini M, Collins AR, Riboni R, Klaude M, Botta E, Mitchell DL, Nuzzo F (1991): Novel Chinese hamster ultraviolet-sensitive mutants for excision repair form complementation groups 9 and 10. Cancer Res. 51:3965-3971.

Stefanini M, Lagomarsini P, Arlett CF, Marinoni S, Borrone C, Crovato F, Trevisan Getal (1986): Xeroderma pigmentosum (complementation group D) mutation is present in patients affected by trichothiodystrophy with photosensitivity. Hum. Genet. 74:107-112.

Strathdee CA, Duncan AM, Buchwald M (1992a): Evidence for at least four Fanconi anaemia genes including *FACC* on chromosome 9. Nature Genet. 1:196-198.

Strathdee CA, Gavish H, Shannon WR, Buchwald M (1992b): Cloning of cDNAs for Fanconi's anaemia by functional complementation. Nature 356:763-767.

Sung P, Bailly V, Weber C, Thompson LH, Prakash L, Prakash S (1993): Human xeroderma pigmentosum group D gene encodes a DNA helicase. Nature 365:852-855.

Sung P, Prakash S, Prakash L (1990): Mutation of cysteine-88 in the Saccharomyces cerevisiae RAD6 protein abolishes its ubiquitin-conjugating activity and its various biological functions. Proc. Natl. Acad. Sci. U. S. A. 87:2695-2699.

Svoboda DL, Taylor JS, Hearst JE, Sancar A (1993): DNA repair by eukaryotic nucleotide excision nuclease. Removal of thymine dimer and psoralen monoadduct by HeLa cell-free extract and of thymine dimer by *Xenopus laevis* oocytes. J. Biol. Chem. 268:1931-1936.

Takao M, Abramic M, Moos MJr, Otrin VR, Wootton JC, McLenigan M, Levine AS, Protic M (1993): A 127 kDa component of a UV-damaged DNA-binding complex, which is defective in some xeroderma pigmentosum group E patients, is homologous to a slime mold protein. Nucleic Acids Res. 21:4111-4118.

Takayama K, Salazar EP, Lehmann AR, Stefanini M, Thompson LH, Weber CA (1995): Defects in the DNA repair and transcription gene *ERCC2* in the cancer-prone disorder xeroderma pigmentosum group D. Cancer Research submitted.

Tanaka K, Miura N, Satokata I, Miyamoto I, Yoshida MC, Satoh Y, Kondo S, Yasui A, Okayama H, Okada Y (1990): Analysis of a human DNA excision repair gene involved in group A xeroderma pigmentosum and containing a zinc-finger domain. Nature 348:73-76.

Tanaka K, Satokata I, Ogita Z, Uchida T, Okada Y (1989): Molecular cloning of a mouse DNA repair gene that complements the defect in group-A xeroderma pigmentosum. Proc. Natl. Acad. Sci. U.S.A. 86:5512-5516.

Tano K, Shiota S, Collier J, Foote RS, Mitra S (1990): Isolation and structural characterization of a cDNA clone encoding the human DNA repair protein for O^6-alkylguanine. Proc. Natl. Acad. Sci. U. S. A. 87:686-690.

Tebbs RS, Zhao Y, Tucker JD, Scheerer JB, Siciliano MJ, Hwang M, Liu N, Legerski RJ, Thompson LH (1995): Correction of chromosomal instability and sensitivity to diverse mutagens by a cDNA of the *XRCC3* DNA repair gene. Proc. Natl. Acad. Sci. U.S.A. 92:in press.

Teo IA, Arlett CF, Harcourt SA, Priestley A, Broughton BC (1983): Multiple hypersensitivities to mutagens in a cell strain (46BR) derived from a patient with immunodeficiencies. Mutat. Res. 107:371-386.

Thacker J (1989): Inherited sensitivity to X-rays in man. Bioessays 11:58-62.

Thacker J, Tambini CE, Simpson PJ, Tsui L-C, Scherer SW (1995): Localization to chromosome 7q36.1 of the human *XRCC2* gene, determining sensitivity to DNA-damaging agents. Human Mol. Genet. 4:113-120.

Thacker J, Wilkinson RE (1991): The genetic basis of resistance to ionising radiation damage in cultured mammalian cells. Mutat. Res. 254:135-142.

Thompson LH, Brookman KW, Dillehay LE, Mooney CL, Carrano AV (1982): Hypersensitivity to mutation and sister-chromatid-exchange induction in CHO cell mutants defective in incising DNA containing UV lesions. Somat. Cell. Genet. 8:759-773.

Thompson LH, Brookman KW, Jones NJ, Allen SA, Carrano AV (1990): Molecular cloning of the human *XRCC1* gene, which corrects defective DNA strand-break repair and sister chromatid exchange. Mol. Cell. Biol. 10:6160-6171.

Thompson LH, Brookman KW, Weber CA, Salazar EP, Reardon JT, Sancar A, Deng Z, Siciliano MJ (1994): Molecular cloning of the human nucleotide-excision-repair gene *ERCC4*. Proc. Natl. Acad. Sci. U.S.A. 91:6855-6859.

Thompson LH, Busch DB, Brookman KW, Mooney CL, Glaser DA (1981): Genetic diversity of UV-sensitive DNA repair mutants of Chinese hamster ovary cells. Proc. Natl. Acad. Sci. U.S.A. 78:3734-3737.

Thompson LH, Jeggo PA (1995): Nomenclature of human genes involved in ionizing radiation sensitivity. Mutat. Res. in press.

Troelstra C, Hesen W, Bootsma D, Hoeijmakers JH (1993): Structure and expression of the excision repair gene *ERCC6*, involved in the human disorder Cockayne's syndrome group B. Nucleic Acids Res. 21:419-426.

Troelstra C, Jasper NGJ (1994): Ku starts at the end. Current Biol. 4:1149-1154.

Troelstra C, Landsvater RM, Wiegant J, van der Ploeg M, Viel G, Buys CH, Hoeijmakers JH (1992a): Localization of the nucleotide excision repair gene *ERCC6* to human chromosome 10q11-q21. Genomics 12:745-749.

Troelstra C, van Gool A, de Wit J, Vermeulen W, Bootsma D, Hoeijmakers JH (1992b): *ERCC6*, a member of a subfamily of putative helicases, is involved in Cockayne's syndrome and preferential repair of active genes. Cell 71:939-953.

van Duin M, de Wit J, Odijk H, Westerveld A, Yasui A, Koken MHM, Hoeijmakers J, Bootsma D (1986): Molecular characterization of the human excision repair gene *ERCC-1*: cDNA cloning and amino acid homology with the yeast DNA repair gene *RAD10*. Cell 44:913-923.

van Duin M, Koken MHM, van den Tol J, ten Dijke P, Odijk H, Westerveld A, Bootsma D, Hoeijmakers JHJ (1987): Genomic characterization of the human DNA excision repair gene *ERCC-1*. Nucleic Acids Res. 15:9195-9213.

van Duin M, Vredeveldt G, Mayne LV, Odijk H, Vermeulen W, Klein B, Weeda G, Hoeijmakers JHJ, Westerveld A (1989): The cloned human DNA reapir gene *ERCC-1* fails to correct xeroderma pigmentosum complementation groups A through I. Mutat. Res. 217:83-92.

van Hoffen A, Natarajan AT, Mayne LV, van Zeeland AA, Mullenders LH, Venema J (1993): Deficient repair of the transcribed strand of active genes in Cockayne's syndrome cells. Nucleic Acids Res. 21:5890-5895.

van Vuuren AJ, Appeldoorn E, Odijk H, Yasui A, Jaspers NGJ, Bootsma D, Hoeijmakers JHJ (1993): Evidence for a repair enzyme complex involving ERCC1 and complementing activities of ERCC4, ERCC11 and xeroderma pigmentosum group F. EMBO J 12:3693-3701.

van Vuuren AJ, Vermeulen W, Ma L, Weeda G, Appeldoorn E, Jaspers NG, van der Eb AJ, Bootsma D, Hoeijmakers JH, Humbert S, et al (1994): Correction of xeroderma pigmentosum repair defect by basal transcription factor BTF2 (TFIIH). EMBO J. 13:1645-1653.

Venema J, van Hoffen A, Natarajan AT, van Zeeland AA, Mullenders LH (1990): The residual repair capacity of xeroderma pigmentosum complementation group C fibroblasts is highly specific for transcriptionally active DNA. Nucleic Acids Res. 18:443-448.

Venema J, van Hoffen A, Karcagi V, Natarajan AT, van Zeeland AA, Mullenders LH (1991): Xeroderma pigmentosum complementation group C cells remove pyrimidine dimers selectively from the transcribed strand of active genes. Mol. Cell. Biol. 11:4128-4134.

Vermeulen W, Scott RJ, Rodgers S, Muller HJ, Cole J, Arlett CF, Kleijer WJ, Bootsma D, Hoeijmakers JH, Weeda G (1994): Clinical heterogeneity within xeroderma pigmentosum associated with mutations in the DNA repair and transcription gene *ERCC3*. Am. J. Hum. Genet. 54:191-200.

Vermeulen W, Stefanini M, Giliani S, Hoeijmakers JH, Bootsma D (1991): Xeroderma pigmentosum complementation group H falls into complementation group D. Mutat. Res. 255:201-208.

Vickers MA, Vyas P, Harris PC, Simmons DL, Higgs DR (1993): Structure of the human 3-methyladenine DNA glycosylase gene and localization close to the 16p telomere. Proc. Natl. Acad. Sci. U. S. A. 90:3437-3441.

Weber CA, Salazar EP, Stewart SA, Thompson LH (1990): *ERCC2*: cDNA cloning and molecular characterization of a human nucleotide excision repair gene with high homology to yeast *RAD3*. EMBO J. 9:1437-1447.

Weber CA, Salazar EP, Stewart SA, Thompson LH (1988): Molecular cloning and biological characterization of a human gene, *ERCC2*, that corrects the nucleotide excision repair defect in CHO UV5 cells. Mol. Cell. Biol. 8:1137-1146.

Weeda G, Ma LB, van Ham RC, van der Eb AJ, Hoeijmakers JH (1991): Structure and expression of the human *XPBC/ERCC-3* gene involved in DNA repair disorders xeroderma pigmentosum and Cockayne's syndrome. Nucleic Acids Res. 19:6301-6308.

Weeda G, van Ham RCA, Vermeulen W, Bootsma D, van der Eb AJ, Hoeijmakers JHJ (1990): A presumed DNA helicase encoded by *ERCC-3* is involved in the human repair disorders xeroderma pigmentosum and Cockayne's syndrome. Cell 62:777-791.

Westerveld A, Hoeijmakers JHJ, van Duin M, de Wit J, Odijk H, Pastink A, Wood RD, Bootsma D (1984): Molecular cloning of a human DNA repair gene. Nature 310:425-429.

Yates JL, Warren N, Sugden B (1985): Stable replication of plasmids derived from Epstein-Barr virus in various mammalian cells. Nature 313:812-815.

Yoshimura Y, Morita T, Yamamoto A, Matsushiro A (1993): Cloning and sequence of the human RecA-like gene cDNA. Nucleic Acids Res. 21:1665.

Zelle B, Lohman PH (1979): Repair of UV-endonuclease-susceptible sites in the 7 complementation groups of xeroderma pigmentosum A through G. Mutat. Res. 62:363-368.

Genetics and Cancer Susceptibility:
Implications for Risk Assessment, pages 201–209

FROM HOST FACTORS TO GENETIC SUSCEPTIBILITY

Paul Kleihues and Bernard W. Stewart

International Agency for Research on Cancer, 150 Cours Albert-Thomas, 69372 Lyon Cedex 08 France.
Children's Leukaemia and Cancer Research Centre, University of New South Wales, Prince of Wales Children's Hospital, Sydney, New South Wales 2031, Australia.

BACKGROUND TO A CURRENT PERSPECTIVE

Epidemiological data may be used to infer that a major proportion of human cancer is preventable. This knowledge was initially interpreted with reference to the impact of specific chemical carcinogens occurring in a variety of environmental contexts (Higginson, 1969). It was subsequently recognised that life style factors and chronic inflammatory states variously contribute to the distribution of cancer (Doll, Peto, 1981; Preston-Martin et al., 1990). In recent years, a new layer of complexity has been added to our understanding of the distribution of human cancer, with evidence that endogenous risk factors and genetic makeup may determine the consequences of carcinogen exposure. These considerations make estimation of risk increasingly sophisticated. In offering the following perspective, we wish to examine findings from both human and experimental animal studies which are relevant to this increased understanding of risk determination.

'CARCINOGENIC FOR HUMANS': BUT FOR *WHICH* HUMANS?

Since 1972, the International Agency for Research on Cancer (IARC) has conducted a data assessment program, the results of which are published as 'IARC Monographs on the Evaluation of Carcinogenic Risks to Humans' (IARC, 1972). The program, which was recently extended to allow consideration of biological risk factors including certain infectious agents (IARC, 1994) has predominantly concerned a range of chemicals, certain complex mixtures and some occupational exposures (IARC, 1987). In respect of any agent being evaluated, data considered specifically include epidemiological findings (where available), chronic toxicity bioassay in experimental animals and laboratory findings indicative of mechanism of action. The evaluation process requires discrimination between agents definitively established to cause cancer in humans (categorized Group 1), those which probably cause cancer (Group 2A), possibly cause cancer (Group 2B) and other categories for which evidence of carcinogenicity falls short of that already described (Groups 3 and 4). Given a positive evaluation (ie. classification to Group 1 or 2), there is an implicit opportunity (arguably, an obligation) to prevent the likelihood cancer by reducing or precluding human exposure to the agent in question. From a biological perspective, however, it is clear that not all humans exposed to unequivocally carcinogenic agents will, in fact, develop malignancy. Indeed, it is probable that only a minority of such exposed persons will be so affected. Thus, in respect of carcinogenicity data, an important question may be expressed by reference to the notion of an agent being carcinogenic for humans: the question is: 'Carcinogenic for *which* humans?'

CANCER RISK VIEWED AS AN INTERACTION BETWEEN HOST FACTORS AND CARCINOGEN EXPOSURE

That individual characteristics may determine tumorigenic outcome following carcinogen exposure has long been recognised in the understanding of 'host factors' relevant to experimental or human populations (IARC, 1982). Manipulation of experimental systems has allowed the extent to which populations may be either resistant or susceptible to carcinogens to be demonstrated. Susceptibility to tumorigenesis may vary considerably depending upon the carcinogenic agent: some agents override host defences, while the outcome of exposure to others is determined by such host factors. Since *N*-nitrosodiethylamine-induced tumors are evident in all fourteen species tested thus far (ranging from non-human primates to fish) (Preussmann, Stewart, 1984), it would appear that no species is resistant to this compound. Moreover, under some experimental conditions, all (ie. 100%) members of the exposed experimental population may develop tumors following administration of a nitrosamine carcinogen (Swann, McLean, 1971).

Thus biological factors operating to reduce susceptibility to carcinogens may be overcome and rendered irrelevant. In other circumstances 'host factors' primarily determine response of experimental animals to carcinogen treatment. Malkinson (1991) categorises strains of mice according to lung tumor number and incidence following treatment of the animals with urethane. 'Sensitive' strains (NGP, SWR) exhibit 100% incidence of multiple tumors whilst some 'resistant' strains (SJL, AKR) approach no demonstrable carcinogen-induced response. Other strains of mice are known to develop a high incidence of lung, liver or other tumors spontaneously: ie. in the absence of any defined external carcinogenic stimuli (Drinkwater, Bennett, 1991). The genetic basis of such phenomena is described comprehensively in the present volume. These studies taken together indicate that strain differences in susceptibility to tumorigenesis provides a basis for chromosomal mapping and the characterisation of associated genes. The extent to which these genes provide an basis for understanding human susceptibility to environmental carcinogens remains to be determined.

Observations in humans provide equally clearcut illustration of the dynamic interaction between (external) carcinogenic stimuli and individual susceptibility. At one extreme, carcinogens such as 2-naphthylamine have caused bladder cancer in all (ie. 100%) of those occupationally exposed (Doll, 1977). X-irradiation may be universally carcinogenic at high exposure. At the other, tumorigenesis may occur in the apparent absence of external stimuli. In the past, such observations formed an *ad hoc* spectrum of observations regarding, for example, 'cancer prone' families. Currently, these phenomena may be described with reference to specific genes. The estimated risks for breast or ovarian cancer because of the BRCA1 mutation in one family (195 members) were 40% by age 50 and 90% by age 70 (Goldgar et al., 1994). Within affected families, the BRCA1 and related cancer susceptibility genes are known to exhibit up to 100% penetrance which is synonymous with cancer development in all 'at-risk' individuals (Eeles et al., 1994).

These various examples from both human and experimental situations may be considered to be extremes in terms of the spectrum of carcinogen-host interactions. In such extreme circumstances either genetic predisposition or carcinogenic potency may result in cancer irrespective of other variables. Most instances of cancer in the human population, however, are dependent upon both to carcinogens exposure and genetic susceptibility. Granted the inevitability of some level of human exposure to environmental carcinogens, it is obviously desirable to determine differences in individual susceptibility and whether such differences may be associated with particular genes.

INDICATORS OF CARCINOGEN EXPOSURE/HOST GENOME RESPONSE PATTERNS

The Li-Fraumeni syndrome involves greatly increased risk for a number of tumor types, and is consequent upon mutation of the tumor suppressor gene p53 (Malkin, 1994). Moreover, it is evident that p53 is relevant to many instances of human cancer outside Li-Fraumeni families. Approximately half adult cancers of colon, stomach, lung, oesophagus, breast, brain and liver contain mutant p53 (Greenblatt et al., 1994). The typical pattern is point mutation of one allele and loss of heterozygosity in the other. The pattern of mutation may be indicative of particular environmental factors (ultraviolet radiation, aflatoxin, etc). The role of p53 in determining susceptibility to environmental carcinogens is complicated, nevertheless, as indicated at one level by the gene's apparent influence in both late and early stages of tumorigenesis. Mutation of p53 is considered to be a late event in some cancers including those of liver and ovary (Nishida et al., 1993; Teneriello et al., 1993). However p53 overexpression in anal, oesophageal and bronchial lesions is evident with progressive dysplasia, suggestive of a role in the early stages in transformation (Reichel et al., 1994; Sauter et al., 1994; Chang et al., 1994).

Current indications are that the BRCA1 gene is not mutated in 'spontaneous' breast cancer. However, in affected families, the influence of the gene is evident in breast cancer patients of young age (Eeles et al., 1994). It is possible that environmental exposures may be relevant to tumor development in such individuals. Women with a family history of breast cancer have a slightly greater risk associated with oral contraceptive use than those without (Romieu et al., 1989). Use of the injectable contraceptive Depot-medroxyprogesterone acetate (Depo-Provera) is not a risk factor for breast cancer when data for 'all ages' are analysed, but two studies have suggested increased risk in respect of younger women developing cancer (WHO Collaborative Study of Neoplasia and Steriod Contraceptives, 1991; Paul et al., 1989). More recent observations, including metanalysis, confirm this trend.

BRCA1 and p53 are illustrative of human cancer susceptibility genes. Such genes provide a basis for experimental examination of the possibility that the risk posed by at least some environmental carcinogens may be genetically influenced.

INVOLVEMENT OF SPECIFIC GENES IN DETERMINING CARCINOGEN-INDUCED RISK

Experimental manipulation of the genome, in the context of transgenic and 'null' mice, has provided evidence that single genes may determine responses to tumor-inducing stimuli. The potential of transgenic mouse models to enhance understanding of chemical carcinogenesis specifically is well recognised and already an extensive literature exists (Tennant et al., 1994). By germ-line modification, all cells in an animal can be modified and the effect of such change on carcinogenesis may be determined. Thus, studies with p53 heterozygotes (+/-) mice have demonstrated increased tumorgenesis in response to x-irradiation. A single dose of 4Gy radiation dramatically decreases the latency for tumor development in these animals. Moreover, the pattern of mutation at the remaining wildtype allele in these tumors differs substantially from the pattern in spontaneous tumors from similar mice, indicating that p53 itself may have been a target for radiation-induced mutation (Kemp et al., 1994). Extending this line of investigation to chemical carcinogens, there is evidence that mice hemizygous for p53 (+/-) exhibit a markedly reduced latency period for mutagenic, but not for non-mutagenic carcinogens (RW Tennant, personal communication). Such results have clear inferences for humans, but these remain to be fully evaluated.

The first human cancer susceptibility gene identified was the reintoblastoma gene which has been the vehicle for current understanding of a tumor susceptibility gene (Knudson, 1978). There are indications that this gene determines tumorigenic response to environmental stimuli. Relevant data involve second tumors in retinoblastoma patients. In one study (Eng et al., 1993), cumulative mortality in these patients from second primary neoplasms was 26% of bilateral patients *vs* 1.5% of unilateral retinoblastoma patients. Second tumors were predominantly bone & connective tissue (300-fold excess), melanoma (100-fold) and brain (24-fold). Children with bilateral disease (whose 'normal' tissue harbors a defective RB allele) who are irradiated manifest a 3-fold higher mortality from second tumors compared to non-irradiated patients. The possibility that status of the RB gene may determine response to irradiation has wide implications since mutation of RB has been detected in a variety of cancers including sarcomas, breast cancer, lung cancer and genitourinary cancers (Goodrich, Lee, 1993). In the immediate context of chemotherapy for retinoblastoma, the efficacy of protocols involving cyclophosphamide, platinum compounds, epipodophyllotoxins, doxorubicin and vincristine (Doz et al.,) suggests that data on second cancers consequent upon chemically-induced, rather than irradiation-induced, genomic damage will become available.

INTERACTIONS BETWEEN CANCER SUSCEPTIBILITY GENES

Multistep carcinogenesis has been recognised and well defined (in some cancers) using gene markers (Bodmer et al., 1994). The notion of multiple genetic alterations contributing to malignant transformation was initially understood in terms of dominant oncogenes. There is now evidence which is at least consistent with cooperativity between tumor suppressor genes (Williams et al., 1994). Appropriate crossing of 'knockout' mice has yielded animals mutant for both RB and p53 (RB+/-, p53-/-) which spontaneously exhibit novel tumors including pinealoblastomas and islet cell tumors; notably no retinoblastomas were observed. Hypotheses which may explain tumorigenesis in these animals include the suggestion that in the absence of p53 there is more rapid loss of the wildtype allele in RB +/- cells. If valid, this would exemplify an early stage involvement p53 mutation in multistage carcinogenesis.

Involvement of multiple genes in the evolution of metatstatic cancer may be a basis for proposing the 'mutator phenotype': the understanding that the rate of mutation may itself be subject to genetic control. Such a notion may be readily related to DNA repair which, by dint of xeroderma pigmentosum and other conditions, provides a basis for associating lack of genomic integrity with increased likelihood of (ultraviolet radiation-induced) malignant transformation (Cleaver, 1994). The risk of breast cancer is elevated in carriers of the ataxia-telangectasia gene (Swift et al., 1991). The finding that the length of selected CA repeats is variable in hereditary non-polyposis coli colon cancer (HNPCC) provided the first definitive demonstration of a mutator phenotype in contributing to the evolution of metastatic cancer cells (Bodmer et al., 1994). Loeb (1994) has discussed the broader aspects of this principle, suggesting that early mutations may occur in a range of 'stability' genes (DNA repair, mismatch repair) leading to mutations of 'cancer-associated' genes. Interestingly, in terms of this model, p53 was deemed to be a 'late-stage' cancer-associated gene.

GENETIC DETERMINATION OF LUNG CANCER IN HUMANS

The distribution of human lung cancer does not appear to be explicable primary on the basis of cancer susceptibility genes. Early appreciation that metabolic activation is critical for (most) chemical carcinogenesis, provided a basis for investigating genetic susceptibility to this specific tumor type (Kellerman et al., 1973). However, initial optimism has not been matched by definitive knowledge that simple genetic analysis may allow determination of individual risk for lung cancer. Indeed, a recent 'twin' study failed to provide evidence for such susceptibility (Braun et al., 1994). However, a more complex genetic basis for disease is evident, and specifically implicates the role of environmental carcinogens (Sellers et al., 1990; Amos et al., 1992). Thus, in a Japanese population, risk for squamous cell carcinoma of the lung is associated with two polymorphisms (Msp 1 cleavage and replacement of Ile by Val at residue 462) of CYP1A1 gene together with deficiency of a subclass of glutathione S-transferase (GST1). These findings were studied in relation to smoking consumption (Nakachi et al., 1993). Individuals with the susceptible Msp1 or Ile-Val genotype combined with deficient GST1 were at high risk. However, the difference in susceptibility for combined genotype of Ile-Val and GST(-) was much larger (odds ratio of 41) for the group categorised as having low cigarette consumption than for the high smoking group (odds ratio 2). A similar finding, that the impact of genetically-determined predisposition is much more appreciable at low levels of exposure, was made by Vineis *et al* () who determined DNA adducts in bladder cells and 4-aminobiphenyl-hemoglobin, the N-acetylation non-inducible phenotype and urinary nicotine-cotinine levels in random groups of smokers and non-smokers. Among the slow acetylators, 4-aminobiphenyl adducts were higher in rapid acetylators than in the low or null nicotine-cotinine group whereas the difference was less evident at increasing nicotine-cotinine levels. The data thus suggested that the clearance of low-dose carcinogens is decreased in the genetically based slow-acetylator phenotype.

RISK DETERMINATION: COMPLEXITY AT EVERY LEVEL

Data of the type summarised above are consistent with the notion of genetic determination of risk, whilst at the same time indicating the likely complexity of such a relationship. If genetic determinants of risk are confirmed, it is probable that quantitative risk assessment will be rendered more complex. Such a perspective cannot be allowed to imply that such quantitative determinations are currently simple, by comparison. On the contrary, mathematical analyses for modelling the impact of exogenous chemicals on an organism are already bewildering to all but the non-expert (Tardiff, Rodricks, 1987; Garrett, 1987). Quantitative determinations of risk are typically subject to wide 'confidence intervals'. Determination of risk based on available biological parameters has been discussed by Lucier et al (1993), specifically in relation to receptor-mediated carcinogenesis by 2,3,7,8-tetrachlorodibenzo-*p*-dioxin (TCDD). Using different models, exposure standards for TCDD as determined by various regulatory authorities yield a range of values extending over four orders of magnitude. It is possible that knowledge based upon genotypic characterisation of TCDD effects may allow the development of more stringent models of carcinogenesis in this case and in respect of other agents.

The deceptively simple question of 'carcinogenic for humans, but for which humans' which introduced this discussion cannot be resolved on the basis of available knowledge. In respect of carcinogenicity *per se*, a singular, if not unique, contribution by the IARC has been the establishment of a context for data assessment. This has been achieved through the IARC Monographs on the Evaluation of Carcinogenic Risks to Humans. As a consequence, the collective implications of diverse observations have been elevated to authoritative statements regarding the degree of hazard posed by many hundreds of diverse agents. With the development of new methods for characterising cancer susceptibility, specifically including molecular genetics, the perspective from the IARC is that the Agency will continue to strive to provide a forum for the evaluation of data at the highest level of international authority.

CONCLUSION

In the past, estimation of risk for tumorigenesis was concerned almost entirely with the identity of carcinogenic agents, their potency and their metabolism in animals and humans. It is now appreciated that these parameters constitute only part of the spectrum of complex issues determining individual carcinogenic risk in humans. Genetic determination of susceptibility is now known to be a significant factor not only in the context of single gene disease (ie. familial cancer), but also as an aspect of complex genetic traits which may determine susceptibility in relation to many environmental risk factors. Such aspects of individual susceptibility raise the question as to whether estimations of carcinogenic risk should continue to be made with reference to whole populations or should be determined for the genetically most susceptible ('weakest') group or groups within the population. These latter determinations will require a new level of sophistication in risk assessment: one which takes into account human genetic data and which may also include knowledge of susceptibility genes from genetically manipulated animals.

REFERENCES

Amos CI, Caporaso NE, Weston A (1992): Host factors in lung cancer risk: A review of interdisciplinary studies. Cancer Epidemiol Biomarkers Prevent 1:505-513.

Bodmer W, Bishop T, Karran P (1994): Genetic steps in colorectal cancer. Nature Gen 6:217-219.

Braun MM, Caporaso NE, Page WF, Hoover RN (1994): Genetic component of lung cancer: Cohort study of twins. Lancet 344:440-443.

Chang F, Syrjanen S, Tervahauta A, Kurvinen K, Wang L, Syrjanen K (1994): Frequent mutations of p53 gene in oesophageal squamous cell carcinomas with and without human papillomavirus (HPV) involvement suggest the dominant role of environmental carcinogens in oesophageal carcinogenesis. Br J Cancer 70:346-351.

Cleaver JE (1994): It was a very good year for DNA repair. Cell 76:1-4.

Doll R (1977): Strategy for detection of cancer hazards to man. Nature 265:589-596.

Doll R, Peto R (1981): The causes of cancer: quantitative estimates of avoidable risks of cancer in the United States today. J Natl Cancer Inst 66:1192-1308.

Doz F, Khelfaoui F, Mosseri V, Validire P, Quintana E, Michon J, Desjardins L, Schlienger P, Neuenschwander S, Vielh P, Putterman M, Dufier J-L, Zucker J-M (1994): The role of chemotherapy in orbital involvement of retinoblastoma. Cancer 74:722-732.

Drinkwater NR, Bennett LM (1991): Genetic control of carcinogenesis in experimental animals. Pro Exp Tumor Res 33:1-20.

Eeles RA, Stratton MR, Goldgar DE, Easton DF (1994): The genetics of familial breast cancer and their practical implications. Eur J Cancer 30A:1383-1390.

Eng C, Li FP, Abramson DH, Ellsworth RM, Wong L, Goldman MB, Seddon J, Tarbell N, Boice JD Jr (1993): Mortality from second tumors among long-term survivors of retinoblastoma. J Natl Cancer Inst 85:1121-1128.

Garrett, E.R. (1987): Toxicokinetics. In Tardiff RG, Rodricks JV: (eds.). Toxic Substances and Human Risk. Principles of Data Intepretaton New York: Plenum Press (pp. 153-235).

Goldgar DE, Fields P, Lewis CM, Tran TD, Cannon-Albright LA, Ward JH, Swensen J, Skolnick MH (1994): A large kindred with 17q-linked breast and ovarian cancer: Genetic, phenotypic and genealogical analysis. J Natl Cancer Inst 86:200-209.

Goodrich DW, Lee W-H (1993): Molecular characterisation of the retinoblastoma susceptibility gene. Biochim Biophys Acta 1155:43-61.

Greenblatt MS, Bennett WP, Hollstein M, Harris CC (1994): Mutations in the p53 tumor suppressor gene: Clues to cancer etiology and molecular pathogenesis. Cancer Res 54:4855-4878.

Higginson J (1969): Present trends in cancer epidemiology. Proc Can Cancer Res Conf 8:40-75.

International Agency for Research on Cancer (1972): IARC Monographs on the Evaluation of Carcinogenic Risk of Chemicals to Man. Volume 1. Lyon: IARC.

International Agency for Research on Cancer (1982): Host Factors in Human Carcinogenesis. Bartsch H, Armstrong B (eds): IARC Scientific Publication No. 39. Lyon: IARC.

International Agency for Research on Cancer (1987): IARC Monographs on the Evaluation of Carcinogenic Risks to Humans. Supplement 7. Overall evaluations of carcinogenicity: An updating of *IARC Monographs* Volumes 1 to 42. Lyon: IARC.

International Agency for Research on Cancer (1994): IARC Monographs on the Evaluation of Carcinogenic Risks to Humans. Volume 59: Hepatitis viruses. Lyon: IARC.

Kellerman G, Shaw CR, Luyten-Kellermann M (1973): Aryl hydrocarbon hydroxylase inducibility and bronchogenic carcinoma. New Engl J Med 289:934-937.

Kemp CJ, Wheldon T, Balmain A (1994): p53-deficient mice are extremely susceptible to radiation-induced tumorigenesis. Nature Genetics 8:66-69.

Knudson AG (1978): Retinoblastoma: A prototypic hereditary neoplasm. Semin Oncol 5:57-60.

Loeb LA (1994): Microsatellite instability: Marker of a mutator phenotype in cancer. Cancer Res 54:5059-5063.

Lucier GW, Portier CJ, Gallo MA (1993): Receptor mechanisms and dose-response models for the effects of dioxins. Environ Hlth Perspect 101:36-44.

Malkin D (1994): p53 and the Li-Fraumeni syndrome. Biochim Biophys Acta 1198:197-213.

Malkinson AM (1991): Genetic studies on lung tumor susceptibility and histogenesis in mice. Environ Hlth Perspect 93:149-159.

Nakachi K, Imai K, Hayashi S, Kawajiri K (1993): Polymorphisms of the CYP1A1 and glutathione S-transferase genes associated with susceptibility to lung cancer in relation to cigarette dose in a Japanese population. Cancer Res 53:2994-2999.

Nishida N, Fukuda Y, Kokuryu H, Toguchida J, Yandell DW, Ikenega M, Imura H, Ishizaki K (1993): Role and mutational heterogeneity of the p53 gene in hepatocellular carcinoma. Cancer Res 53:368-372.

Paul C, Skegg DCG, Spears GFS (1989): Depot medroxyprogesterone (Depo-Provera) and risk of breast cancer. Brit Med J 299:759-762.

Preston-Martin S, Pike MC, Ross RK, Jones PA, Henderson BE (1990): Increased cell division as a cause of human cancer. Cancer Res 50:7415-7421.

Preussmann R, Stewart BW (1984): N-nitroso carcinogens. In Searle CE: (ed.). Chemical Carcinogens 2nd ed. Washington DC: American Chemical Society (pp. 643-828).

Reichel MB, Ohgaki H, Petersen I, Kleihues P (1994): p53 mutations in primary human lung tumors and their metastases. Mol Carcinogenesis 9:105-109.

Romieu I, Willett WC, Colditz GA, Stampher MJ, Hennekens CH, Speizer FE (1989): Prospective study of oral contraceptive use and risk of breast cancer in women. J Natl Cancer Inst 81:1313-1321.

Sauter ER, Cleveland D, Trock B, Ridge JA, Klein-Szanto AJP (1994): p53 is overexpressed in fifty percent of pre-invasive lesions of head and neck epithelium. Carcinogenesis 15:2269-2274.

Sellers TA, Bailey-Wilson JE, Elston RC, Wilson AF, Elston GZ, Ooi WL, Rothschild H (1990): Evidence of mendelian inheritance in the pathogenesis of lung cancer. J Natl Cancer Inst 82:1272-1279.

Swann PF, McLean AEM (1971): Cellular injury and carcinogenesis. The effect of protein-free high-carbohydrate diet on the metabolism of dimethylnitrosamine in the rat. Biochem J 124:283-289.

Swift M, Morrell D, Massey RB, Chase CL (1991): Incidence of cancer in 161 families affected by ataxia-telangiectasia. New Engl J Med 325:1831-1836.

Tardiff, R.G. & Rodricks, J.V. (1987): Comprehensive risk assessment. In Tardiff RG, Rodricks JV: (eds.). Toxic Substances and Human Risk. Principles of Data Interpretation New York: Plenum Press (pp. 391-434).

Teneriello MG, Ebina M, Linnoila RI, Henry M, Nash JD, Park RC, Birrer MJ (1993): p53 and Ki-ras gene mutations in epithelial ovarian neoplasms. Cancer Res 53:3103-3108.

Tennant RW, Hansen L, Spalding J (1994): Gene manipulation and genetic toxicology. Mutagenesis 9:171-174.

Vineis P, Bartsch H, Caporaso N, Harrington AM, Kadlubar FF, Landi MT, Malaveille C, Shields PG, Skipper P, Talaska G, Tannenbaum SR (1994): Genetically based *N*-acetyltransferase metabolic polymorphism and low-level environmental exposure to carcinogens. Nature 369:154-156.

WHO Collaborative Study of Neoplasia and Steriod Contraceptives (1991): Breast cancer and depot-medroxyprogesterone acetate: A multinational study. Lancet 338:833-838.

Williams BO, Remington L, Albert DM, Mukai S, Bronson RT, Jacks T (1994): Cooperative tumorigenic effects of germline mutations in Rb and p53. Nature Genetics 7:480-484.

Genetics and Cancer Susceptibility:
Implications for Risk Assessment, pages 211–222

EPIDEMIOLOGY OF HUMAN AFLATOXIN EXPOSURES AND THEIR RELATIONSHIP TO LIVER CANCER

John D. Groopman, Peter Scholl and Jia-Sheng Wang

Department of Environmental Health Sciences
The Johns Hopkins University
School of Hygiene and Public Health
615 North Wolfe Street
Baltimore, MD 21205, U.S.A.

INTRODUCTION

For decades, veterinary practitioners recognized the linkage between the consumption of certain moldy grains and the rapid onset of hepatotoxicity in many animal species. With the structural identification of the aflatoxins as a major principle in these toxic events, there have now been thousands of scientific publications characterizing the toxicology of these mycotoxins. Within a few years of the identification of the aflatoxins, these agents had been demonstrated to be very potent carcinogens. Since human liver cancer is very prevalent in regions of the world that are hot and humid, a number of investigators sought to link dietary exposure to aflatoxins with human disease. Initially, these studies were compromised by the lack of adequate dosimetry data on aflatoxin intake, excretion and metabolism in people, as well as by the general poor quality of world-wide cancer morbidity and mortality statistics. In the ensuing three decades, a number of new technologies to assess exposure status and risk for aflatoxins have been devised and these agents are among the few environmental carcinogens for which quantitative risk assessments have been attempted. Indeed, aflatoxin risk assessments are intensively debated because of the major economic consequences of high aflatoxin levels in stable grains. In many countries, the price of corn and peanuts is dictated by aflatoxin levels. Thus, these risk assessments have hastened the development of preventive intervention methods that will try to lower the human health impact from aflatoxin exposures. Primary prevention methods have included the development of aflatoxin resistant plants, the building of better storage facilities for grains and the dramatic increase in aflatoxin testing in the world market. Secondary prevention, including chemoprevention protocols, has been facilitated by the development of many different mechanistically derived biomarkers to identify high-risk individuals and then apply these biomarkers to epidemiologic investigations. Hopefully, the combination of both primary and secondary prevention techniques will lower human exposure to this potent carcinogen. In fact, limiting intake of aflatoxins is a readily obtainable public health goal requiring the allocation of appropriate economic resources to assure minimal mold contamination of foods and grains.

This article will highlight some of the current epidemiologic and biomarker studies that were used to associate dietary aflatoxin exposure with human liver cancer. In 1972, in the first monograph on the evaluation of the carcinogenic risk of chemicals to man published by the International Agency for Research on Cancer (IARC), the aflatoxins were classified as suspect human carcinogens. The aflatoxins were reevaluated several times and in the most recent IARC evaluation, aflatoxin B_1 was reclassified as a Category I known human carcinogen (1993). Both epidemiologic and toxicologic information were used by the expert panel in its deliberations and the aflatoxins are among the very few chemical agents that have been classified as known human carcinogens. A comprehensive review of the literature on the toxicology of aflatoxins can be found in chapters in a recent book (Eaton and Groopman, 1994).

RECENT EPIDEMIOLOGICAL STUDIES OF AFLATOXIN AND HUMAN LIVER CANCER

Since the discovery of the aflatoxins in the early 1960's, many traditional epidemiologic studies have been conducted to explore the aflatoxin/human liver cancer link (reviewed by Wild and Hall, 1994). These studies ranged from cross-sectional surveys to case-control studies. Most of these investigations suffered from a lack of good data on aflatoxin exposure and/or poor information on cancer incidence. Assessment of dietary exposure to aflatoxins is a very difficult task that generally requires split-bowl studies to measure aflatoxin contents in the diet. Food questionnaire data is a poor predictor of exposure because of the heterogeneity of mold growth. Thus, a person's daily exposure may come from a single food in one meal rather than being equally distributed across all meals. In fact, as the diet of the individual becomes more complex the degree of difficulty in measuring aflatoxin exposures increases. This problem alone was responsible for the development of the individually based biomarkers to be described in the following sections. A further complexity to understanding human liver cancer etiology was that prior to 1980 the studies suffered from the inability to accurately test cases for hepatitis B viral (HBV) status. The availability of a rapid test for HBV was extremely valuable; however, in 1989, the hepatitis C virus was first characterized. This viral agent is thought to be responsible for many liver cancers in Japan following blood transfusion with contaminated blood products. Several assays are now available for this virus and these will be tested in future epidemiologic investigations. Despite the overwhelming potency of the aflatoxins and hepatitis viruses as carcinogens, there are a number of risk factors that also contribute to human liver cancer, including nutritional status, tobacco smoking and alcohol. All of these risk factors are present in widely ranging levels across different populations.

Given the complexity of the etiology of human liver cancer, the aflatoxin-human liver cancer link remained unclear until the simultaneous application of aflatoxin molecular dosimetry and accurate hepatitis B virus assessment methods to epidemiologic studies. Since epidemiological studies cannot reveal information about an individual's risk to develop disease, it is hoped that the use of molecular biomarkers of aflatoxin exposures in individuals can provide information for the prediction of individual risk for liver cancer. A start towards this goal was the initiation of a prospective epidemiological study in Shanghai where healthy people were followed until the diagnosis of disease. A nested case-control study initiated in 1986 in Shanghai examined the relation between markers for aflatoxin and hepatitis B virus and the development of liver cancer (Ross, et al., 1992; Qian, et al., 1994). In this study, 18,244 urine samples were collected from healthy males between the ages of 45 and 64. In the subsequent seven years, fifty of these individuals developed liver cancer. The urine samples for 50 of these cases were age-matched and residence-matched with 267 controls and analyzed for both aflatoxin biomarkers and hepatitis B virus surface antigen status. The data revealed a highly significant increase in the relative risk (RR=3.4) for those liver cancer cases where urinary aflatoxins were detected. The relative risk for people who tested positive for the hepatitis B virus surface antigen was also about seven, but individuals with both urinary aflatoxins and positive HBV surface antigen status had a relative risk for developing liver cancer of about 59. These results show for the first time a relationship between presence of carcinogen specific biomarkers and cancer risk. Moreover, these findings provide for the first time a demonstration of a multiplicative interaction between two major risk factors for liver cancer, hepatitis B virus and AFB_1 exposure. Finally, when individual aflatoxin metabolites were stratified for liver cancer outcome, the presence of the aflatoxin-nucleic acid adduct in urine always resulted in a two- to three-fold elevation in risk of developing liver cancer. These findings extend the conclusions from the rodent chemoprotection studies that monitoring levels of this biomarker may be very useful for assessing individual risk.

Taken together, these epidemiological results provide the scientific basis for the reclassification of aflatoxin as a known human carcinogen. Biologically, the indication that hepatitis virus and aflatoxin can act in a concerted fashion to increase cancer risk has been clearly shown. However, aflatoxin exposure in the absence of chronic hepatitis B infection is also etiologically associated with liver cancer. These findings provide the compelling basis to increase efforts both in hepatitis B virus immunization programs and in the development of concerted programs to lower dietary aflatoxin exposure as means of lowering human cancer risk.

BIOMARKERS OF BIOLOGICALLY EFFECTIVE DOSE IN TRANSITIONAL HUMAN EPIDEMIOLOGICAL STUDIES

The development of biomarker methods to monitor human exposure to aflatoxins requires techniques which are sensitive, specific and amenable to large numbers of samples. Among the various possible biomarkers of aflatoxin exposure, the measurement of carcinogen-DNA and protein adducts are of major interest because they are direct products of (or surrogate markers for) damage to a critical cellular macromolecular target. The chemical structures of the major aflatoxin macromolecular adducts have been identified (Essigmann, et al., 1977; Sabbioni, et al., 1987). The interest in using the major aflatoxin-nucleic acid adduct in urine as a biomarker was enhanced by the finding that this metabolite is excreted exclusively in urine of exposed rats (Bennett, et al., 1981). This finding obviates the potential pharmacokinetic problem of biliary and urinary excretion. The serum albumin adduct has also been examined as a biomarker of exposure and because of the longer half-life in vivo of albumin compared to the urinary DNA adduct, the serum albumin adduct can integrate exposures over longer time periods. Further, data from human exposure studies have shown that the excretion of the urinary aflatoxin nucleic acid adduct and formation of the serum albumin adduct are highly correlated (data from Gan, et al., 1988; Groopman, et al., 1992a).

Over the past ten years many systematic evaluations of these molecular biomarkers in several human populations have been undertaken. Early studies by Autrup, et al., (1983; 1987) used synchronous fluorescence spectroscopy for the analysis of AFB-DNA adducts in human urine samples in Kenya. Over a thousand urine samples were analyzed and nearly 13% of the urines were positive for excreted aflatoxin-nucleic acid adducts. These data provided important evidence that humans had the metabolic capacity to produce the aflatoxin-DNA adducts previously detected in experimental animals.

Subsequent studies conducted in an area in the People's Republic of China with a high-incidence of liver cancer determined both dietary intake of aflatoxin as well as the levels of urinary aflatoxin biomarkers. The average dietary intake of aflatoxins, primarily from contaminated corn consumption, was approximately 275 μg and 540 μg in males and females, respectively, over the seven-day monitoring period (Groopman, et al., 1992a). Total 24 hr urine samples were collected starting on the fourth day of the study as consecutive twelve hour fractions. Using a radioimmunoassay, immunoreactive aflatoxins in the urine samples were measured and the relation between AFB_1 intake per day determined. These studies showed that levels of total immunoreactive aflatoxin equivalents in urine did not correspond with aflatoxin intake indicating that using this type of immunoassay approach was not an appropriate dosimeter for determining individual exposure status.

These results prompted an immunoaffinity-HPLC analysis to determine individual aflatoxins in the samples. AFB-N^7-gua, aflatoxin M_1 (AFM_1), AFP_1, and AFB_1 were the aflatoxins most commonly detected. However, only AFB-N^7-gua and AFM_1 showed a dose-dependent relationship between aflatoxin intake and urinary levels indicating that these two metabolites might be useful biomarkers of exposure. Interestingly, these studies also demonstrate that the formation and excretion of AFB-N^7-gua in urine is similar in the rat and human, thereby adding an important confirmation of the rat to human extrapolation for risk analysis.

Using the same study population, Gan, et al. (1988) monitored levels of aflatoxin-serum albumin adducts. A highly significant association between adduct level and intake was observed. Further, it was calculated that about 2% of the ingested AFB_1 became covalently bound to serum albumin, a value very similar to that observed when rats are administered AFB_1. When the data for DNA adduct excretion in urine (Groopman, et al., 1992a) and serum albumin was compared, a statistically significant relationship was seen with a correlation coefficient of 0.73. Thus, both of these markers appear to be useful in human monitoring studies.

Similar studies examining the relationship between aflatoxin exposure and DNA adduct excretion and serum albumin adduct formation have been conducted in The Gambia, West Africa (Wild, et al., 1992; Groopman, et al., 1992b). These studies revealed similar relationships between dietary exposure and adduct levels, as seen in China. Thus, the utility of these dosimetry markers as effective monitors of exposure to aflatoxins has been confirmed in two populations at high risk for liver cancer. From a practical perspective pertinent to epidemiologic studies, the measurement and quantification of the aflatoxin-serum albumin adduct offers a rapid, facile approach that can be used to screen very large numbers of people. This method has been extensively validated in experimental and human sample analyses and the technique is described in detail in Wild, et al. (1990a). To date extensive geographic surveys have been carried out on hundreds of samples (Wild, et al., 1990b) showing that the measurement of the serum albumin adduct is probably the most practical biomarker for epidemiologic studies.

In Qidong, P.R.C., liver cancer accounts for 10% of all adult deaths and both HBV and aflatoxin exposures are common. As described above, the development of molecular biomarkers of aflatoxins has proven to be very valuable for epidemiologic studies; however, our knowledge base about temporal patterns of formation and persistence of aflatoxin-macromolecular adducts in human samples is limited. We have designed a longitudinal study to address these questions in a population in Qidong (Wang, et al., 1995). For this study, 120 adults (60 males and 60 females) ranging in age from 19 to 73 (mean age = 44.5) were recruited. Blood samples were drawn from these people every other week for 3 months starting in mid-September, 1993. In addition, complete food surveys and urine collections were done. At the end of the study, 115 people still remained (57 males and 58 females) and of these people 57 were HBV antigen positive and 58 were HBV antigen negative. Aflatoxin-albumin adducts were determined in 825 serum samples by immunoassay and HPLC with a range of aflatoxin-albumin adducts from 0.3 - 4.6 p mole aflatoxin per mg albumin. These are levels comparable to those detected in other high risk populations. This investigation is being followed up to determine tracking parameters across time in individuals and this population is currently being studied for chemoprevention intervention.

LINKAGE BETWEEN AFLATOXIN EXPOSURES AND MUTATIONS IN THE TUMOR SUPPRESSOR GENE P53

Some of the most exciting prospects for markers of biological effect or pre-clinical disease arise from tools developed in the field of molecular biology. The increasing mechanistic understanding of the genetic alterations underlying the progression from initiation to tumor formation has permitted the beginning development of sensitive tests for diagnosis of tumors. One example of this emerging field is the studies of the tumor suppressor gene, p53, that is the most common mutated gene detected in human cancers. The number and type of mutations in this gene are not equally distributed, but occur in specific hotspots that vary with tumor type (Hollstein, et al., 1991). Different patterns in mutation patterns between tumors are consistent with different etiologies for the specific tumor types. This area of research has been comprehensively reviewed recently by Greenblatt, et al. (1994) and Aguilar, et al. (1994). The initial results from two independent studies of p53 mutations in hepatocellular carcinomas (HCCs) occurring in populations exposed to aflatoxin found high frequencies of G-->T transversions, with clustering at codon 249 (Hsu, et al., 1991; Bressac, et al., 1991; Li, et al., 1993). On the other hand, studies of p53 mutations in HCCs from Japan and other areas where there is little exposure to aflatoxin, revealed no mutations at codon 249 (Ozturk, et al., 1991). Previous data in bacteria had shown that AFB_1 exposure causes almost exclusively G-->T transversions (Foster, et al., 1983). Also recent work has shown that aflatoxin-epoxide can bind to this particular codon 249 of p53 in a plasmid in vitro, providing further indirect evidence for a putative role of aflatoxin exposure in p53 mutagenesis (Puisieux, et al., 1991). This information provided the circumstantial, but as yet unproven, linkage between this signature mutation of aflatoxin exposure and the events detected in p53 in liver tumors from China and southern Africa. In the past three years these studies have been greatly expanded and are summarized in the following.

Ng, et al. (1994) assessed the expression and point mutation of the p53 gene in 31 patients with hepatocellular carcinomas by using Northern blotting, immunohistochemical methods, and DNA sequencing. All patients were ethnic Chinese, and 90.3% were positive for hepatitis B surface antigen (HBsAg). The p53 transcript or protein was found in 14 (48.4%) of the 31 patients. Detectable p53 mRNA transcripts were found in 10 patients, and p53 protein was detected in 8 patients. In most cases of patients who had detectable p53 mRNA transcripts, the transcripts in the tumors were exhibited at a higher level than they were in the corresponding non-tumorous livers. No p53 protein was detected in the non-tumorous livers in all 31 patients. Six (23.1%) of the 26 tumors sequenced showed point mutation scattered in exons 5-9. Of these, only two were at codon-249, and were G-->T transversions. All but one of the six patients with point mutations had overexpression of the gene. These results showed that scattered point mutations are not uncommon in hepatocellular carcinomas in patients from Hong Kong. The distribution pattern of the mutations seems to have no particular correlation with HBsAg status despite a high prevalence rate of HBsAg positivity in these patients. These researchers suggest that aflatoxin-related specific mutation at codon-249 is much less related to the pathogenesis of hepatocellular carcinoma in Hong Kong Chinese people than in other regions of China with a high aflatoxin exposure.

Fujimoto, et al. (1994) further examined the hypothesis that exposure to aflatoxin B1 either alone or coincident with other environmental carcinogens might be associated with allelic losses occurring during development of human hepatocarcinogenesis in China. The HCCs were obtained from two different areas in China: Qidong, where exposure to HBV_1 and aflatoxin B_1 is high; and Beijing, where exposure to HBV is high but that of aflatoxin B_1 is low. They analyzed the tumors for mutations in the p53 gene and loss of heterozygosity for the p53, Rb, and APC genes and at marker loci on chromosomes 4, 13, and 16. The frequencies of mutation, loss, and aberration (mutation and loss) of the p53 gene in 25 HCCs from Qidong were 60, 58, and 80%, respectively. The frequencies in 9 HCCs from Beijing were 56, 57, and 78%; however, the frequency of a G-->T transversion at codon 249 in HCCs from Qidong and Beijing were 52 and 0%, respectively. These data indicate that mutation and/or loss of heterozygosity in the p53 gene, independent of the 249 mutation, play a critical role in the development of hepatitis B virus-associated HCCs in China. Loss of the Rb and APC genes was observed in 44 and 7% of HCCs from Qidong, respectively. Allelic losses on chromosome 4 and especially on chromosome 16 were frequent in HCCs from Qidong but were not observed in HCCs from Beijing, while loss of heterozygosity on chromosome 13 occurred at similar frequency in both Qidong and Beijing. These results show distinct differences in the pattern of allelic losses between HCCs in Qidong and Beijing and suggest that aflatoxin B_1 and/or other environmental carcinogens may contribute to this difference.

The observation of the codon 249 mutation in p53 with aflatoxin exposure is not limited only to China and southern Africa. Senegal is a country where liver cancer incidence is one of the highest in the world and where people are highly exposed to aflatoxin. In this country 15 liver cancer samples were examined for mutation at codon 249 of the p53 gene (Coursaget, et al., 1993). Non-tumoral DNA from the patients showed a wild type genotype. Mutation at codon 249 of the p53 gene was detected in 10 of the 15 tumor tissues tested (67%). This frequency of mutation in codon 249 of the p53 gene is the highest described to date in the literature and the authors suggest that these results confirm that there is an association between countries of high aflatoxin intake and a high frequency of mutation in codon 249 of p53 gene, and that HBV alone does not contribute to these base changes.

The timing of the occurrence of the p53 mutation in human cancer is of importance in the pathogenesis of the disease. Recent data from Aguilar, et al. (1994) examined the role of AFB_1 and p53 mutations in hepatocellular carcinomas and in normal liver samples from the United States, Thailand, and Qidong, where AFB_1 exposures are negligible, low and high, respectively. The frequency of the AGG to AGT mutation at codon 249 paralleled the level of AFB_1 exposure, which supports the hypothesis that this toxin has a causative and probably early role in hepatocarcinogenesis.

Experimental studies have also been done to link aflatoxin as a causative agent in the described p53 mutations (Cerutti, et al., 1994a). In this study both point mutations in ras protooncogenes and in the p53 tumor suppressor gene, that are common in many forms of human cancer, were examined. To do this work, a restriction fragment length polymorphism/polymerase chain reaction method for genotypic mutation analysis was devised and applied to the study of the mutability of hot-spot codons in c-H-ras1 and p53 genes with human carcinogens. In particular, they studied the mutability of codons 247-250 of p53 with AFB_1 in human hepatocytes. AFB_1 preferentially induced the transversion of guanosine to thymidine in the third position of codon 249, generating the same mutation which is found in a large fraction of hepatocellular carcinomas from regions of the world with AFB_1-contaminated food. These experimental results are in support of AFB_1 as an etiological factor for hepatocellular carcinoma in AFB_1-contaminated areas. In an ongoing study these researchers compared the load of mutations in hot-spot codon 12 of c-H-ras1 in urinary bladder carcinoma and in normal tissue, by restriction fragment length polymorphism/polymerase chain reaction and observed moderately elevated abundances of guanosine to thymidine transversions in the middle position of codon 12 in tumor DNA. These results may reflect a mutator phenotype of the tumor tissue or they could be the consequence of the heterogeneity of the biopsies which were analyzed.

Finally, Aguilar et al, 1993 studied the mutagenesis of codons 247-250 of p53 by rat liver microsome-activated AFB_1 in human HCC cells HepG2 using a similar restriction fragment length polymorphism/polymerase chain reaction genotypic strategy. They found that AFB_1 preferentially induced the transversion of G-->T in the third position of codon 249; however, AFB_1 also induced G-->T and C-->A transversions into adjacent codons, albeit at lower frequencies. Since the latter mutations are not observed in HCC it follows that both mutability on the DNA level and altered function of the mutant serine 249 p53 protein are responsible for the observed mutational hotspot in p53 in HCC from AFB_1-contaminated areas.

In summary, the work on p53 mutations in human liver cancer has provided important evidence linking for the first time exposures to an environmental carcinogen with mutations in an important regulatory gene in cell-cycle homeostasis. These studies pioneer the development of future investigations where other specific genes relevant to the cancer process will be examined.

A FUTURE DIRECTION FOR LIVER CANCER PREVENTION

Several approaches can be considered for the prevention of liver cancer. A first approach is vaccination against HBV. Unfortunately, many people living in high-risk areas for liver cancer acquire the HBV infection before age three. Thus, an immunization program for total population protection would minimally have to occur over a 20-30 year period, provided that mutant strains of hepatitis B virus do not arise, thereby eliminating the utility of current vaccines. Despite these problems, vaccination programs for HBV should be implemented with the required long-term follow-up. A second approach for cancer prevention would be the elimination of aflatoxin exposures. Primary prevention of aflatoxin exposures could be accomplished through large expenditures of resources for proper crop storage and handling; however, this approach is not economically feasible in many areas of the world. Thus, chemoprotective interventions may provide a near-term alternative for some very high-risk populations. Indeed, clinical trials of selenium in such populations are presently underway.

Cancer prevention trials that use biological markers as intermediate endpoints provide the ability to assess the efficacy of promising chemoprotective agents in an efficient manner by reducing sample size requirements as well as the time required to conduct the studies compared to trials that have cancer incidence or mortality as endpoints (Lippman, et al., 1990). These intermediate markers are particularly valuable when investigating chemoprotective agents such as oltipraz that may have an effect at early, preclinical stages of carcinogenesis. The key issue in trials that use biomarkers as the outcome of interest is to have a marker that is directly associated with the evolution or development of neoplasia. These biomarkers are typically organ site-specific genomic, proliferation, and differentiation markers that reflect different intermediary stages of the neoplastic process. As an adjunct to these process-dependent markers it may also be possible to devise markers specific to interventions in selected groups at high risk for carcinogen exposure. These agent-dependent approaches would be based upon knowledge of the etiologic agent(s) in the study population.

The long-term goal of the research described herein is the application of biomarkers to the development of preventive interventions for use in human populations at high risk for cancer. Several of the aflatoxin-specific biomarkers have been validated in epidemiologic studies and are now available to use as intermediate biomarkers in prevention studies. The development of these aflatoxin biomarkers has been based upon the knowledge of the biochemistry and toxicology of aflatoxins gleaned from both experimental and human studies. These biomarkers have been subsequently utilized in experimental models to provide data on the modulation of these markers under different situations of disease risk. This systematic approach provides encouragement for preventive interventions and should serve as a template for the development, validation and application of other chemical-specific biomarkers to cancer or other chronic diseases.

ACKNOWLEDGMENTS

This work was supported by grants from the USPHS P01 ES06052, NIEHS Center Grant ES 03819, and Training Grant T32 ES07141.

REFERENCES

Aguilar F, Harris CC, Sun T, Hollstein M, Cerutti P (1994): Geographic variation of p53 mutational profile in nonmalignant human liver. Science 264:1317-1319.

Aguilar F, Hussain SP, Cerutti P (1993): Aflatoxin B1 induces the transversion of G-->T in codon 249 of the p53 tumor suppressor gene in human hepatocytes. Proc Natl Acad Sci USA 90:8586-8590.

Autrup H, Seremet T, Wakhisi J, Wasunna A (1987): Aflatoxin exposure measured by urinary excretion of aflatoxin b_1-guanine adduct and hepatitis b virus infection in areas with different liver cancer incidence in Kenya. Cancer Res 47:3430-3433.

Autrup H, Bradley KA, Shamsuddin AKM, Wakhisi J, Wasunna A (1983): Detection of putative adduct with fluorescence characteristics identical to 2,3-dihydro-2-(7' guanyl)-3-hydroxyaflatoxin B1 in human urine collected in Murang'a district, Kenya. Carcinogenesis 4(9):1193-1195.

Bennett RA, Essigmann JM, Wogan GN (1981): Excretion of an aflatoxin-guanine adduct in the urine of aflatoxin B_1-treated rats. Cancer Res 41:650-654.

Bressac B, Kew M, Wands J, Ozturk M (1991): Selective G to T mutations of p53 gene in hepatocellular carcinoma from Southern Africa. Nature 350:429-431.

Cerutti P, Hussain P, Pourzand C, Aguilar F (1994): Mutagenesis of the H-ras protooncogene and the p53 tumor suppressor gene. Cancer Res 54:1934s-1938s.

Coursaget P, Depril N, Chabaud M, Nandi R, Mayelo V, LeCann P, Yvonnet B (1993): High prevalence of mutations at codon 249 of the p53 gene in hepatocellular carcinomas from Senegal. Br J Cancer 67:1395-1397.

Eaton DL, Groopman JD (eds.) (1994): "The Toxicology of Aflatoxins: Human Health, Veterinary and Agricultural Significance." New York: Academic Press, p. 556.

Essigmann JM, Croy RG, Nadzan AM, Busby WF, Jr, Reinhold VN, Buchi G, Wogan GN (1977): Structural identification of the major DNA adduct formed by aflatoxin B_1 in vitro. Proc Natl Acad Sci USA 74:1870-1874.

Foster PL, Eisenstadt E, Miller JH (1983): Base substitution mutations induced by metabolically activated aflatoxin B_1. Proc Natl Acad Sci USA 80:2695-2698.

Fujimoto Y, Hampton LL, Wirth PJ, Wang NJ, Xie JP, Thorgeirsson SS (1994): Alterations of tumor suppressor genes and allelic losses in human hepatocellular carcinomas in China. Cancer Res 54:281-285.

Gan L-S, Skipper PL, Peng X-C, Groopman JD, Chen J-S, Wogan GN, Tannenbaum SR (1988): Serum albumin adducts in the molecular epidemiology of aflatoxin carcinogenesis: Correlation with aflatoxin B_1 intake and urinary excretion of aflatoxin M_1. Carcinogenesis 9:1323-1325.

Greenblatt MS, Bennett WP, Hollstein M, Harris CC (1994): Mutations in the p53 tumor suppressor gene: clues to cancer etiology and molecular pathogenesis. Cancer Res 54:4855-4878.

Groopman JD, Zhu J, Donahue PR, Pikul A, Zhang L-S, Chen J-S, Wogan GN (1992a): Molecular dosimetry of urinary aflatoxin DNA adducts in people living in Guangxi Autonomous Region, People's Republic of China. Cancer Res 52: 45-51.

Groopman JD, Hall A, Whittle H, Hudson G, Wogan GN, Montesano R, Wild CP (1992b): Molecular dosimetry of aflatoxin-N^7-guanine in human urine obtained in The Gambia, West Africa. Cancer Epidemiol, Biomarkers Prev 1:221-228.

Hollstein M, Sidransky D, Vogelstein B, Harris CC (1991): p53 Mutations in human cancers. Science 253:49-53.

Hsu IC, Metcalf RA, Sun T, Wesh JA, Wang NJ, Harris CC (1991): Mutational hotspot in the p53 gene in human hepatocellular carcinomas. Nature 350:427-428.

IARC Monographs on the Evaluation of Carcinogenic Risks to Humans (1993): Volume 56: "Some Naturally Occurring Substances: Food Items and Constituents, Heterocyclic Aromatic Amines and Mycotoxins." Lyon: IARC Monographs, p. 599.

Li D, Cao Y, He L, Wang NJ, Gu J (1993): Accelerated Paper. Aberrations of p53 gene in human hepatocellular carcinoma from China. Carcinogenesis, 14:169-173.

Lippman SM, Lee JS, Lotan R, Hittleman W, Wargovich MJ, Hong, WK (1990): Biomarkers as intermediate end points in chemoprevention trials. J Natl Cancer Inst 82:555-562.

Ng IO, Srivastava G, Chung LP, Tsang SW, Ng MM (1994): Overexpression and point mutations of p53 tumor suppressor gene in hepatocellular carcinomas in Hong Kong Chinese people. Cancer 74:30-37.

Ozturk, M and collaborators (1991): p53 Mutation in hepatocellular carcinoma after aflatoxin exposure. The Lancet 338:1356-1359.

Puisieux A, Lim S, Groopman JD, Ozturk M (1991): Selective targeting of p53 gene mutational hotspots in human cancers by etiologically defined carcinogens. Cancer Res 51:6185-6189.

Qian G-S, Yu MC, Ross R, Yuan J-M, Gao Y-T, Wogan GN, Groopman JD (1994): A follow-up study of urinary markers of aflatoxin exposure and liver cancer risk in Shanghai, P.R.C. Cancer Epidemiol, Biomarkers Prev 3:3-11.

Ross R, Yuan J-M, Yu M, Wogan GN, Qian G-S, Tu J-T, Groopman JD, Gao Y-T, Henderson BE (1992): Urinary aflatoxin biomarkers and risk of hepatocellular carcinoma. The Lancet 339:943-946.

Sabbioni G, Skipper P, Buchi G, Tannenbaum SR (1987): Isolation and characterization of the major serum albumin adduct formed by aflatoxin B_1 in vivo in rats. Carcinogenesis 8:819-824.

Wang J-S, Qian G-S, Zhu Y-R, Zarba A, Munoz A, Kensler TW, Groopman JD (1995): Temporal patterns and persistence of aflatoxin-albumin adducts in residents of Daxin Township, Qidong, P.R.C. Proc Am Assoc Cancer Res 36:282.

Wild CP, Hall A (1994): Epidemiology of human liver cancer. In Eaton DL, Groopman JD (eds): "The Toxicology of Aflatoxins: Human Health, Veterinary and Agricultural Significance." New York: Academic Press, p. 556.

Wild, CP, Hudson G, Sabbioni G, Wogan GN, Whittle H, Montesano R, Groopman JD (1992): Correlation of dietary intake of aflatoxins with the level of albumin bound aflatoxin in peripheral blood in The Gambia, West Africa. Cancer Epidemiol, Biomarkers Prev 1:229-234.

Wild CP, Jiang YZ, Sabbioni G, Chapot B, Montesano R (1990a): Evaluation of methods for quantitation of aflatoxin-albumin adducts and their application to human exposure assessment Cancer Res. 50:245-251.
Wild CP, Jiang YZ, Allen SJ, Jansen LA, Hall AJ, Montesano, R (1990b): Aflatoxin-albumin adducts in human sera from different regions of the world. Carcinogenesis 11:2271-2274.

Genetics and Cancer Susceptibility:
Implications for Risk Assessment, pages 223–234

DIET INTERVENTION FOR MODIFYING CANCER RISK

Diane F. Birt, Jill C. Pelling, Satish Nair and Denise Lepley

Eppley Institute for Research in Cancer and Department of Biochemistry and Molecular Biology, University of Nebraska Medical Center, Omaha, NE 68198-6805

ABSTRACT

Considerable evidence suggests that dietary differences between populations account for a significant proportion of the variation in cancer occurrence in different parts of the world. A major problem has been identifying the particular dietary components which predispose or protect individuals against cancer. For example, the high rates of breast and colon cancer in the United States have been associated with numerous dietary patterns including high fat, high dietary energy, and low fruit and vegetable intakes. Our laboratories have attempted to identify mechanisms whereby diet may modify cancer and it is anticipated that future studies will determine which of these potential mechanisms may be relevant in humans. A promising lead in understanding the mechanism of high dietary fat/high dietary energy promotion of cancer was the impact of these diets on cellular protein kinase C (PKC). PKC is important in cellular signaling events which are critical to tumor promotion. Our studies demonstrated increased PKC activity and/or protein expression observed in epidermis and pancreatic epithelial cells of rodents fed high fat/energy diets. The inverse association between cancer at a number of sites and fruit and vegetable intake may be due to both micronutrient and non-nutrient components of fruits and vegetables. We have studied the prevention of skin tumor promotion by apigenin, a plant flavonoid. Apigenin may block several points in the process of tumor promotion, including inhibiting kinases, reducing transcription factors and regulating cell cycle. The complexity of our diets and the multitude of potential dietary effects which may be important in cancer development make this a fertile area for future study.

INTRODUCTION

Diets rich in fat and energy and low in fruits and vegetables are associated with elevated rates of cancer at several sites including the breast, colon, prostate, and pancreas (Willett, 1990; Potter et al., 1993). The particular dietary constituents involved are being investigated and mechanisms responsible have not been identified. Considering the complexity of the human diet it is likely that numerous factors contribute to the observed relationship between diet and cancer and research suggests that factors interact.

There is considerable controversy surrounding the role of dietary fat in cancer. It appears that high fat diet may be a factor in the etiology of some forms of cancer such as colon but not in others such as breast (Willett et al., 1992; Giovannucci et al., 1995). Experimental animal studies suggest that some of the relationship between high fat diet and elevated cancer rates may be due to the high dietary energy contribution of a high fat diet (Birt, 1987). Dietary energy intake has not been adequately studied in humans and considering the difficulties with estimating energy intake, data will probably be hard to interpret once it is gathered. However, epidemiological studies have shown reduced risk of breast and colon cancer in physically active individuals in comparison with sedentary controls (Whittemore et al., 1990). These data suggest that energy use, or potentially energy balance, is an important factor in human cancer.

Diets rich in fruits and vegetables have also been associated with reduced cancer rates in a number of epidemiological studies. It is not entirely clear if this association is due to the fact that such diets tend to be lower in energy and fat or that the specific components of fruits and vegetables are responsible. Epidemiological studies have observed reduced rates of cancer is association with high vegetable and/or fruit intake when the subjects were stratified according to energy and or fat intake suggesting that fruits and vegetables contain compounds which are important in cancer prevention (Hunter et al., 1993). Furthermore, studies with cultured cells and with laboratory animals have clearly supported a role for numerous plant compounds in the prevention of cancer (Birt and Bresnick, 1991). In particular, a number of isothiocyanates have been identified in vegetables with potent anti-cancer activity (Zhang, Talalay, 1994). One mechanism whereby these agents may prevent cancer is through induction of enzymes which detoxify reactive species and thus prevent DNA damage which is believed to be important for the induction of cancer (Zhang, Talalay, 1994). Other potential mechanisms include control of cell cycle which is often deranged in the rapidly proliferating pre-cancerous state and in full blown cancer. Several flavonoids and isoflavonoids have been identified which have the potential to block cell cycle events as described below.

It is certainly possible that dietary factors will be of particular importance in individuals with genetic sucpetibility to cancer. Clearly, considering differences in strain and species responses to individual carcinogens, all rodent cancers can be considered genetic susceptibilities. However, we presently do not know the nature of the particular genetic susceptibility. As we learn more regarding mechanisms for genetic susceptibility and mechanisms for dietary modulation of carcinogenesis it should become possible to use diet to intervene and reduce risk in the genetically susceptible groups.

STUDIES ON BIOCHEMICAL MECHANISMS FOR DIETARY INTERVENTION IN CANCER

It is important to identify mechanisms whereby diet may alter cancer to identify the optimal intakes of foods and nutrients for cancer prevention in animals and to allow us to translate these findings to human diets. It will be particularly important to understand mechanisms of dietary intervention in cancer to assess how diet may intervene in the process of genetic predisposition to cancer. In the remainder of this paper we will describe work in our laboratories and by others which lead to biochemical and molecular understanding of the impact of high energy and particular plant components on carcinogenesis in rodents. Future studies will be required to determine the applicability of these mechanisms to human cancer intervention and to determine particular genetic susceptibilities to cancer which can be attacked by dietary intervention.

ENERGY RESTRICTION INHIBITION OF CANCER

Rodent studies on the impact of dietary intake and cancer have generally used a dietary restriction protocol. In most cases less diet has been fed to the restricted animals in comparison with freely fed controls. Dietary restriction protocols have been widely used and shown to inhibit numerous models of cancer including chemically induced, radiation induced and viral carcinogenesis (Birt, 1987). In general, the most severe restriction used is a 40% reduction in intake in comparison with control animals. Restrictions of as little as 20% has been effective in the inhibition of mammary carcinogenesis (Klurfeld et al., 1989). In diet restriction studies the rodents receive less of all dietary components including reduced intakes of vitamins and minerals. Such studies do not clearly indicate the dietary component which is most effective in reducing cancer rates.

A number of laboratories, including our own, have used a dietary energy (calorie) restriction protocol where the diets are reformulated to reduce the intake of energy from some combination of protein, carbohydrate and fat. Such studies indicate that the inhibition of carcinogenesis in diet restricted animals is probably due to the reduction in energy intake. In studies from our laboratory we have demonstrated that restriction of energy from fat or from carbohydrate were both effective in the inhibition of skin carcinogenesis but fat restriction reduced cancer to a greater extent than carbohydrate restriction (Birt et al., 1993).

Skin

Numerous mechanisms have been suggested for dietary restriction inhibition of carcinogenesis including reduction in the secretion of hormones which are important in cell proliferation, reduction in the immune responses which enhance inflammation, reduced oxygen radical damage and increases in apoptosis with reductions in cell proliferation (Moriguchi et al., 1989; Rao et al., 1990; Schulte-Hermann et al., 1994). Research in our laboratory has focused on important events in skin tumor promotion by the phorbol ester tumor promoters since this model is particularly well developed with mechanisms of carcinogenesis better understood than with other forms of cancer (Yuspa, 1994). We were particularly interested in the impact of dietary fat and energy on protein kinase C activation and protein expression in the skin because this family of proteins was found to be the cellular binding site for phorbol ester tumor promoters and also to be important in cellular proliferation and differentiation (Nakamura, Nishizuka, 1994). Furthermore, PKC is distinctive in that these kinases are lipid regulated and it seemed reasonable that dietary fat and energy might modify lipid metabolism in a manner such that PKC activation would be altered. PKC is a family of at least 12 members which have been grouped according to their regulation. Common PKC (cPKC) are both diacylglycerol/phorbol ester and calcium regulated (PKC α, βI, βII, and γ). Novel PKC (nPKC) are diacylglycerol/phorbol ester regulated (PKC δ, ∈, η, and θ). Atypical PKC (aPKC) are neither diacylglycerol/phorbol ester nor calcium regulated (PKC ζ and λ).

Our first studies assessed dietary fat intake (dietary levels of 5% and 24% of the diet) as a mediator of PKC activity. We measured the phosphorylation of lysine-rich histone in the particulate and cytosolic compartments of epidermal cells isolated from mice pre-fed experimental diets for a period of 6-7 weeks. We noted a near doubling of particulate PKC activity in the epidermis of Sencar mice pre-fed high fat diet (Choe et al., 1992). In parallel studies we assessed the impact of 40% dietary energy restriction (ER) on PKC activity and observed about a 50% reduction in PKC activity in the particulate fraction from epidermal cells from ER mice (Kris et al., 1994). Further studies assessed the impact of reduction of fat or carbohydrate calories and determined that restriction of fat calories, feeding a high carbohydrate diet, was somewhat more effective in the inhibition of PKC activity than the reduction of carbohydrate calories (Kris et al., 1994). These studies complemented the studies on the inhibition of skin carcinogenesis since the reduction in PKC activity was greatest in the group with the fewest skin tumors (Birt et al., 1993).

We have gone on to assess the impact of dietary energy restriction and high fat diet on the expression of PKC proteins in mouse epidermis to determine if some of the impact of dietary restriction is due to reduced expression of particular PKC proteins (Birt et al., 1994). We detected the presence of PKC α, δ, ∈ and ζ in the mouse epidermis. Our studies demonstrated a reduced expression of PKC α and PKC ζ in the energy restricted mouse epidermis. PKC δ and ∈ were not significantly modified. Feeding high fat diet did not modify the expression of any of the detected PKC proteins. A representative western blot and graphic representation of our series of experiments are shown in figures 1 and 2.

Using receptor binding assay approaches to determine the ability of phorbol ester binding to epidermal cells we have determined that epidermal cells from dietary energy restricted mice have reduced binding to phorbol dibutyrate. This observation may relate to the reduction in PKC α expression in epidermal cells since PKC α has phorbol ester binding domains and PKC α was reduced in the epidermis of the ER mouse (Birt et al., 1994). The reduction in PKC ζ would not be expected to cause a reduction in phorbol binding because this PKC isoform does not have phorbol binding domains.

We have also assessed the impact of dietary energy restriction and high fat diet on the metabolism of lipids which are potentially important in PKC activation. We first assessed the generation of 1,2-diacylglycerol (DAG) in epidermal cells from mice pre-

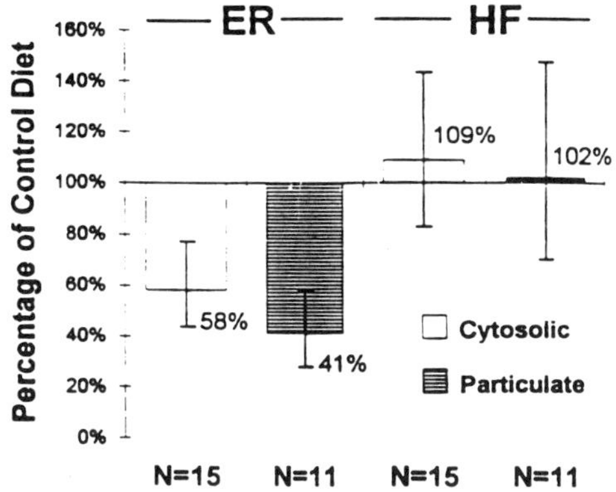

Figure 1: Influence of ER and HF diets on immunoreactive PKC ζ relative to control. Epidermis was pooled from 2-4 mice for each observation, the number of observations is indicated below the bars. Variability is shown as 95% confidence intervals. Mice were pre-fed diet for 6-29 weeks; there was no significant influence of the time the mice were pre-fed the experimental diets on PKC ζ in either fraction, and so values were pooled across time. Energy restriction decreased PKC ζ immunoreactivity in the cytosolic ($P<0.0006$) and particulate fractions ($P<0.0001$). HF diet did not significantly influence PKC ζ immunoreactivity. From: Birt DF, et al (1994) Carcinogenesis: 15:2727-2732 with permission of Oxford University Press.

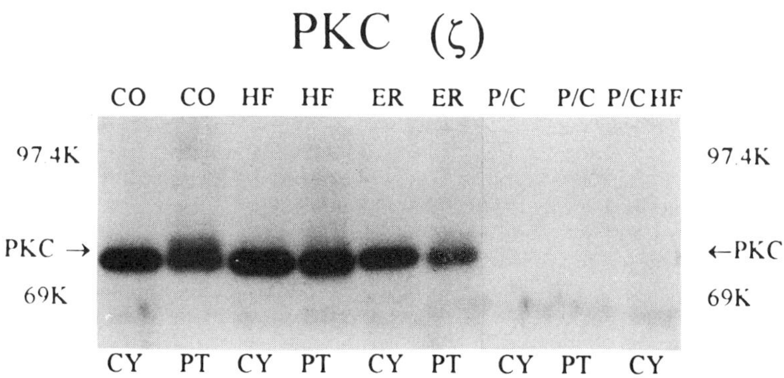

Figure 2: Representative Western blot of PKC ζ antibody in epidermis from mice fed control, ER and HF diets. C, control; HF, high fat; ER, energy restricted; P/C, peptide competed; CY, cytosolic fraction PT, particulate fraction. Normalized densities for lanes were: CO/CYT = 1.0; CO/PT = 1.0; HF/CYT = 1.2; HF/PT = 1.1; ER/CYT = 0.7; ER/PT = 0.4. From: Birt DF, et al (1994) Carcinogenesis: 15:2727-2732 with permission of Oxford University Press

fed high fat and energy restriction diets. Our results indicated an elevation in DAG in both cells from animals pre-fed high fat diet and energy restricted mice (Choe et al., 1992; Kris et al., 1994). The elevated DAG may help explain the increased PKC activity in the epidermis of mice fed high fat diet, but it certainly does not explain the reduced PKC activity in the epidermis from ER mice. It is possible that a compensatory increase in DAG was observed because of the striking reduction in the expression of certain isoforms of PKC. We have gone on to demonstrate that the increase in DAG in the ER epidermis may come from increased turnover of phosphatidylinositol (Kris et al., 1994). The DAG in the mice fed high fat diet however, does not come from this source (Choe et al., 1992).

Our data at present suggests that high fat diets increase epidermal PKC activity through increasing the availability of DAG, the endogenous activator of PKC. Dietary energy restriction decreased PKC activity through decreasing specific isoenzymes of PKC. We believe the elevation in PKC activity is relevant to the enhancement of skin carcinogenesis in mice fed high fat diet and the reduction in ER mice is relevant to the inhibition of cancer by these diets because of the importance of the interaction between TPA and PKC. Although the aspects of the interaction between TPA and PKC which are important to tumor promotion have not been clearly worked out, It is clear that the interaction appears to be important for tumor promotion (Weinstein, 1991).

Pancreas

Epidemiological studies have shown that the high fat, high energy diet consumed by a large proportion of Western society is associated with elevated rates of pancreatic cancer (Haddock, Carter, 1990). Experimental animal studies have suggested that high fat diets may certainly increase the rate of pancreas cancer and the enhancement does not appear to be due to elevated energy intake of rodents fed high fat diet. For example, studies from this laboratory compared freely fed syrian hamsters fed control and high fat diets with control fed hamsters fed control and high fat diet (Birt et al., 1989). Control fed hamsters were given allotments of food equivalent to a 16% reduction in comparison with control freely fed hamsters. The control fed control and high fat animals received the same dietary energy intake. Pancreatic carcinogenesis was initiated by a single dose of N-nitroso-bis (2-oxopropy)lamine (BOP) given at 8 weeks of age. The cumulative incidence of pancreatic cancer and the mean latency in hamsters in the four groups is shown in Table 1. Dietary fat enhanced pancreatic carcinogenesis in both freely fed and control fed hamsters to a similar extent, but the control-fed hamsters on high fat diet developed cancer, on average, 8 weeks later than the freely fed animals on high fat diet.

This result, and the prior observation of Craven-Giles et al. (1994) indicated that dietary energy restriction would be expected to inhibit or delay the induction of pancreatic carcinogenesis. Recent studies in our laboratory have determined the impact of dietary energy restriction on PKC isozyme expression in the pancreas to determine if the expression of pancreatic PKC is reduced similar to the reduction of skin PKC discussed above. Our first studies assessed the expression of PKC isoforms

Table 1. Survival and pancreatic ductular carcinoma yield in hamsters fed low- and hgh-fat diets by ad litibum or control-fed protocol

Carcinogen treatment	Type of feeding	Level of fat	% surviving at 95 wk.	Overall incidence (%)	No of CRC[b]/EAN	Av. survival of CRC-bearing hamsters (wk ± SD)
With	ad libitum	Low	27	8 (A)	0.2(A	75 ± 22
With		High	26	30 (B)	0.6 (B)	80 ± 18
With	Control-fed	Low	27	18 (C)	0.2 (A)	75 ± 4
With		High	33	52 (D)	0.8 (B)	88 ± 10

All hamsters were treated with 20 mg BOP/100 gm body weight at 8 weeks of age.

[a] x2 test comparisons on age-adjusted data within each column: A<B , C< D , (P<0.05). Number effective hamsters = 24 – 33.

[b] CRC, carcinoma; EAN, effective animal. Data from (Birt et al., 1989) with permission.

in the hamster pancreas. We observed little evidence of expression of PKC α, β, γ, δ, or ∈ (Nair et al., 1995a) but PKC ζ was well expressed by normal hamster pancreas, hamster pancreatic carcinoma cells (PC-1) and human pancreatic carcinoma cells (PANC-1) (Nair et al., 1995a). We went on to assess the impact of graded dietary restriction (ER) (10, 20, and 40% reduction in comparison with control) on pancreatic PKC ζ expression for hamsters restricted for a period of 8 or 16 weeks (Nair et al., 1995b). In general, all levels of dietary ER reduced the expression of PKC ζ in a similar manner with 8 weeks of ER reducing PKC ζ by 30-50% and with 15 weeks of ER depressing PKC ζ expression by 70-80%. The impact of these levels of dietary restriction on pancreatic carcinogenesis by BOP is currently under investigation.

FLAVONOID INHIBITION OF SKIN CANCER

Numerous chemicals from fruits and vegetables are probably responsible for the reduced rate of cancer observed in people consuming diets rich in fruits and vegetables (Birt, Bresnick, 1991). Classes of chemicals with cancer prevention properties in fruits and vegetables include carotenoids, terpenes, isothiocyanates, organo sulfur compounds, flavonoids and ioflavonoids (Birt, Bresnick, 1991). Studies in our laboratory have focused on one particular flavonoid, apigenin [5,7,4'-trihydroxyflavone] (figure 3). While apigenin is found ubiquitously in fruits and vegetables, little is know regarding its ability to modify cancer.

Our initial studies assessed the impact of apigenin on ornithine decarboxylase activity induction by TPA in mouse skin. We used this system to screen for anti-promotion activity of a number of chemicals present in fruits and vegetables. Apigenin at doses

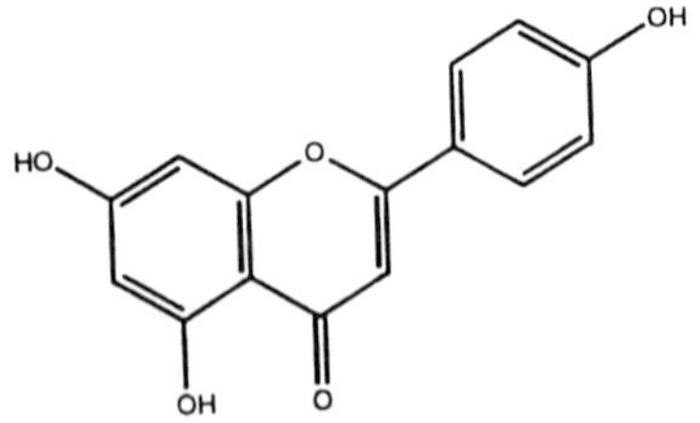

Figure 3: Structure of apigenin

of 5 μmole/200 acetone inhibited ODC activity to about 40% (Wei et al., 1990). Further studies demonstrated that when given 30 minutes prior to TPA, apigenin effectively inhibited the development of papillomas and carcinomas in DMBA initiated mouse skin (Wei et al., 1990). In more recent studies we have determined that apigenin also inhibits uv-light induced squamous cell carcinomas in the epidermis of SKH-1 hairless mice (Birt et. al., unpublished).

Studies in other laboratories have assessed the impact of a number of flavonoids and isoflavonoids with anticancer activity on cell cycle regulation in tumor cells. In particular, genistein, an isoflavonoid, was found to inhibit in a dose dependent manner the progression of HGC-27 cells (human gastric cancer cells) through G2-M (Matsukawa et al., 1993). Furthermore, quercetin, a widely occurring flavonoid, blocked human leukemic T-cells in late G1 phase of the cell cycle (Yoshida et al., 1992). Quercetin treatment of several cancer cell lines induced apoptosis as indicated by DNA fragmentation analysis and by the appearance of hypodiploid cells as assessed by flow cytometry (Wei et al., 1994). Apigenin was shown to induce differentiation and G2-M arrest in rat neuronal cells (Sato et al., 1994). These observations suggest that a number of flavonoids and isoflavonoids may inhibit tumor growth and cell proliferation through cell cycle blockage.

We have recently found that doses of apigenin which give cellular concentrations of apigenin in cultured cells similar to the concentrations observed in our in-vivo studies are effective in blocking cell cycle at G2/M (Lepley, et. al., unpublished). An example of a representative experiment is provided in table 2. We also determined the impact of apigenin on p34 cdc2 kinase which regulates passage through G2-M. Preliminary results suggest that apigenin inhibits this kinase activity in the range of doses where it blocks cell cycle (see table 2 for representative data). Since p34 cdc2 kinase requires association with cyclin B, with associated phosphorylation and dephosphorylation events for activation, our recent studies have assessed the impact of apigenin on the presence of cyclin B protein. Table 2 shows preliminary results which suggest that apigenin may reduce the expression of cyclin B protein in C50 cells. Our observations on apigenin inhibition of p34 cdc2 kinase activity are consistent with the inhibition of this kinase in human breast cancer cells by quercetin, genistein and a potent flavonoid analog L86-8275 (Losiewicz et al., 1995). These provocative findings suggest that several flavonoids and isoflavonoids with cancer prevention properties may function through a common pathway to block aberrant cell proliferation.

Table 2. Effect of Apigenin on Cell Cycle, p34 cdc2 Kinase Activity and Cyclin B Protein in C50 Mouse Epidermal Cells.

Apigenin Dose	% of Cells in G2/M	Relative Cyclin B-Associated p34cdc2 Kinase Activity	Level of Cyclin B Protein Relative to % of Cells in G2/M
0mM	31	1	1
5mM	37	0.94	0.90
15mM	49	1.07	0.64
30mM	74	1.62	0.36
45mM	69	0.41	0.15

The normal mouse epidermal cell line, C50, was cultured to 30-50% confluency before re-feeding with fresh media and adding apigenin in DMSO to reach the desired final concentration. All cultures contained the same concentration of DMSO. The cells were cultured with apigenin for 24 hours in all experiments. Data in Table 2 are from separate experiments that have been repeated at least once.

POTENTIAL ROLE OF DIET IN THE INTERVENTION OF GENETIC RISK FOR CANCER

Animal models for cancer are essentially models of genetic susceptibility. It is clear that some strains and species are more susceptible to carcinogenesis by a given agent than other species and strains. It has been the practice in nutritional carcinogenesis studies to use only the more susceptible strain to reduce the size and expense of experiments. Unfortunately this means that we generally conduct our experiments on diet and cancer in only the most susceptible strains, without a control for genetic differences. This will certainly change as we uncover mechanisms for genetic susceptibility which will allow us to determine the impact of dietary intervention in a particular genetic background and compare the impact of diet in models with different genetic lesions.

A better understanding of mechanisms for dietary modification of cancer will allow us to better design and optimize studies on dietary intervention in genetic susceptibility. We will be able to attack the particular genetic deficit with a diet with a known biochemical/molecular effect. Considering the complexity of genetic factors in cancer and the complexity of the human diet, studies on the impact of diet on genetic susceptibility will be a fertile area for research for many years to come.

REFERENCES

Birt DF (1987): Fat and calorie effects on carcinogenesis at sites other than the mammary gland. Am J Clin Nutr 45:203-209.

Birt DF, Julius AD, White LT, Pour PM (1989): Enhancement of pancreatic carcinogenesis in hamsters fed a high-fat diet *ad libitum* and at a controlled calorie intake. Cancer Res 49:5848-5851.

Birt DF, Pinch HJ, Barnett T, Phan A, Dimitroff K (1993): Inhibition of skin tumor promotion by restriction of fat and carbohydrate calories in SENCAR mice. Cancer Res 53:27-31.

Birt DF, Copenhaver J, Pelling JC, Anderson J (1994): Dietary energy restriction and fat modulation of protein kinase C isoenzymes and phorbol ester binding in Sencar mouse epidermis. Carcinogenesis 15:2727-2732.

Birt DF, Bresnick E (1991): Chemoprevention by nonnutrient components of vegetables and fruits. In: Alfin-Slater R, Kritchevsky D (eds): "Human Nutrition: A Comprehensive Treatise." New York, NY: Plenum, pp 221-261.

Choe M, Kris ES, Luthra R, Copenhaver J, Pelling JC, Donnelly TE, Birt DF (1992): Protein kinase C is activated and diacylglycerol is elevated in epidermal cells from Sencar mice fed high fat diets. J Nutr 122:2322-2329.

Craven-Giles T, Tagliaferro AR, Ronan AM, Baumgartner KJ, Roebuck BD (1994): Dietary modulation of pancreatic carcinogenesis: Calories and energy expenditure. Cancer Res 54 Suppl.:1964s-1968s.

Giovannucci E, Ascherio A, Rimm EB, Colditz GA, Stampfer MJ, Willett WC (1995): Physical activity, obesity, and risk for colon cancer and adenoma in men. Ann Intern Med 122:327-334.

Haddock G, Carter DC (1990): Aetiology of pancreatic cancer. Br J Surg 77:1159-1166.

Hunter DJ, Manson JE, Colditz GA, Stampfer MJ, Rosner B, Hennekens CH, Speizer FE, Willett WC (1993): A prospective study of the intake of vitamins C, E, and A and the risk of breast cancer. N Engl J Med 329:234-240.

Klurfeld DM, Welch CB, Davis MJ, Kritchevsky D (1989): Determination of degree of energy restriction necessary to reduce DMBA-induced mammary tumorigenesis in rats during the promotion phase. J Nutr 119:286-291.

Kris ES, Choe M, Luthra R, Conway H, Barnett T, Yaktine A, Birt DF (1994): Protein kinase C activity is reduced in epidermal cells from energy-restricted SENCAR mice. J Nutr 124:485-492.

Losiewicz M, Carlson B, Kaur G, Sausville E, Worland P (1995): Potent inhibition of cdc2 kinase activity by the flavonoid L86-8275. Biochem Biophys Res Commun 201:589-595.

Matsukawa Y, Marui N, Sakai T, Satomi Y, Yoshida M, Matsumoto K, Nishino H, Aoike A (1993): Genistein arrests cell cycle progression at G_2-M. Cancer Res 53:1328-1331.

Moriguchi S, Toba M, Kishino Y (1989): Effects of dietary restriction on cellular immunity in rats. J Nutr Sci Vitaminol 35:49-59.

Nair S, Pour P, Lawson T, Kolar C, Vaughn R, Birt DF (1995a): Identification of protein kinase C zeta isozyme in the hamster pancreas and pancreatic carcinoma cell lines. Molecular Carcinogenesis In Press.

Nair S, Toshkov I, Yaktine A, Barnett T, Chaney W, Birt DF (1995b): Dietary energy restriction-induced modulation of Protein Kinase C zeta isozyme in the hamster pancreas. Molecular Carcinogenesis in press.

Nakamura S, Nishizuka Y (1994): Lipid mediators and protein kinase C activation for the intracellular signaling network. J Biochem (Tokyo) 115:1029-1034.

Potter JD, Slattery ML, Bostick RM, Gapstur SM (1993): Colon cancer: A review of the epidemiology. Epidemiol Rev 15:499-545.

Rao G, Xia E, Nadakavukaren MJ, Richardson A (1990): Effect of dietary restriction on the age-dependent changes in the expression of antioxidant enzymes in rat liver. J Nutr 120:602-609.

Sato F, Matsukawa Y, Matsumoto K, Nishino H, Sakai T (1994): Apigenin induces morphological differentiation and G2-M arrest in rat neuronal cells. Biochem Biophys Res Commun 204:578-584.

Schulte-Hermann R, Grasl-Kraupp B, Bursch W (1994): Tumor development and apoptosis. Int Arch Allergy Immunol 105:363-367.

Wei H, Tye L, Bresnick E, Birt DF (1990): Inhibitory effect of apigenin, a plant flavonoid, on epidermal ornithine decarboxylase and skin tumor promotion in mice. Cancer Res 50:499-502.

Wei Y, Zhao X, Kariya Y, Fukata H, Teshigawara K, Uchida A (1994): Induction of apoptosis by quercetin: Involvement of heat shock protein. Cancer Res 54:4952-4957.

Weinstein IB (1991): Cancer prevention: Recent progress and future opportunities. Cancer Res 51 Suppl.:5080s-5085s.

Whittemore AS, Wu-Williams AH, Lee M, Shu Z, Gallagher RP, Deng-ao J, Lun Z,

Xianghui W, Kun C, Jung D, Teh C-Z, Chengde L, Yao XJ, Paffenbarger RS,Jr., Henderson BE (1990): Diet, physical activity, and colorectal cancer among Chinese in North America and China. JNCI 82:915-926.

Willett WC (1990): Epidemiologic Studies of Diet and Cancer. Med Oncol &Tumor Pharmamother 7:93-97.

Willett WC, Hunter DJ, Stampfer MJ, Colditz G, Manson JE, Spiegelman D, Rosner B, Hennekens CH, Speizer FE (1992): Dietary fat and fiber in relation to risk of breast cancer. An 8-year follow-up. JAMA 268:2037-2044.

Yoshida M, Yamamoto M, Nikaido T (1992): Quercetin arrests human leukemic T-cells in late G_1 phase of the cell cycle. Cancer Res 52:6676-6681.

Yuspa SH (1994): The pathogenesis of squamous cell cancer: Lessons learned from studies of skin carcinogenesis—Thirty-third G. H. A. Clowes Memorial Award Lecture. Cancer Res 54:1178-1189.

Zhang Y, Talalay P (1994): Anticarcinogenic activities of organic isothiocyanates: Chemistry and mechanisms. Cancer Res 54 Suppl.:1976s-1981s.

Genetics and Cancer Susceptibility:
Implications for Risk Assessment, pages 235–247

GENETIC VARIATION IN SUSCEPTIBILITY AS A KEY PARAMETER IN RISK ASSESSMENT AND RISK COMMUNICATION: POLICY ASPECTS

Gilbert S. Omenn, M.D., Ph.D.

School of Public Health and Community Medicine
University of Washington
Seattle, Washington 98195-7230

INTRODUCTION

Risk assessment provides an essential framework for organizing, evaluating, and characterizing scientific information on the nature and magnitude of hazards from specific chemicals, as well as complex exposures. Qualitative and quantitative characterization of risk is needed for risk communication and for risk reduction/risk management. In light of the diversity of human populations (and other target populations in the environment), there are major policy implications of the variability of response in the "host" or "target" species.

This Conference and its Proceedings address an under-investigated variable in the risk assessment paradigm: genetic variation within species and genetic variation across species in the biotransformation of chemicals and in target site susceptibility to their actions. Previous relevant documents include a book from the Banbury Conference on "Genetic Variability in Responses to Chemical Exposure" (Omenn & Gelboin, 1984) and a book from the UCLA/Keystone Symposium on "Biotechnology and Human Genetic Predisposition to Disease" (Cantor et al., 1990). The concept of "ecogenetics" emerged in the 1970s from the principles and mechanistic findings in "pharmacogenetics", which began in the late 1950s. Pharmacogenetics and ecogenetics stress the interaction between the host and the environmental exposure, between nature and nurture, and the reasons for desirable or adverse effects resulting from such interactions. Led by Dr. Arno Motulsky, a pioneer in pharmacogenetics, the Division of Medical Genetics and later the University of Washington School of Public Health & Community Medicine, through our Charles A. Dana Program in Genetics and Environmental Health, have been in the forefront of ecogenetics research, training, and policy analysis.

Policy ramifications of variation in susceptibility were highlighted in the National Research Council report "Science and Judgment in Risk Assessment" (NRC, 1994), which carefully distinguished variability from uncertainty (below). This distinction is important also in the charge to the presidential/congressional Commission on Risk Assessment and Risk Management (Omenn, 1994a).

Rapid advances in molecular genetics and human genome research add a dimension of gene finding and knowledge of gene sequence variability before we have knowledge of the functional effects of many of those genes (Andrews et al., 1994). Surely some or many of these genes which are associated epidemiologically with higher risk (predisposition) or lower risk (resistance) to various diseases and disorders will prove to have their effects mediated through interaction with environmental exposures. Testing for such genes, especially workplace or community-based screening outside the clinical setting, raises important ethical and policy issues of privacy, confidentiality, and equity in employment and insurance.

The Place of Eco-Genetics in the Framework for Risk Assessment

In a framework that was developed for the federal Interagency Regulatory Liaison Group in 1979 and published from the White House Office of Science and Technology Policy in 1980, host variation in susceptibility to environmental agents was recognized explicitly as a prominent variable in the characterization of risk. This framework is applicable to diverse health endpoints--carcinogenicity, mutagenicity, birth defects, reproductive, immunologic, neurobehavioral, and other organ-specific toxicity (Calkins et al., 1980):

Table 1. Framework for Risk Assessment and Risk Management

Hazard Identification	Epidemiology
	Lifetime rodent bioassays
	Short-term, in vitro/in vivo tests
	Structure-activity relationships
Risk Characterization	Potency (dose/response)
	Exposure analysis
	Variation in susceptibility
Risk Reduction	Information
	Substitution
	Regulation/Prohibition

Subsequently, the "Red Book" from the National Research Council (NRC, 1983) established four steps for the risk assessment part (top two-thirds) of this risk assessment/risk management framework: hazard identification, dose-response assessment, exposure assessment, and risk characterization. Host variability was embedded in the risk characterization step. The present Conference Proceedings succeed in re-emphasizing the importance of variation in susceptibility.

Intra-Species Variation In Humans

We need to investigate the marked variation among humans for clinical, regulatory, and scientific reasons. In occupational and environmental medicine, physicians are often asked, "Why me, Doc?", when we inform the patient that hazards on the job might explain the clinical problem. The patient may claim that "I am no less careful than others who have no such problems". There is an ethical imperative to utilize our scientific knowledge and methods to address such reasonable and logical questions from patients and workers.

We are expected under the Clean Air Act and the Occupational Safety and Health Act to promulgate standards that protect, respectively, the most susceptible subgroups or most susceptible individuals in the population. In the case of the Clean Air Act National Ambient Air Quality Standards for ozone and for lead, the Environmental Protection Agency postulated that the most susceptible subgroups would be children and adults with asthma, chronic bronchitis, or emphysema in the case of ozone (photochemical oxidants) and all children, especially low-income urban children, in the case of lead. Of course, the ozone proposal could have focussed on children with cystic fibrosis, but did not. How do we know who the most susceptible are? What level of protection will be appropriate? Do we obtain data, or do we simply make "safety factor" assumptions?

By focussing investigations on definitely or possibly highly susceptible individuals with relevant exposures, we may have a much better chance to identify significant adverse effects than among the much larger number exposed, only a small proportion of whom typically show any effects. Once exposures and effects are associated, we can more effectively proceed to elucidate the underlying mechanisms (Omenn et al., 1990).

Besides genetics, people vary in susceptibility because of differences in gender, age, nutrition, co-existent exposures, pre-existing illness and organ dysfunction, lifestyle/behavioral factors like cigarette smoking and diet, medications, and use of protective gear. All of these factors deserve careful investigation as independent risk factors and for potential interaction with specific genetic factors and mechanisms. Here we are focussed on the genetic predispositions. We already have excellent examples of genetic variation in susceptibility to many kinds of environmental agents (see Table 2) (Omenn & Motulsky, 1978; Vogel & Motulsky, 1986).

Table 2. Eco-Genetics: Known Inherited Predispositions

Drug chemicals
Pesticides
Inhaled pollutants
Foods
Food additives
Sensory stimuli
Allergic and sensitizing agents
Infectious agents

It is useful to distinguish differences in metabolism of a chemical agent from differences in susceptibility at the cellular and molecular level to the action of the agent. Examples are listed in Table 3. Moreover, in an increasing number of cases, we are finding genetic "markers" for disease predisposition for which we do not yet know the function; therefore, we need more information in order to classify these genes' predisposition by such category of mechanism.

Table 3. Classification and Examples of Eco-genetic Predispositions

Variations in Biotransformation Enzymes	
	N-acetyl transferase
	Cytochrome P450 monooxygenases
	Epoxide hydrolase
	Glutathione-S-transferases
	Paraoxonase
Variation in Cellular/Tissue Susceptibility to Chemical Action	
	Glucose-6-phosphate dehydrogenase deficiency (red blood cells)
	Alpha-1 anti-trypsin (protease inhibitor) deficiency (lung)
	Ah receptor and arylhydrocarbon hydroxylase induction (liver and other tissues)
Inherited Variation in Genes of Unknown Function Associated with Diseases	
	BRCA 1 (chromosome 17q21), BRCA 2 (chromosome 13q12-13)

The biotransformation polymorphisms have been described in detail elsewhere (Omenn et al., 1990; Nebert, 1991; Eaton & Gallagher, 1994), as have the tissue-based polymorphisms (Vogel & Motulsky, 1986; 1996). The identification of genes predisposing to various cancers--including the BRCA 1 predisposition to breast and ovarian cancer--is moving ahead rapidly (Andrews et al., 1994; Mimi et al., 1994; Futreal et al., 1994; Wooster et al., 1994). A few selected highlights are included here.

N-acetyl transferase (NAT). A polymorphism of this liver enzyme was reported 35 years ago to account for marked differences in blood levels of the anti-TB drug isoniazid after a standard dose. The difference was shown by family studies to be due to a single gene, with the recessive slow acetylator phenotype associated with higher levels of active, unacetylated drug and, therefore, propensity to adverse effects. Not surprisingly, some environmentally-encountered chemicals are metabolized by this same enzyme; prominent examples are the potent human bladder carcinogens beta-naphthylamine, benzidine, and 4-amino-biphenyl.

There is support for the hypothesis that slow acetylators would be at higher risk for bladder cancers from these agents than are rapid acetylators (Hein, 1988). For example, in Huddersfield, UK, 22/23 cases of bladder cancer among dyestuff workers were slow-acetylators (the 23rd case was atypical), compared with 44% among clerical workers. Cigarette smoking appears to be an independent risk factor, unassociated with acetylator phenotype.

The enzyme is rather complex, with both N-acetylating and O-acetylating activities. In bladder epithelia, the NAT activity predominates. In contrast, the hydroxamic O-acetyl transferase activity (OAT), which generates DNA-adduct-forming intermediates, predominates in colon, where heterocyclic arylamines may be found as pyrolysis products from charbroiled meat or fish. It is possible that slow acetylator phenotype thereby predisposes to colon cancer. Thus, any genetic screening or monitoring must be related to important risk factor exposures for bladder or colon cancer.

Phenotyping the NAT polymorphism has long relied upon administration of sulfamethazine or isoniazid; more recently, consumption of coffee or tea, with measurement of an acetylated metabolite of caffeine has proved convenient. The frequency of the slow acetylator phenotype is about 50% in Caucasian and Black populations, but only 10-15% in Asian populations. Gene probes for the NAT polymorphism have been reported, but still are being refined. Variants of this NAT gene have been shown to have two or three nucleotide transitions each (Vatsis et al., 1991). The Weber laboratory also has developed a useful mouse model with congenic rapid and slow acetylators in C57BL6 and A/J strains, but the location and effect of the single missense mutation are different from those identified in the human polymorphism (Martell et al., 1991).

Cytochrome P450 monooxygenases. These microsomal enzymes are a highly heterogeneous set of gene products with overlapping substrate specificity, responses to inducers, susceptibility to inhibitors, and patterns of expression in different tissues of the same organism. A classic substrate is benzo(a)pyrene, which is activated by P450s to reactive epoxides, then converted by epoxide hydrolase to a diol which is further activated by P450s to the highly carcinogenic electrophile BP-7,8-diol-9,10-epoxide. In turn, this compound is detoxified by pathways utilizing glutathione transferase or epoxide hydrolase (Omenn et al., 1990). Another prominent chemical activated by multiple P450s (and detoxified by conjugation with glutathione) is aflatoxin B1 (Eaton & Gallagher, 1994).

Despite the complexity, several specific P450s have been identified that are expressed polymorphically in humans and significant functional differences. Examples are P450s that catalyze the metabolism of the drugs debrisoquine, mephenytoin, and nifedipine, respectively.

The debrisoquine polymorphism affects alicyclic hydroxylation of debrisoquine, aromatic hydroxylation of guanoxan, oxidation dealkylation of phenacetin, and N-oxidation of sparteine--all due to a single gene difference in a quite minor P450, now designated P450 (CYP)2D6. The range of substrates is broad, and the difference in activity can be large. There is fairly consistent evidence that extensive metabolizers (activators) are at higher risk than poor metabolizers for lung cancer, though the relevant substrates have not been identified; at least expression of the debrisoquine P450 has been demonstrated in lung. Probe-based tests for this polymorphism are well-developed, but a multiplex assay is required to test for several different variants associated with low metabolic activity.

Epoxide hydrolase (EH). Only one isozyme of epoxide hydrolase acts on xenobiotics, a microsomal enzyme whose gene has been mapped to chromosome 1q. Thus, the analysis of EH is much less complex than analyses of variation in P450s or glutathione-S-transferases. This EH inactivates electrophilic epoxides by hydration to dihydrodiols. However, as noted above, the 7,8-diol of benzo(a)pyrene is a substrate for a P450 which produces a new highly carcinogenic epoxide. EH can be induced by phenobarbital, trans-stilbene oxide, and acetylaminofluorene.

Glutathione-S-transferases (GST). These detoxifying enzymes form inactive conjugates with glutathione. Numerous isozymes are known, classified in 6 families (Eaton &

Gallagher, 1994), some of which are inducible. Nevertheless, Seidegard et al. (Seidegard, 1985) identified a very common polymorphism of lymphocyte GST activity; about 45-50% of Caucasians are deficient in GST activity against the substrate trans-stilbene oxide (TSO). Following the reports from Pero's group in Sweden and Mantle in Dublin, a research team in our Charles A. Dana Program for Genetics and Environmental Health investigated the role of GST-mu in smoking-related and non-smoking related cancers, both in leukocytes (Heckbert et al., 1992) and in lung (Nazr-Stewart et al., 1993). The leukocyte results were consistent with, but not strongly supportive of, the earlier conclusion that GST-mu protected against smoking related cancers (odds ratio = 0.6, 95%CI 0.3-1.1). Fortunately, enzyme, antigen, and DNA probe assays in lung tissue from a new set of patients and controls showed striking protection associated with high GST-TSO activity and GST-mu antigen (relative risk = 0.30; 95%CI 0.11-0.79), as well as in a subgroup with both maternal and paternal copies of the GST-mu DNA intact (RR = 0.35, CI 0.06-2.1), compared with smokers lacking GST-mu activity, antigen, or DNA. High GST-mu activity was associated with a greater decrease in lung cancer risk among 38 heavy cigarette smokers (RR = 0.15; CI 0.03-0.64) than among 38 light smokers with lung cancer (RR = 0.61; CI 0.14-2.6).

Paraoxonase. This serum phosphotriesterase is highly active in detoxifying the active metabolite, paraoxon, of the common organophosphorus pesticide, parathion. About half of the Caucasian population has the phenotype of low activity and half has the phenotype of high activity, with a mean difference of three-fold. This difference is sufficient to make the low-activity individuals susceptible to neurotoxic effects of the pesticide at exposures which might have no discernible effect on those with the high activity. A preclinical early effect marker is inhibition of red blood cell cholinesterase activity, which has long been recommended for monitoring of workers exposed to this class of pesticides.

Cancer Predisposing Genes

The recent, highly-publicized capture of the BRCA1 gene and identification of mutants that predispose young women to high risk of breast and ovarian cancers has opened the prospect of genetic testing of asymptomatic women with a family history of these cancers (Miki et al., 1994). Much work needs to be done to define the spectrum of predisposing BRCA1 mutations (Futreal et al., 1994) and the cancer risks associated with each of the many mutations. To date, the emphasis has been entirely on clinical applications and associated technical and ethical challenges. Identifying the gene product and learning the function of the normal gene and the functional consequences of numerous mutations will be crucial to efficient diagnosis and to devising mechanism-based new therapeutic and preventive interventions. Meanwhile, those of us interested in environmental and eco-genetic aspects should begin to examine hypotheses about specific environmental influences that might act differentially through these specific mutations. For example, there is intense interest in xenoestrogens and, of course, endogenous estrogens, and in the role of dietary fat in the causation and promotion of breast cancer in humans. These and other hypotheses can be focussed in studies on women genotyped for BRCA1 and other breast cancer-predisposing genes. Additional prospects already identified are BRCA2 (chromosome 13q) and the ataxia-telangiectasia gene.

Analogous approaches may be fruitful with the familial polyposis gene and other genes with inherited variation in the pathway to colon cancer, and genes presently being investigated roles in melanoma and other cancers.

CRITICAL VARIATION ACROSS SPECIES: ARE SOME RODENT CARCINOGENS NOT HUMAN CARCINOGENS?

Lifetime rodent bioassays are hardly themselves a "gold standard", given their statistical and biological limitations and the observation that congruence of results between rats and mice is only 70 percent (Haseman & Lockhart, 1993). It is unlikely that rodent/human congruence would be higher (Lave et al., 1988). Detailed knowledge of molecular mechanisms and cellular and organ system responses can guide us to make better decisions about which chemicals that produce cancers, neurotoxicity, birth defects, or other adverse effects in rodents really represent significant risks of doing the same in humans. As summarized by McClain (1993), we now have quite a list of rodent carcinogenic responses that probably have no similar effect in humans (Table 4).

Table 4. Rodent Carcinogenic Responses Not Likely to Apply in Humans

Tumor Site	Illustrative Chemical Agents
male rat kidney	D-limonene, unleaded gasoline
male bladder	saccharin, nitriloacetic acid
rat thyroid	EBDC fungicides, goitrogens
forestomach-only (after gavage)	BHA, propionic acid, ethyl acrylate
lung	various particles
mouse liver	certain classes of liver carcinogens

Mechanistic understanding of some of these site-specific responses has been discussed in this Conference. The male rat kidney has been demonstrated to respond with a nephropathy mediated by alpha-2 euglobulin for which there is no significant counterpart in humans or in other animals. Formal EPA action to recognize this distinction is, I believe, still in process. The thyroid and other hormone-dependent tumors in rodents reflect marked species differences in the stimulating and feedback systems; sustained, excessive levels of TSH and 7lack of serum thyroid hormone-binding globulin are the key elements in the hyperplasia and tumors of the rat thyroid (McClain & Harbison, 1992/3). The incidence of spontaneous thyroid follicular cell neoplasia is also much higher in rats in the laboratory (e.g., Fischer 344) and in endemic areas of iodine deficiency where many people have goiters but rarely is thyroid cancer found in the humans. Local necrosis and reactive hyperplasia in the bladder and in the forestomach represent responses to very high local concentrations of the cytotoxic agent, and lung tumors have occurred with a variety of essentially inert particles when the clearance capacity is markedly exceeded. The mouse liver cancer picture is considerably more complicated, with a half-dozen different mechanisms, some of which do have definite counterparts in humans.

These mechanism-based differences between species and sometimes between strains within rodent species are of great policy importance. The regulatory agencies may be able to make qualitative judgments that certain animal responses can be excluded in the hazard identification step of the risk assessment and risk characterization.

Elucidation of a major interspecies difference has been accomplished by Eaton and colleagues in the case of aflatoxin B1 (see Eaton & Gallagher, 1994). Rats are 100,000 times more sensitive than mice to liver cancers from aflatoxin B1. The activation of the aflatoxin to the reactive epoxide is just as active in the rat as in the mouse; the difference in risk is fully explained by the much greater glutathione-S-transferase activity of the mouse, especially when AFB1-8,9-epoxide is used as the substrate. Humans seem to be closer to the rat than the mouse in the biochemical studies.

Environmental exposures act on highly variable people and rodent species/strains. Perhaps the strategy of testing chemicals as independent, sufficient causative agents for carcinogenesis and other adverse health effects is flawed. It may be necessary to consider a chemical a risk factor with dependence on host organism response features and other environmental factors (W. Farland, personal communication). These environmental factors may be chemical, infectious, physical, or behavioral. The relationship of cigarette smoking to coronary heart disease is an example of interaction of a chemical (mixture) with other known host and environmental risk factors, with modest attributable risk and relative risk less than two.

Variability and Uncertainty

The National Research Council (1994) carefully distinguished variability from uncertainty. Variability reflects currently or potentially measurable differences in exposure, co-existing factors, and host responses, as discussed above. Biomarkers of exposure, effect, and susceptibility are certain to assist in characterizing variability within populations (NRC, 1989a, b; 1992a, b). Currently, the regulatory agencies tend to rely on factor-of-10 safety factor approaches for health effects in threshold models, generating a margin of safety in extrapolating from a No-Observed-Adverse-Effect-Level or a Benchmark Dose in a sensitive test species (Faustman & Omenn, 1995). Actual data on variability in susceptibility will improve on the default assumption of a factor of 10 for variation among humans and another factor of 10 for the extrapolation to humans from the most sensitive test species.

Uncertainty, in contrast, reflects mostly unmeasureable parameters, due to assumptions in the threshold or no-threshold models for the dose-response relationship. Uncertainty also reflects variation in technical measurements and stochastic events underlying occurrence of endpoints.

The NRC report takes the position that "uncertainty is always with us" that we should learn ways to conduct risk assessments in the face of uncertainty and then to explain the significance of the uncertainty to risk managers and other interested persons. A quantitative approach, with probability distributions for numerous specific variables, was proposed

(NRC, 1994). Such formal uncertainty analyses might guide future work to reduce sources of uncertainties.

The Presidential/Congressional Commission on Risk Assessment and Risk Management

The same section of the 1990 Clean Air Act Amendments which mandated the National Research Council report "Science and Judgment in Risk Assessment" mandated a presidential/congressional commission to consider the social process of risk management. Ten members were appointed, three by the Senate, three by the House, three by the President, and one by the National Academy of Sciences. The Commission's mandate is to address the following five general areas or issues:

1. The uses and limitations of risk assessment in establishing emissions and effluent standards, ambient standards, exposure standards, acceptable concentration levels, tolerances or other environmental criteria for hazardous substances that present a risk of carcinogenic effects or other chronic health effects and reductions in the number of persons exposed at various levels of risk; the incidence of cancer; and other public health factors.
2. The most appropriate methods for measuring and describing cancer risks or risks of other chronic health effects from exposure to hazardous substances, considering such alternative approaches as the lifetime risk of cancer or other effects to the individual or individuals most exposed to emissions from a source or sources on both an actual and worst case basis; the range of such risks; the total number of health effects avoided by exposures standards, acceptable concentration levels, tolerances and other environmental criteria; reductions in the number of persons exposed at various levels of risk; the incidence of cancer; and other public health factors.
3. Methods to reflect uncertainties in measurement and estimation techniques; the existence of synergistic or antagonistic effects among hazardous substances; the accuracy of extrapolating human health risks from animal exposure data; and the existence of unquantified direct or indirect effects on human health in risk assessment studies.
4. Risk management policy issues including the use of lifetime cancer risks to individuals most exposed; incidence of cancer; the cost and technical feasibility of exposure reduction measures and the use of site specific actual exposure information in setting emissions standards; and other limitations applicable to sources of exposure to hazardous substances.
5. The degree to which it is possible or desirable to develop a consistent standard of acceptable risk, among various Federal programs.

The Commission will review carefully the risk assessment approaches and risk communication needs related to cancer and non-cancer health effects, and will focus much of its effort on the risk-based decision-making processes which good science can assist. Commission meetings are being held around the country. All meetings are open to the public. These policy issues have become major items of legislative interest in the Congress.

The deliberations are not at all limited to the Clean Air Act or the EPA, since issues about appropriate uses of risk assessment, the extrapolation to "acceptable risk" levels, the explanation of findings to stakeholders and decision makers, and the incorporation of parameters important to local citizens, Indian Nations, and environmental organizations apply to numerous other laws and many other federal and state agencies. A leading example is the Environmental Restoration and Waste Management Program of the U.S. Department of Energy (DOE), which is responsible for cleanup of the DOE's nuclear weapons production sites (Omenn, 1994b).

CONCLUSION

Research advances in molecular genetics and understanding of human and rodent genetic variability will surely bring mechanism-based information to the risk assessment process. Such knowledge and use of biomarkers in individual workers or other exposed individuals to estimate exposure, detect early non-clinical effects, and identify variation in susceptibility will help make risk communication and risk management more comprehensible for individuals and communities. Meanwhile, appreciation of striking differences between rodents and humans in certain biological responses can help the regulatory agencies make biologically and clinically sound judgments in setting health-based standards. Conversely, demonstration of similarity in response between rodents and humans will serve to reinforce the general assumption that regulatory action can be based on results from non-human studies. As risk assessments are used more widely, there will be increasing interest in comparisons of similar and different types of health and environmental risks and in cost-benefit analyses of proposed risk management actions.

REFERENCES

Andrews LB, Fullarton, JE, Holtzman NA, Motulsky AG (1994): “Assessing Genetics Risks: Implications for Health and Social Policy”, Washington DC: National Academy Press.

Calkins DR, Dixon RL, Gerber CR, Zarin D, and Omenn GS (1980): Identification, characterization, and control of potential human carcinogens: a framework for federal decision-making. JNCI 61:169-175.

Cantor CR, Caskey CT Hood LE, Kamely D, Omenn GS (1990): “Biotechnology and Human Genetic Predisposition to Disease: Proceedings of a UCLA Symposium Held at Steamboat Streams, Colorado, March 27-April 3, 1989.” New York: Wiley-Liss, Inc.

Colborn T, vom Saal FS, Soto AM (1993): Developmental effects of endocrine-disrupting chemicals in wildlife and humans. Environ Health Perspect 101: 378-384.

Davis DL, Bradlow HL, Wolff M, Woodruff T, Woodruff T, Hoel DG, et al. (1993): Medical hypothesis: xenoestrogens as preventable causes of breast cancer. Environ Health Perspect 101:372-377.

Eaton DL, Gallagher EP (1994): Mechanisms of aflatoxin carcinogenesis. Annu Rev Pharmacol Toxicol 34:135-172.

Faustman EM, Omenn GS (1995): Risk assessment. In C. Klaassen (ed), Casarett & Doull's Toxicology, 5th ed. New York: Pergamon Press (In press).

Futreal PA, Liu Q, Shattuck-Eidens, Cochran C, Harshman K, Tavtigian S, et al. (1994): BRCA1 mutations in primary breast and ovarian carcinomas. Science 266:120-122.

Haseman JK, Lockhart AM (1993): Correlations between chemically related site-specific carcinogenic effects in long-term studies in rats and mice. Environ Health Perspectives 101:50-54.

Heckbert SR, Weiss NS, Hornung SK, Eaton DL, Motulsky AG (1992): Glutathione S-transferase and epoxide hydrolase activity in human leukocytes in relation to risk of lung cancer and other smoking-related cancers. JNCI 84:414-422.

Hein DW (1988): Acetylator genotype and arylamine-induced carcinogenesis. Biochimica et Biophysica Acta 948:37-66.

Lave LB, Ennever FK, Rosenkranz HS, Omenn GS (1988): Information value of the rodent bioassay. Nature, 336: 631-633.

Martell KJ, Vatsis, KP, Weber WW (1991). Molecular genetic basis of rapid and slow acetylation in mice. Mol Pharmacol 40: 218-227.

McClain RM (1993): Mechanistic considerations in the regulation and classification of chemical carcinogens. In Kotsonis FN, Mackey M, Hijele J (eds.): "Nutritional Toxicology." New York: Raven Press Ltd., pp 273-304.

McClain RM, Harbison ML (1992/3): Receptor mediated cell proliferation and thyroid neoplasia. BGA Schriften, 49.

Miki Y, Swensen J, Shattuck-Eidens D, Futreal PA, Harshman K, Tavtigian S, et al. (1994): A strong candidate for the breast and ovarian cancer susceptibility gene BRCA1. Science 266:66-71.

Mumtaz MM, Sipes IG, Clewell HJ, Yang RSH (1993): Risk assessment of chemical mixtures: biologic and toxicologic issues. Fundamental and Applied Toxicology 21:258.

National Research Council (1994): Science and Judgment in Risk Assessment. Washington DC: National Academy Press.

National Research Council (1992a): Environmental Neurotoxicology. Washington DC: National Academy Press.

National Research Council (1992b): Biological Markers in Immuno-toxicology.

Washington DC: National Academy Press.

National Research Council (1989a): Biological Markers in Reproductive Toxicology. Washington, DC: National Academy Press.

National Research Council (1989b): Biological Markers in Pulmonary Toxicology. Washington, DC: National Academy Press.

National Research Council (1983): Risk Assessment in the Federal Government: Managing the Process (referred to as "The Red Book"). Washington, DC: National Academy Press.

Nazr-Stewart V, Motulsky AG, Eaton DL, White E, Hornung SK, Leng ZT, et al. (1993): The glutathione S-transferase μ Polymorphism as a marker for susceptibility to lung carcinoma. Cancer Research 53:2313-2318.

Nebert DW, Petersen DD, Puga A (1991): Human Ah locus polymorphism and cancer: inducibility of CYP1A1 and other genes by combustion products and dioxin. Pharmacogenetics:1:68-78.

Omenn (1994a): Progress in science-based risk assessment and risk management. Technology: Journal of the Franklin Institute 331:21-27.

Omenn GS (1994b): Can Systematic, Integrated Risk Assessment With Full Stakeholder Participation Enhance Cleanup at DOE's Sites? The 1994 Herbert M. Parker Lecture the Thirty-Third Hanford Symposium on Health and the Environment. In Gee GW, Wing R, (eds): "In-situ remediation: scientific basis for current and future technologies." Columbus, OH: Battelle Press, Part I, pp xv-xxx.

Omenn GS, Goodman G, Grizzle J, Thornquist M, Rosenstock L, Barnhart S, et al. (1992): Recruitment for CARET, the ß-carotene and retinol efficacy trial to prevent lung cancer in smokers and in asbestos-exposed workers. West J Med, 156: 540.

Omenn GS, Omiecinski CJ, Eaton DL (1990): Eco-genetics of chemical carcinogens. In Cantor CR, Caskey CT, Hood LE, Kamely D, Omenn GS (eds.): "Biotechnology and Human Genetic Predisposition to Disease," New York: Wiley-Liss, Inc. pp 81-93.

Omenn GS, Lave LB (1988): Scientific and cost-effectiveness criteria in selecting batteries of short-term tests. Mutation Research 205: 41-49.

Omenn GS, Gelboin HV (eds) (1984): "Genetic Variability in Responses to Chemical Exposure." Banbury Report 16. New York: Cold Spring Harbor Laboratory.

Omenn GS, Motulsky HG (1978): Eco-genetics: genetic variation in susceptibility to environmental agents. In Cohen BH, Lilienfeld AM, Huang PC (eds): "Genetic issues in public health and medicine." Springfield, IL: CC Thomas, pp 83-111.

Seidegard J, DePierre JW, Pero RW (1985): Hereditary interindividual differences in the glutathione transferase activity towards trans-stilbene oxide in resting human mononuclear leukocytes are due to a particular isozyme(s). Carcinogenesis 6:1211-1216.

Vatsis KP, Martell KJ, Weber WW (1991): Diverse point mutations in the human gene for polymorphic N-acetyltransferase. Proc Natl Acad Sci US 88: 6333-6337.

Vogel F, Motulsky AG (1986 & 1996): "Human Genetics: Problems and Approaches," (2nd & 3rd ed.). Heidelberg, Germany: Springer-Verlag.

Wooster R, Neuhausen SL, Mangion J, Quirk Y, Ford D, Collins N, et al. (1994): Localization of a breast cancer susceptibility gene, BRCA2, to chromosome 13q12-13. Science 265:2088-2090.

Index